Handbook of Vitamins, Minerals and Hormones

SECOND EDITION

Handbook of Vitamins, Minerals and Hormones

SECOND EDITION

Roman J. Kutsky, Ph. D.

Consultant and Professor
World Open University
Vancouver, Washington

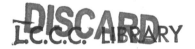

VAN NOSTRAND REINHOLD COMPANY
NEW YORK   CINCINNATI   ATLANTA   DALLAS   SAN FRANCISCO
LONDON   TORONTO   MELBOURNE

Van Nostrand Reinhold Company Regional Offices:
New York   Cincinnati   Atlanta   Dallas   San Francisco

Van Nostrand Reinhold Company International Offices:
London   Toronto   Melbourne

Library of Congress Catalog Card Number: 80-29483
ISBN: 0-442-24557-2

Manufactured in the United States of America

Published by Van Nostrand Reinhold Company
135 West 50th Street, New York, N.Y. 10020

Published simultaneously in Canada by Van Nostrand Reinhold Ltd.

15 14 13 12 11 10 9 8 7 6 5 4 3 2 1

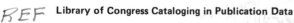

Library of Congress Cataloging in Publication Data

Kutsky, Roman J   1922-
    Handbook of vitamins, minerals, and hormones.

    First ed. published in 1973 under title: Handbook
of vitamins and hormones.
    Includes bibliographies and index.
    1. Vitamin therapy.   2. Minerals in human nutrition.
3. Hormone therapy.   I. Title.   [DNLM: 1. Hormones.
2. Vitamins.   3. Minerals.   QU 160 K97h]
    RM259.K88   1981   612'.399   80-29483
    ISBN 0-442-24557-2

Introduction

Recent research in tissue culture, physiology, and biochemistry has demonstrated a need for an all-inclusive compendium on minerals as well as vitamins and hormones, as growth factors. In addition, great interest has been generated in presentation of properties of the actual controlling agents which accurately blend all the cellular enzyme systems and organelles to produce a living cell, and, from that, a living multicellular organism. It is precisely in this area of control mechanisms that the minerals, vitamins, and hormones play such a key role, because they are controlling agents.

This book is written primarily from the standpoint of the vitamin, mineral and hormone requirements and contents of individuals of the *human* species. It should be understood that requirements and contents differ from species to species, in general becoming simpler as one goes down the evolutionary scale. For the purposes of this book, a *vitamin* is defined as a biologically active, organic compound, a controlling agent essential for an organism's (human's) normal health and growth (its absence causing a deficiency disease or disorder), not synthesized within the organism, available in the diet in small amounts, and carried in the circulatory system in small concentrations to act on target organs or tissues. A *hormone* is defined as a biologically active, organic compound, a controlling agent essential for normal health and growth (its absence causing a deficiency disease or disorder), synthesized within the organism (human being) in ductless glands which release the agent in very small concentrations into the circulatory system to act on the target organs or tissues.

The chief differences between a vitamin and a hormone seem to be the site of biosynthesis, the types of organic compounds present in vitamins as opposed to the hormones, and some of the modes of action. These differences between vitamins and hormones in essential properties are small compared to their similarities and explain why both vitamins and hormones are combined into one book.

In the light of new evidence, it is becoming difficult to differentiate certain vitamins from some hormones. For example, both vitamin D and niacin are synthesized (but in an inadequate amount) in the human, thus conferring on them a hormonal quality. Similarly, the human requirement for the hormone thyroxine can be partially satisfied by a dietary intake of iodine, and some of the steroid hormones are active in a dietary form, thus giving them a vitamin quality. Moreover, the fat-soluble vitamins (A, D, E, K) show many similarities in biosynthesis, structure, properties and function to the fat-soluble hormones (steroids). Finally, the same molecule can function as a hormone or as a vitamin, depending on the species involved. For example, vitamin C functions as a vitamin in primates because they cannot synthesize it, but it functions as a hormone in cows because they can synthesize it.

We can see that the concept of vitamins and hormones, as defined here, could be extended to all organisms with circulatory systems and would therefore include all vertebrates, many invertebrates, and the higher plants, excepting mainly the lower plants and animals and unicellular organisms. The concept of vitamin is therefore very much dependent on the species concerned. Vitamins seem to have arisen very early in the evolution of life as judged by their presence and requirement in some of the most primitive forms of life known today. Hormones, according to our original definition, however, denote a much later period of emergence, becoming prominent mainly with the evolution of the various animals. They, therefore, reflect a shorter evolutionary history. In view of their primitive nature, vitamins would be expected to have, in general, a simpler structure than hormones, and this is indeed the case, with a few exceptions.

As we compare modes of action of vitamins and hormones, we should compare their chemical structures. The vitamins consist of a fat-soluble series and a water-soluble series. The fat-soluble vitamins (A, D, E, K) consist of derivatives of partially cyclized isoprenoid polymers, somewhat similar to the intermediates in cholesterol (steroid) synthesis. These vitamins seem to act by virtue of their lipid solubility in various cell membranes to affect permeability or transport, and by virtue of their chemical groups as redox agents (A, E, K), as coenzymes or enzyme activators (D, K, A). The water soluble vitamins (B_1, B_2, B_6, B_{12}, niacin, pantothenic acid, folic acid, biotin, C) consist, in general, of derivatives or substituted derivatives of sugars (C), pyridine (niacin, B_6), purines and pyrimidines (folic acid, B_2, B_1), amino acid-organic acid complexes (folic acid, biotin, pantothenic acid), and a porphyrin-nucleotide complex (B_{12}). These structurally diverse water-soluble vitamins act as enzyme activators and coenzymes (B_1, B_2, B_6, B_{12}, pantothenic acid, folic acid, biotin, niacin), as redox agents on enzyme reactions (C, B_2, B_{12}, folic acid, niacin), as nuclear agents (folic acid, B_{12}, C, biotin), and probably as mitochondrial agents (B_2, C, niacin).

The hormones also include a fat-soluble, steroid series (estradiol, progesterone, aldosterone, testosterone, cortisol) which seems to act (1) by virtue of lipid solubility to stabilize and change permeability of the cell membranes, (2) to regulate enzyme activity and membrane polarization, (3) to regulate redox potential, and (4) to affect RNA transcription in the nucleus. The water-soluble hormones consist of a protein series (STH, TSH, FSH, LH, prolactin) which seems to act on the cell membrane to stimulate cyclic AMP production (except STH and prolactin) enzyme activation, and to activate certain genes in the nucleus. The peptide series of water-soluble hormones (insulin, glucagon, ACTH, MSH, oxytocin, ADH, PTH, T4, TCT, and relaxin) acts similarly to the proteins and also has an effect on the mitochondria by T4 and PTH. The amine, water-soluble hormone series (epinephrine, norepinephrine) seems to act chiefly by the cyclic AMP mechanism on the membrane, with consequent enzyme activation. The very extensive role of cyclic AMP as an intracellular mediator of hormonal activity is most noteworthy.

It can be seen that the fat-soluble vitamins and hormones act similarly on membranes, on redox potentials, and as enzyme activators, the only difference being in a demonstrated action on the nucleus by the steroids. Comparison of the water-soluble series of hormones with that of the vitamins again shows a basic similarity in action, the vitamins acting as direct enzyme activators and coenzymes, and the hormones acting as indirect activators via cyclic AMP. Both act on the nucleus but differ in that only some of the water-soluble vitamins have redox properties. Again here, the differences between the two water-soluble series of vitamins and hormones lie chiefly in their differing structures and in some of their properties, such as redox regulation and presence of cyclic AMP intermediates.

The subject of vitamin requirements requires comment. There is now sufficient evidence to indicate that the concept of biochemical individuality has much merit. Thus the recommended allowances as stated in this book (NRC data) should be considered only as average figures, and variations (increase or decrease) of twentyfold or more in individual human requirements may be found, depending on the genetic and physiological state of the individual. Germane to this are the topics of subclinical vitamin deficiencies and megavitamin therapy, i.e., large overdosages of one or more vitamins such as are now being used as treatment of colds and schizophrenia.

The existence of subclinical vitamin deficiencies is extremely difficult to prove without adequate statistical data, but, undoubtedly, if we accept the principle of biochemical individuality, they do exist. In like manner, the use of megavitamins may be helpful to those individuals whose systems for some reason destroy these vitamins rapidly or require these vitamins in large quantity owing to their biochemical individuality. However, in view of the fact that accurate data are lacking, one should treat and use megavitamins as drugs with competent medical advice, being wary of possible unexpected individual toxicity.

A perusal of the miscellaneous section for each factor will indicate to the reader the enormous amount of interplay occurring among vitamins, hormones, and minerals. This includes both antagonisms and synergisms occurring simultaneously among various vitamins, minerals, and hormones. Undoubtedly there exists an optimal set of levels for each factor which, presumably, is that which has been found in "normal" human values. But maximum optimization of levels at "normal" human values has not been proved experimentally; perhaps the human system could run more efficiently at a different set of values. More research is needed to determine this. In any case, optimum amounts and ratios of all vitamins and hormones are important to get full benefits of these agents.

A section is now included on the trace elements and mineral cofactors required for functioning of most coenzyme systems as well as some hormones, e.g., magnesium, iron, copper, iodine, selenium, cobalt, and so on. These trace elements should be present in correct amounts and ratios in any balanced diet containing adequate vitamins.

In relation to requirements, the subject of undiscovered or unaccepted factors should be mentioned. This book has included only those minerals, vitamins and hormones with widespread acceptance. In addition to the 13 vitamins listed here, there are at least another 13 compounds with various acceptabilities as vitamins, plus possibly other vitamins still undiscovered. In view of individual requirements, and the mutual interdependence of vitamins mentioned above, it would still be advisable to rely for one's vitamin requirement chiefly on rich natural sources in the diet, since these would most likely contain the undiscovered vitamins and minerals. However, because of the possible extreme losses of vitamin potency even in our richest dietary sources caused by our present methods of processing, storing, and cooking of food, it would be advisable to consider vitamin supplementation of certain vitamins, especially if one's diet has not been carefully planned.

As far as the hormones are concerned, at least another 23 compounds, in addition to the 23 listed here, are known with various degrees of acceptance as true hormones. No doubt many more remain to be discovered. This book has not listed the insect or plant hormones, because human requirements and levels are being stressed.

Presentation of Data

This book will serve as a ready reference to four major groups of readers, inasmuch as the data for each factor are presented in several separate sections, as follows: "General Information" and "Miscellaneous Information" for the general reader and all other groups; "Medical and Biological Role" mainly for the biologists, physicians, nurses, and pharmacologists; "Chemical Properties" and "Metabolic Properties" for the biochemists and physiologists; and "Nutritional Role" for dietitians and nutritionists. However, it is hoped that parts of all sections will be useful to all the groups. Insofar as possible, the format is similar for all factors for ease of reference. A list of abbreviations is given at the beginning of the book.

The minerals, vitamins, and hormones chosen for coverage in this book are those that have the widest acceptance by the various workers in these fields. Only the most active of the steroid hormones in each category of mineralocorticoids, glucocorticoids, and sex hormones in the human is being covered (out of the 40 plus already discovered).

Chapters on Vitamins, Hormones and Minerals
General Information Section
"Active analogs and related compounds" includes vitamers, isotels, etc.
"Antagonists" and "Synergists" may be the same chemical species but in different concentrations. Interaction at the target site is used as a criterion of antagonism or synergism.

"Sources for Species" (Essentiality) indicates degree of requirement for various species including man. Endogenous = made within organism. Exogenous sources include intestinal bacteria.

Chemical Properties Section

"Reactions" refers to those carried out with standard laboratory conditions and reagents and not under extreme conditions, unless otherwise noted. i.e., heat $\leqslant 100°C$, weak acids or alkalies, reactivity with water, atmospheric or mild oxidation agents, mild reducing agents, bright daylight.

Isolation method gives a typical procedure now in use.

Medical and Biological (Nutritional) Section

This provides, in general, clinical information. Contents of vitamins and minerals are per 100-g edible portion

Antigenicity is defined as the ability to act as an antigen creating an immune response when administered to an organism. Specificity is here defined as the degree of restriction of biological activity to a certain species.

Metabolic Role Section

"Enzyme Reactions" lists enzyme systems affected by the vitamin, mineral, or hormone, organ location, and effects on enzymes, where known.

"Mode of Action" subdivides functions on both a cellular basis (anabolic, catabolic, etc.) and an organismal basis. Anabolic denotes synthetic processes; catabolic denotes degradative reactions and includes most energy-yielding reactions.

Miscellaneous Information Section

"Relationships to other Vitamins, Hormones" attempts to indicate the mutual involvement of both vitamins and hormones in most actions of both groups either together or within the group; similarly for minerals.

"Unusual Features" includes various chemical, biological, and pharmacological features that could not be listed elsewhere.

"Possible Relationships" attempts to draw a parallel between the action of a mineral, a vitamin, or a hormone and its deficiency symptoms.

The tables presented list some of the data already given and some new data in an attempt to indicate fundamental similarities and dissimilarities in structure and function of vitamins, minerals, and hormones.

References are presented in numbered form at the end of sections, and are subdivided into two categories: general and specific. An effort has been made to cite only the latest available handbooks, compendia, journal references, and texts.

Abbreviations

A.A. . . . . amino acid
Absn. . . . . absorption
Acet. . . . . acetone
ACH . . . . acetyl choline
ACTH . . . . . . adrenocorticotrop(h)ic
      hormone
ADH . . . . antidiuretic hormone
      (vasopressin)
Ala. . . . . alanine
Aldos. . . . . aldosterone
Alc. . . . . (ethyl) alcohol
Alk. . . . . alkaline
AMP . . . . adenosine monophosphate
$_c$AMP . . . . . . cyclic adenosine mono-
      phosphate
Approx. . . . . approximately
Aq. . . . . aqueous
Arg. . . . . arginine
Asn. . . . . asparagine
Asp. . . . . aspartic acid
ATP . . . . adenosine triphosphate

Benz. . . . . benzene

Bio. . . . . .biotin
BMR . . . . basal metabolic rate
CDPG . . . .cytidine diphosphoglucose
CF . . . . .citrovorum factor
Chl. . . . . chloroform
CHO . . . . .carbohydrate
Chromatog. . . . . . . chromatograph
CMC, CM cell . . . . . . .carbosymethyl
      cellulose
CNS . . . . central nervous system
CoA . . . . coenzyme A
Conc. . . . . .concentrated
Conv. . . . . converted
CoQ . . . . Coenzyme Q
Cort. . . . . .cortisol
CRH . . . . . .corticotrop(h)in-releasing
      hormone
Cys. . . . . cysteine

DDT . . . . dichloro-diphenyl-trichloro-
      ethane (insecticide)
DEAE . . . . diethylaminoethyl
      (cellulose)

Defic. . . . . .deficiency

Dil. . . . . .dilute

DOPA . . . . dihydroxyphenylalanine

DPN . . .diphosphopyridine nucleotide

DNA. . . . . . . .deoxyribonucleic acid

Enz. . . . . enzyme

Ep., Epi. . . . . .epinephrine

Equiv. . . . . .equivalent

Esp. . . . . especially

Est. . . . . .estradiol

Eth. . . . . .ether

Ext. . . . . .extract

F.A. . . . . folic acid

FAD . . . . .flavin adenine dinucleotide

FMN. . . . . . . .flavin mononucleotide

FRH . . . . FSH-releasing hormone

FSH . . . .follicle-stimulating hormone

Fluoresc. . . . . fluorescent

GH . . . . .growth hormone (STH)

G.I. . . . . gastro-intestinal

Gln. . . . . glutamine

Glu. . . . . .glutamic acid

Gluc(ag). . . . . .glucagon

Gly. . . . . .glycine

GPU . . . . .guinea pig unit

GRH. . . . . growth (somatotrop(h)in

releasing hormone

GTF . . . . . . .glucose tolerance factor

HCG . . . . . .human chorionic gonado

trophin

HGH. . . . . . human growth hormone

His. . . . . .histidine

HMG. . human menopause gonadotro-

phin (mixture of FSH and LH)

HMP . . . . . . .hexose monophosphate

Hyp. R.F., HRH .hypothalamic-releas-

ing factor (hormone)

Ile. . . . . isoleucine

In. . . . . insulin

Insol. . . . . .insoluble

IRC . . . . ion exchange resin

Irrad. . . . . irradiated

I.U. . . . . .international unit

I.V. . . . . .intravenous

Leu. . . . . .leucine

LH . . . . luteinizing hormone

LLD . . . . L. lactis Dorner

LRH . . . . .LH-releasing hormone

Lys. . . . . .lysine

Max. . . . . .maximum

me. . . . . .methyl

Met. . . . . methionine

Metab. . . . . .metabolism

MIH . . . . . MSH-inhibiting hormone

Monocl. . . . . monoclinic

MP . . . . .melting point

MRH. . . . . . .MSH-releasing hormone

MSH .melanocyte-stimulating hormone

MW. . . . . molecular weight

NAD(P) . . . . nicotinamide adenine di-

nucleotide (phosphate)

NADPH. . . . . .reduced NADP

Nia. . . . . .niacine

NIH . . . National Institutes of Health

Nor., Norepi. . . . . . . norepinephrine

NRC . . . . . National Research Council

OAA. . . . . .oxaloacetic acid

Oxy. . . . . .oxytocin

P.A., Pant. . . . . . . pantothenic acid

PBI . . . . protein-bound iodine

Pet. . . . . .petroleum

PGA . . . . .pteroyl glutamic acid, folic

acid

Phe. . . . . phenylalanine

pI . . . . .isoelectric point

PIH. . . . prolactin-inhibiting hormone

PMSG . . . . .pregnant mare serum
gonadotrophin

Ppt. . . . . precipitate

PRH . . . . prolactin-releasing hormone

Pro. . . . . .proline

Prog. . . . . progesterone

Prol. . . . . .prolactin

PTH . . . . parathormone

RBC . . . . red blood cell

Relax. . . . . relaxin

RNA . . . . .ribonucleic acid

$_m$RNA . . . messenger ribonucleic acid

Ser. . . . . .serine

Serot. . . . . serotonin

Sl. . . . . .slightly

Sol. . . . . .soluble

Soln. . . . . solution

St. . . . . .standard

STH . . . . .somatotrop(h)in (GH)

T3 . . . . triiodothyronine

T4 . . .tetraiodothyronine (thyroxine)

TCA . . . . . tricarboxylic acid (cycle),
Krebs (cycle)

TCT . . . . thyrocalcitonin

Test., Testos. . . . . testosterone

Thr. . . . . threonine

TPN . . triphosphopyridine nucleotide
(NADP)

TRH . . . . TSH-releasing hormone

Try. . . . . tryptophan

TSH . . . thyroid-stimulating hormone

Tyr. . . . . tyrosine

UDP . . . . uridine diphosphate

USP . . . . *United States Pharmacopeia*

UV . . . . .ultraviolet

v . . . . volt

Val. . . . . .valine

Vaso. . . . . vasopressin

Vit. . . . . .vitamin

Contents

Part II: INTRODUCTION TO THE VITAMINS   179

Part III: INTRODUCTION TO THE HORMONES   296

Part 1

The following 15 mineral elements consist of 5 macro or bulk essential elements (Ca, Mg, Na, K, P) and 10 micro or trace elements (Fe, Cu, Mn, Zn, I, Se, Mo, Cr, Co, F). Not all of the latter have been proved essential for life in man, but they have been proved essential for some living system or for normal health and longevity in humans. On the basis of present ongoing research, it is most likely that the elements in question (Se, Mo, Mn, Cr, F) will be shown to be essential for the human system in the near future. Need for the bulk essential elements has already been demonstrated. Several other elements (e.g., Sn, Si, V, As, and Ni) may also be found to be essential in extremely small amounts, but much research remains to be done before such determinations can be made.

It should be noted that under physiological conditions (i.e., in aqueous solution) 10 of the 15 elements (Ca, Mg, Na, K, Fe, Cu, Mn, Zn, Cr, Co) are positively charged (cations). Five elements (P, I, Se, Mo, F) are negatively charged (anions), three of them occur as oxide complexes (PO_4, SeO_4, MoO_4). Four elements (Na^+, K^+, F^-, I^-) are univalent in physiological solutions; ten elements (Ca^{2+}, Mg^{2+}, Fe^{2+}, Cu^{2+}, Co^{2+}, Mn^{2+}, Zn^{2+}, SeO_4^{2-}, MoO_4^{2-}, HPO_4^{2-}) are divalent; one is trivalent (Cr^{3+}).

These elements can and do interact with one another as shown in the solubility table where the physiological forms of the minerals and other physiological ions present in the gastrointestinal tract are charted (as negative ions against positive ions). It will be noted that the divalent negative ions tend to form more insoluble products when in the presence of oppositely charged

Solubility Table

	I^-	Cl^-	SeO_4^{2-}	SO_4^{2-}	CO_3^{2-}	F^-	PO_4^{3-}	OH^-	MoO_4^{2-}
H^+	S	S	S	S	S	S	S	S	sa
NH_4^+	S	S	S	S	S	S	S	S	S
Na^+	S	S	S	S	S	S	S	S	S
K^+	S	S	S	S	S	S	S	S	S
Mg^{2+}	S	S	S	S	sa	sa	sa	la	sa
Ca^{2+}	S	S	sa	sa	sa	sa	sa	S	la
Co^{2+}	S	S	S	S	la	S	la	la	—
Fe^{2+}	S	S	—	S	sa	sa	la	la	—
Cu^{2+}	—	S	S	S	lsa	sa	la	la	—
Mn^{2+}	S	S	S	S	sa	la	la	la	—
Zn^{2+}	S	S	S	S	sa	la	la	la	—
Cr^{3+}	S	I	—	I	S	la	I	la	—

S = soluble in water; sa = sparingly soluble in water, soluble in acids; la = insoluble in water soluble in acids; lsa = insoluble in water, sparingly soluble in acids; I = insoluble in water and acids.

divalent positive ions than with univalent ions. Note that most ions are soluble at the acid pH of the stomach, (H^+ row), but when the pH turns alkaline in the intestine, most of the divalent positive metal ions become insoluble (OH^- column) especially trace elements. This property has significance for the human uptake of metallic ions, making it harder for them to be absorbed and necessitating special mechanisms for absorption (e.g., active transport, vitamin D, bile salts, etc.). Although it makes absorption of a toxic excess of metal ions more difficult, it hinders absorption of essential minerals as well. This may explain why practically all essential minerals have a mineralovitamin form that is preferentially absorbed (e.g., vitamin B_{12} and Co, GTF and Cr).

The effective concentrations of some trace elements are very low (parts per million, or micrograms per gram). However, the toxic limits of some are uncomfortably close to the required dosages. This means that a very delicate balance exists for many trace elements between toxicity, vitality, and deficiency. This balance could easily be upset by the presence of excessive trace amounts of precipitating ions, as might occur with incorrect mineral pill supplementation. These precipitates could form in sensitive tissues such as kidney, heart, and brain, with possibly fatal consequences. Moreover, imbalance of ions could disturb intracellular enzyme reactions, and pH, or affect the irritability of muscle or nerve (with resulting tetany or convulsions).

For these and similar physiological considerations, it is definitely not advisable to attempt self-medication with mineral pill supplements without medical supervision. It will be noted that most if not all of the 15 essential trace elements are already present in the average normal American diet in sufficient concentrations, with supplementation indicated only for special conditions such as pregnancy, senescence, and so on. If a deficiency is indeed medically or professionally indicated, it would be far safer to use dietary measures to correct this deficiency, than using pill supplements, using the tables furnished in this book which indicate foods enriched in the particular mineral question. The dangers of exceeding a toxic dose would be minimized, while at the same time one would obtain synergistic vitamins and minerals from the enriched foods.

The picture of the role of essential minerals is by no means clear or complete. With the advent of new, more sensitive analytical methods, discoveries of new functions can be expected in the near future. In addition to the fundamental chemical roles outlined in the succeeding pages there is every likelihood of more basic functions being discovered for several minerals, especially for Cr, Se, Zn, Mo, Mn, and V, such as roles in the fine control of DNA synthesis, mechanisms of development, the onset of senescence, and arteriosclerosis.

Chapter 1. Phosphorus (P)

All body P exists as phosphate (PO_4). Although 80-85% of the P in the body is in structural form in the skeleton, the remainder of the P in the body is chiefly intracellular with four major metabolic functions:

1. Energy transport as a constituent of high-energy phosphate bonds from carbohydrate metabolism, in the form of ATP, ADP, etc.
2. Presence as a key constituent in living membranes, as phospholipids
3. Participation in genetic reactions, as phosphate polymers, DNA, and RNA
4. Buffering, Ca-transport, and osmotic pressure of intracellular fluids

Phosphorus is found in all cells in plants and animals, and is essential for all life and the normal growth, development, and life span of humans and all organisms. Its mode of action is mainly by way of its bonding, polymer formation, hydration, transport properties, sequestering action, and variable acidity. Intracellular fluid containing high P(relative to other anions) may be considered to represent the original fluid (pre-Cambrian seas) in which life evolved. Life as we know it could not have developed without P, which plays a key role in many physiological functions and is associated with several vitamins, hormones, and many enzymes. It is absorbed as the free ion, and its chief synergist is Ca, while its chief antagonists are sulfate and bicarbonate.

There is no evidence that the average American diet includes too little P, since it is present in all foods. However, vegetable diets may contain P in a partially unavailable form (phytate). High P dietary items include seafood, meats, nuts, seeds, dairy products, and grains.

Deficiencies of P may occur in cases of growth, lactation, and pregnancy. Body P is tightly conserved under a system of almost complete homeostasis, and need for replenishment arises only in special physiological situations.

GENERAL INFORMATION

Note: In the following presentation, reference numbers refer to references listed at the end of the minerals section.

1. **Dietary and Medicinal Forms**   18, 49, 53, 54
   Element—Phosphorus nonmetal; not used medicinally
   Inorganic forms—Sodium, potassium phosphates (mono-, di-, tribasic); calcium, magnesium phosphates (mono-, di-, tribasic); phosphoric acid .
   Organic forms—Phosphoproteins (casein, etc.), phospholipids (lecithin, etc.), phosphorylated carbohydrates (glucose-P, etc.), vitamins (B_{12}), bone meal

2. **History of Biological Significance**   18, 21, 35, 50, 53
   1817—Vauqelin: demonstrated P in animal lipids
   1872—Miescher: identified P in salmon sperm nucleic acid
   1906—Harden and Young: discovered DPN and high-energy glucose-P bond
   1927—Eggleton and Eggleton: discovered creatine-P in vertebrate muscle
   1928—Meyerhoff and Lohmann: discovered arginine-P in invertebrate muscle
   1931—Lohmann: isolated ATP from muscle
   1932—Warburg and Christian: discovered TPN (Coenzyme II)
   1935—Lohmann: discovered ATP-creatine-P interaction
   1936—Cori and Cori: discovered glucose-1-phosphate
   1939—Kalckar: discovered oxidative phosphorylation
   1948—Krebs: proposed TCA cycle for production of ATP
   1954—Arnon and Frenkel: discovered photosynthetic phosphorylation

3. **Physiological (Blood) Forms**   18, 21, 50, 51, 53
   HPO_4^{2-}, $H_2PO_4^-$, $NaHPO_4^-$, $CaHPO_4$, $MgHPO_4$, protein-bound P, phospholipids, diphosphoglycerate (RBC), organic-P esters (including eight vitamins)

4. **Synergistic Agents**   30, 35, 39
   Metabolic—Ca^{2+}, Mg^{2+}, TCT (bone), B-complex vitamins
   Absorption—Na^+, K^+, Ca^{2+}, STH, vitamin D, PTH, (H^+)

5. **Antagonistic Agents**   30, 35, 39
   Metabolic—PTH (kidney)
   Absorption—Ba^{2+}, Sr^{2+}, Be^{2+}, Ca^{2+} (excess), $Al(OH)_3$

6. **Physiological Functions (Maintenance of Systems/Components)**   18, 20, 21, 30, 50, 51

   Circulatory—Calcification of vessels involvement

   Excretory—Tubular reabsorption (via vitamin D, PTH)

   Respiratory—O_2 release from RBC (diphosphoglycerate); cellular respiration via ATP

   Digestive—Sugar absorption, Ca excretion (excess P), laxative (excess P)

   Nervous—ATP energy source; component of myelin sheath

   Special sensory—P-component of phospholipid membranes, RNA component

   Endocrine—Interaction with vitamin D, PTH, TCT (Ca absorption)

   Blood—RBC metabolism; lipoproteins, phospholipid components, electrolyte balance, pH

   Muscular—ATP in muscle contraction

   Skeletal—Component of bone, teeth

   Integument—Membrane component (phospholipid in skin, mucous membranes)

   Immune—ATP for leukocytes (energy)

   Metabolic—Ca metabolism, phosphorylation reactions; energy (protein, fat, CHO) via ATP

   Detoxification—Via liver using ATP (energy)

   Growth—++

   Health—+

   Longevity—+

7. **Body Content**   12, 21, 35, 50

   g/70 kg = 780 (500-800); μg/g = 11,000

8. **Relative Organ Concentrations** (80-86% body P in skeleton)   12, 21, 35, 50

   Teeth > skeleton > brain > spleen > kidneys > pancreas, thyroid > liver > muscle > gut > lung > heart > skin > fat

9. **Deficiencies**   18, 21, 23, 30, 36, 50

   Man—Rickets, osteomalacia, osteitis fibrosa cystica, familial hypophosphatemia

   Animals—Pica (ruminants)

10. **Excess Conditions**   18, 21, 23, 30, 36, 38, 39

    Man—Secondary hyperparathyroidism, hypoparathyroidism, hyperphosphatemia (children)

11. **Essentiality**   1, 38, 42

    Man—Vital, normal health and life span

    Other species—All require P for life

12. **Major Commercial Uses (Biological Interface)**   6, 22, 30, 54

Element—(Red P) safety matches, (white P) rat poison, pyrotechnics, munitions

Compounds—Insecticides, pesticides, detergents, fertilizers, nerve gases, acidulants (beverages), gasoline additives (antiknock), baking powders, glass manufacture, enamels

13. **Medicinal Applications**   18, 27, 30, 53, 54

Dentrifice—$(CaHPO_4)$

Dental products—$(CaHPO_4)$, $(Ca_3(PO_4)_2)$, (H_3PO_4)

Mineral supplement—$(CaHPO_4)$, $(Ca(H_2PO_4)_2)$, $(Ca_3(PO_4)_2)$

Urine acidifier—(NaH_2PO_4)

Antacid—$(CaHPO_4)$, $(Mg_3(PO_4)_2)$

Laxative—(Na_2HPO_4), (K_2HPO_4), $(MgHPO_4)$

14. **Hazards and Toxicity**   18, 30, 46, 39, 54

Element (Red P essentially nontoxic, white P extremely toxic)

White P

   Inhalation—Similar to ingestion

   Skin contact—Severe burns

   Ingestion (chronic)—Anemia, anorexia, weight loss, albuminuria, mucous bleeding, bone destruction, infection of jaw

Compounds (salts relatively innocuous; acid and PH_3 see below, PH_3 most toxic

   Inhalation—Acid: irritation; PH_3: weakness, vertigo, dyspnea, bronchitis, edema, lung damage, convulsions, coma, death

   Skin contact—Acid: irritation

   Oral toxicity—See nutrition section, dietary excess

Carcinogenicity/Mutagenicity = —/—

DISTRIBUTION AND SOURCES

1. **Occurrence and Environmental Concentrations (mg/g)**   3, 4, 6, 42

Relative terrestrial abundance—#11

Chief minerals—Phosphorite $[Ca_3(PO_4)_2]$; apatite $[CaF_2 \cdot 3Ca_3(PO_4)_2]$; hydroxyapatite $[Ca_{10}(PO_4)_6(OH)_2]$ (bone)

Earth's crust—1.18

Rocks—0.17-1.05 (sandstone-igneous)

Soils—0.65

Fresh water—5.0

Seawater—70.0

2. Organismal Concentrations (mg/g)   4, 42, 47

Plants—Marine: 3.50; land: 2.30

Animals—Marine: 4.00-18.00; land: 14.00-17.00

Man—11.00-12.00

Special concentrators—Brachiopods (shells), fish (bones), mammals (bones), green algae, protozoa, some fungi (poly-PO_4)

3. Dietary Sources (Variability due to Environment)   5, 12, 26, 27, 36, 48, 52

High (mg/100 g) 200-1200

Seafood—Tuna, mackerel, pike, red snapper, salmon, sardines, whitefish, scallops, shad, smelt, anchovies, bass, bluefish, carp, caviar, eel, halibut, herring, trout

Meat/Organs—Liver (beef, chicken, hog, lamb), rabbit, sweetbreads (beef), turkey, beef brains, chicken, eggs, egg yolk, lamb heart, kidney (beef, pig, lamb)

Nuts/Seeds—Pilinuts, pinon, pistachios, pumpkin, seasame, sunflower, walnuts, almonds, brazils, cashews, filberts, hickory, peanuts, pecans

Vegetables—Chickpeas (dry), garlic, lentils (dry), popcorn, soybeans

Dairy products/Fats—Cheeses (Blue, Brick, Cheddar, Limburger, Parmesan, Swiss)

Grains—Wheat (bran, germ), wildrice, buckwheat, millet, oats, oatmeal, brown rice, rice bran, rye, wheat

Miscellaneous—Chocolate, kelp, yeast (bakers', brewers', torula), bone meal

Medium (mg/100 g) 100-200

Seafood—Perch, shrimp, squid, swordfish, abalone, clams, cod, crab, sole, haddock, lobster, oysters

Meat/Organs—Tongue (beef, pig, lamb), veal, beef, chicken gizzard, heart (beef, chicken, pig), lamb, pork

Nuts/Seeds—Macadamia

Grains—Barley, white rice

Fruits—Prunes (dry), raisins (dry)

Vegetables—Lima beans, corn, cowpeas, peas

Dairy products—Cheese (Camembert, Cottage)

Miscellaneous—Mushrooms

Low (mg/100 g) 50-100

Nuts/Seeds—Chestnuts, coconut

Fruits—Dates (dry), figs (dry)

Vegetables—Collards, watercress, endive, horseradish, kale, kohlrabi, leeks, artichokes, asparagus, broccoli, brussels sprouts, cauliflower, mustard greens, okra, parsley, parsnips, potatoes, spinach, turnip greens, yams

Dairy products—Buttermilk, cheese (cream), cream, milk
Miscellaneous—Molasses (blackstrap, first extract)

CHEMISTRY

1. **Atomic Properties (Element)**   6. 7, 9, 30, 49
   Periodic table group no.—V-A, period 3
   Category of element—Nonmetal
   Atomic weight—30.97
   Atomic number—15
   Atomic radius (metallic)—1.09 Å
   Electron shells—2, 8, 5
   Orbital electrons—$1s^2$, $2s^2$, $2p^6$, $3s^2$, $3p^3$
   Natural isotopes—P^{31} (100%)
   Long-lived radioactive isotopes—P^{32} (14.2 days), P^{33} (24.4 days)

2. **Ionic Properties (Biological Forms)**   6, 7, 9, 30, 49
   Oxidation states (valences)—P^{5+} (PO_4^{3-})
   Ionic radius (Å)—P^{5+} (0.34)
   Oxidation potentials:
   $$P + 2H_2O \rightarrow H_3PO_2 \ (+0.29 \ v)$$
   $$H_3PO_2 + H_2O \rightarrow H_3PO_3 \ (+0.59 \ v)$$
   $$H_3PO_3 + H_2O \rightarrow H_3PO_4 \ (+0.20 \ v)$$

3. **Molecular Properties (Biological Forms)**   6, 7, 9, 30, 49
   Covalent radius (Å)—P^{5+} (0.93-1.20)
   Coordination number—4
   Stereochemistry—4 (tetrahedral)
   Electron transfer compounds—NADH, NADPH, FMN
   Typical molecular complex—$PO(OH)_3$

4. **Analytical Methods**   3, 30, 31, 40, 55
   Physical—Spark mass spectrometry, activation analysis
   Chemical—Spectrophotmetric: phosphomolybdenum blue
   Hair/Nail analysis—Hair by spark mass spectrometry
   Comments—P difficult to analyze by atomic absorption; reference standards
     lacking

5. **Chemical Properties of Compounds**   6, 7, 9, 49, 54
   See Table 1.1.

Table 1.1.   Properties of Phosphorus Compounds

| | REACTIONS | | | SOLUBILITY | | | |
	Heat °C	Air	Water	g/100 cc H_2O	Alc.	Eth.	Acid
Phosphoric acid H_3PO_4	$-H_2O(213°)$	deliq.	acid pH 1.5	548^{20}	S	NA	NA
Na phosphate (monobasic) NaH_2PO_4, H_2O	$-H_2O(100°)$	deliq.	acid pH 4.5	71^{20}	I	SS	NA
Ca phosphate (dibasic) $Ca(H_2PO_4)_2$ $1H_2O$	$-H_2O(100°)$	deliq.	acidic	1.8^{30}	I	NA	S
Ca phosphate (dibasic) $CaHPO_4 \cdot 2H_2O$	$-2H_2O(100°)$	deliq.	acidic	$.03^{18}$	I	NA	S
Ca phosphate (tribasic) $Ca_3(PO_4)_2$	stable	NA	basic	$.002^{20}$	I	NA	S

Table 1.1.   Properties of Phosphorus Compounds (continued)

	Density	MW hyd./anh.	MP °C	XL Form	Color XL/Powd.	Appearance Commercial Form	% Element, hyd./anh.	Odor	Taste	Synonyms
Phosphoric acid H_3PO_4	1.87	—/98.0	29.3	orthor-homb.	col./wh.	C, syrupy liquid	31.6/—	NA	acid	ortho phosphoric acid
Na phosphate (mono) $NaH_2PO_4 \cdot H_2O$	2.04	138.0/120.0	d.	rhomb.	col./wh.	C, P	22.4/25.8	0	NA	sodium biphosphate
Ca phosphate (mono) $Ca(H_2PO_4)_2 \cdot 1H_2O$	2.22	252.1/234.1	d.	triclin.	col./wh.	G, P	12.3/26.5	NA	acid	calcium biphosphate, super-phosphate
Ca phosphate (dibasic) $CaHPO_4 \cdot 2H_2O$	2.31	172.1/136.1	d.	triclin.	col./wh.	C	18.0/22.8	NA	0	NA
Ca phosphate (tribasic) $Ca_3(PO_4)_2$	3.14	—/310.2	1670°	amorph.	col./wh.	P	—/20.0	0	0	tricalcium or tertiary calcium phosphate

Abbreviations: deliq, = deliquesces; Alc. = alcohol; Eth. = ether; I = insoluble; SS =slightly soluble; S = soluble; hyd. = hydrous; anh. = anhydrous; 0 = none; d. = decomposes; orthorhomb. = orthorhombic; rhomb. = rhombic; triclin. = triclinic; amorph. = amorphous; XL = crystal; Powd. = powder; col. = colored; wh. = white; C = crystalline; G = granular; P = powder; MW = molecular weight; MP = melting point; NA = not available.

MEDICINAL AND NUTRITIONAL ROLE

1. **Units of Measurement**
   Weight—μg (microgram); 1 mg (milligram) = 1000 μg = .001 g
   Concentration—ppm (parts per million) = μg/g; mg% = mg/100 ml

2. **Human Body Fluid Levels (Normal) (mg/100 ml)**   1, 2, 4, 12, 23, 35
   Blood—Total P: 34.90; inorg. PO_4: 2.90 (2.40-3.50)
   Plasma/Serum—Total P: 11.40; inorg. PO_4: 3.90 (3.10-4.90)
   Urine—Total P: 57.50; inorg. PO_4: 56.00

3. **Human Tissue Levels (mg/g)**   4, 12, 24, 46
   Hair—0.12
   Bone—50.00
   Liver—1.70
   Muscle—1.30
   Nerve—2.60

4. **Important Dietary Levels**   5, 21, 27, 30, 35, 39, 57
   Recommended dietary allowance—800 mg/day
   Deficiency limits—No data
   Toxic limit—No data

5. **Estimated Human Daily Balance (average American diet, 70 kg ♂, 30 yr)**
   18, 21, 30, 53
   Average intake—1400 mg/day (1395 food, 5 water)
   Average output—1400 mg/day (540 feces, 860 urine, 0.1 sweat)
   Net gain/loss—Balanced normally

6. **Indications for Supplementation of Above Diet**   5, 21, 27, 30, 35, 57
   Healthy normal—None
   Special conditions—Pregnancy, lactation, growth

7. **Factors Affecting Availability from Diet**   18, 21, 27, 51, 53
   Decreased (See absorption section, inhibitors)
       Vegetarian diet
       High calcium, iron, magnesium, aluminum, in diet
       Vitamin D deficiency
   Increased (See absorption section, synergists)
       Vitamin D
       High fat diet
       STH, PTH
       Low calcium diet

8. **Deficiency Symptoms**   18, 21, 23, 30, 36, 51
Man:
  Rickets, osteomalacia, muscle weakness, bone pains, malaise, anorexia

9. **Effects of Dietary Excess** (salts or concentrates)   18, 23, 36, 39, 51
Acute—Hyperphosphatemia, hypocalcemia, hypomagnesemia, tetany, laxative effects
Chronic—Secondary hyperparathyroidism, bone resorption, calcification of heart and kidney, hypocalcemia

METABOLIC ROLE

1. **Intestinal absorption**   13, 18, 30, 35, 39, 44, 51
Chemical forms—Inorganic salts, organic compounds
  Preferred valence—+5
  Poorly absorbed—Phytates, polyphosphates
  Well absorbed—Inorganic salts (except poly-PO_4); organic compounds (except phytates)
Sites—Duodenum, jejunum, ileum
Efficiency—50-70%
Active transport—Yes
Synergizers—Vitamin D, Ca^{2+}, K^+, Na^+, H^+, PTH, STH
Antagonists—Ca^{2+} (excess), $Al(OH)_3$, Ba^{2+}, Sr^{2+}, Be^{2+}, T4, cortisol

2. **Blood carriers**   18, 30, 51
Plasma-protein P (12%), ionic PO_4 (ca. 80%), diphosphoglycerate (RBC), $HPO_4^{2-}/H_2PO_4^- = 5:1$ at physiologic pH (7.35)

3. **Half-life of Element in Blood**   20, 21, 51, 53
Not available; est. 0.83% of PO_4 in plasma excreted per minute at normal plasma levels

4. **Target (Initial) Sites**   30, 51, 53
Tissues—all
Cells—mitochondria

5. **Storage**   21, 30, 35, 51
Sites—Skeleton, (bone), mitochondria
Forms—Hydroxyapatite crystals

6. **Homeostatic Mechanisms**   18, 21, 30, 35, 42, 51, 53
Relative efficiency in element retention—90-100%
Kidney participation—Major controls, reabsorption via vitamin D + PTH
Intestinal participation—Relatively small amount
Liver (bile) participation—Relatively small amount

7. Specific Functions (via Cofactors/Metalloenzymes, Metalloproteins/Ions) 13. 18. 21, 25, 30, 32, 51, 53

Molecular level
  B-complex vitamins—Cofactor
  High-energy bonds—ATP, etc.
  Component of RNA, DNA—Backbone
  Component of phosphoproteins and phospholipids
Cellular level
  Component of membrane phospholipids
  Buffering of intracellular fluids
  Participation in carbohydrate and energy metabolism
  Cellular respiration—Mitochondria
Organismal level
  Buffering of extracellular fluids—Blood
  Component of bones and teeth
  Genetics of RNA and DNA
  Ca metabolism—Homeostasis
  Energy metabolism—via ATP, Krebs cycle
  Muscle contraction—via ATP

8. Metalloenzymes, Cofactors, Metalloproteins, Mineraloproteins   8, 10, 11 15, 18, 25, 30, 32, 35, 50, 51, 53

System Type	Organ	Metallo-Mineralo- Enzyme/Protein	Cofactors (PO_4)	System Function
Cofactors	Various	Pyruvate decarboxylase	Thiamine-P-P	Glucose metabolism
	Various	Dehydrogenases—oxidative phosphorylation	DPN	Energy metabolism
	Liver	Microsomal mixed function oxidases	TPN	Detoxification
	Various	{ Cytochrome C reductase L-amino oxidase	FMN	Oxidation-reduction
	Various	Flavoprotein enzymes	FAD	Oxidation-reduction
	Liver	Transferases	UDPG	CHO metabolism
	Liver	Pyruvate dehase thiokinases, thiolases	CoA	CHO metabolism Fatty acid metabolism
	Various	ATP-ases, phosphorylases, polymerases, synthetases, kinases	ATP	Esp. synthesis of proteins, nucleic acids, energy donor reactions
	Liver	Lecithin synthetases	CDPG	Lecithin synthesis
	Liver	Transmethylases, reductases, mutases, dehydrases	B_{12} coenzymes	Nucleic acid metabolism
	Liver	See vitamin B_6—various enzymes	Pyridoxal-P	Porphyrin, amine, and amino acid metabolism

Mineraloprotein systems—Phosphoproteins include casein (milk), vitellin (egg), nucleoproteins (nuclear)

9. **Excretion**   18, 20, 21, 30, 39, 51
Chemical forms—Urine (inorganic), fecal (phytates, divalent ion, insoluble salts)
Organs—Kidney (urine): 50-70% (tubular reabsorption); intestine (feces): 30-50%; liver (bile, intestine): relatively small amount; skin: very small amount; other: not significant

MISCELLANEOUS

1. **Relationship to Other Minerals**   18, 27, 30, 51, 53
Ca^{2+}—Absorption and metabolic synergist to PO_4; antagonist in excess
Mg^{2+}—Synergist to PO_4 in metabolism
Na^+, K^+—Synergists in PO_4 absorption
Sr^{2+}, Be^{2+}, Ba^{2+}, Al^{3+}—Sequester PO_4 in the gut
Fe^{2+}—Segregates PO_4 in the gut

2. **Relationship to Vitamins**   18, 27, 36, 37, 51, 53
Inositol—Hexaphosphate ester (phytate) segregates divalent ions in gut
B-complex—Most B-complex vitamins require PO_4 for biological activity
Vitamin D—Increases absorption of PO_4 in gut and in kidney

3. **Relationship to Hormones**   18, 20, 27, 50, 51, 53
PTH—Increases PO_4 absorption in gut, increases PO_4 excretion in kidney, and bone resorption
STH—Increases PO_4 absorption in gut and decreases PO_4 excretion in kidney
TCT—Increases PO_4 deposition in bone, increases PO_4 excretion in kidney
C-AMP—Cyclic AMP functions as secondary messenger for hormones
Cortisol, T4—Increase bone resorption

4. **Unusual Features**   18, 21, 27, 30, 36, 50, 51, 53
Central importance of PO_4 to cellular economy—Minerals, energy, growth
High-energy PO_4 bonds chief forms of cellular energy (ATP)
Low content of PO_4 in human milk (high in cow's milk)
Phosphate chains in RNA and DNA
Segregation of PO_4 in mitochondria (with Ca)
Decrease of blood PO_4 with age
Decrease of O_2 binding to Hb in children by higher PO_4 levels in blood

5. **Possible Relationship of Deficiency Symptoms to Metabolic Action**   18, 21, 27, 30, 35, 51, 53

Rickets, osteomalacia—Resorption of bone, ↓ diphosphoglycerate causes ↓ O_2 delivery and loss of ATP

Muscle weakness—lack of PO_4 high-energy compounds

Bone pains—Osteomalacia caused by hypophosphatemia

Malaise ⎱
Anorexia ⎰ —Reduced 2,3 diphosphoglycerate causes ↓ O_2 delivery

Chapter 2. Calcium (Ca)

Although about 99% of the body Ca is in structural form in the skeleton, the remainder of the Ca in the body is chiefly extracellular, with four major metabolic functions:

1. Membrane effects including permeability regulation, Ca pump action, muscular contraction (Ca-binding protein-calmodulin), nerve impulse conduction, intercellular cement.
2. Body fluid regulation including buffering, viscosity, PO_4 transfer, and clotting mechanisms.
3. Regulation of cell division (mitosis)
4. Regulation of hormonal secretion

Calcium is found in all plants and animals, and is essential for all life (except some insects and bacteria), and for normal growth, development, and life span in man and almost all life forms. Its mode of action is mainly by way of its transport properties, alkalinity, conductivity, charge, hydration, and sequestering effects. Without Ca the cell membrane would disintegrate, and life as we know it could not have developed. Extracellular fluid, containing Ca, may be considered to represent the Ca content of the environmental fluid in the post-Cambrian seas, in which animal organisms continued to develop before emergence on dry land. Calcium plays a key role in many physiological functions including cell division and is associated with many hormones and enzyme systems and a few vitamins. Calmodulin is found in most cells, acts as a universal regulator, a Ca transport agent and as a secondary cell messenger similar to C-AMP. It is the object of much research attention. It is absorbed as the free ion, and its chief synergist is phosphate, while its chief antagonist is sodium.

There is some evidence that the average American diet is adequate in Ca for the normal young adult. However, there is also evidence that there are greater calcium losses past middle age and that possibly more dietary calcium is required as senescence approaches. High-Ca dietary items include dairy products, molasses, yeast, whole-body seafoods, (e.g., sardines), and some seeds and nuts.

Deficiencies of Ca are found mainly in cases of vitamin D deficiency, growth, senescence, and individuals with parathyroid defects. Body Ca is well conserved by an efficient homeostatic system, but fecal losses do occur that are due to divalent ion sequestration.

GENERAL INFORMATION

1. **Dietary and Medicinal Forms** 18, 49, 53, 54
   Element—Calcium metal; not used medicinally
   Inorganic salts—Chloride, carbonate, phosphate (mono-, di-, tribasic)
   Chelated forms—Gluconate, lactate

2. **History of Biological Significance** 18, 21, 35, 50, 53
   1905—Delezenne: Ca important in blood clotting and proteolysis
   1920—Höber: smooth muscles require Ca for contraction
   1925—Loew: all animals require Ca in diet
   1926—Höber: Ca decreases permeability of cells
   1927—Gley and Bouckert: nerve cells require Ca for response to stimulus
   1931—Angus: isolation and characterization of vitamin D
   1934—Peters et al: Ca causes increased respiration of mammalian heart
   1941—Heilbrunn and Ashkenaz: skeletal muscle requires Ca for contraction
   1959—Rasmussen: discovery of PTH
   1967—Copp: discovery of calcitonin
   1970—Cheung: first described calmodulin

3. **Physiological (Blood) Forms** 18, 21, 50, 51, 53
   Ca-protein complexes, Ca citrate, Ca phosphate, ionic Ca^{2+} [ionic Ca^{2+} (65%) is only physiologically active form]

4. **Synergistic Agents** 30, 35, 39
   Metabolic—Some functions (Mg, Na, K)
   Absorption—1,25 $(OH)_2D_3$ (vitamin D), PTH, lysine, arginine, lactose

5. **Antagonistic Agents** 30, 35, 39
   Metabolic—Some functions (Mg, Na, K)
   Absorption—Glucocorticoids, calcitonin, T4, phytate, oxalate, PO_4, Mg, F

6. **Physiological Functions (Maintenance of Systems/Components)**   18, 20, 21, 30, 50, 51

Circulatory—Excites heart, constricts arterioles
Excretory—Inhibits diuresis (via ADH)
Respiratory—Stimulates heart respiration
Digestive—Constipative, sequestering agent
Nervous—Nerve impulse transmission (regulates ACH esterase)
Special sensory—Sensitizes neurons
Reproductive—Fertility, gametogenesis, mitosis
Endocrine—TRH, ADH, PTH release inhibited, calcitonin released
Blood—Stimulates hematopoiesis, electrolyte balance, P-transport
Muscular—Irritability, contractility (Ca-binding protein)
Skeletal—Major bone constituent
Integument—Intercellular cement component
Protective/Immune—Blood coagulation mechanisms
Metabolic
    Energy and PO_4 metabolism
    Enzyme catalysis, ↑ BMR (TRH)
Detoxification—Inhibits Pb uptake in gut
Growth—++ (mitotic stimulant)
Health—+
Longevity—+

7. **Body Content**   12, 21, 35, 50
g/70 kg = 1,050-1,200; μg/g = 15,000-17,000

8. **Relative Organ Concentrations**   12, 21, 35, 50
Bone > Thyroid > Uterus > Kidney > Skin > Pancreas > Lungs > Adrenal > Intestine > Liver, Brain > Serum > Spleen > Heart > Testes > Muscle

9. **Deficiencies**   18, 21, 23, 30, 36, 51
Man—Rickets, osteoporosis, osteomalacia, tetany, hypoparathyroidism, hypocalcemia

10. **Excess Conditions**   18, 21, 23, 30, 36, 38, 39
Man—Hypercalcemia, hyperparathyroidism, disuse atrophy (?)

11. **Essentiality**   1, 38, 42
Man—Vital, normal growth and longevity
Other species—All species: vertebrates, Protozoa, algae, fungi, spermatophytes; some species: invertebrates, insects, bacteria

12. **Major Commercial Uses (Biological Interface)**   6, 22, 30, 54
    Element—Deoxidizer and hardener of metals, flints
    Compounds—Preservative, antifreeze, foods, fertilizer, anticaking agents,
    beverages, sewage purification, concrete, glass, acidulants

13. **Medicinal Applications**   18, 27, 30, 53, 54
    Antacid ($CaCO_3$), Ca-deficiency supplement (Ca lactate, Ca gluconate), anti-
    diarrheal ($CaCO_3$), electrolyte replacement ($CaCl_2$), diuretic ($CaCl_2$),
    dentifrices (Ca lactate), acidifier ($CaCl_2$), plaster casts ($CaSO_4$)

14. **Hazards and Toxicity**   18, 30, 46, 39, 54
    Element
        Inhalation—No data
        Contact—Relatively nontoxic
    Compounds
        Inhalation (depends on type of salt)—Possible pneumonia, bronchial
            irriatation, vasomotor disturbances, dyspnea, dermatitis
        Contact (depends on type of salt)—Nontoxic or irritant
        Oral toxicity—See nutrition section, dietary excess
    Carcinogenicity/Mutagenicity = —/—

DISTRIBUTION AND SOURCES

1. **Occurrence and Environmental Concentrations (mg/g)**   3, 4, 6, 42
    Relative terrestrial abundance—#5
    Chief minerals—Limestone ($CaCO_3$), apatite [$Ca_3(PO_4)_2 \cdot CaF_2$], gypsum
    ($CaSO_4$), fluorite (CaF_2), phosphorite [$Ca_3(PO_4)_2$], calcite ($CaCO_3$)
    Earth's crust—36.30
    Rocks—22.10-302.00 (shales-limestones)
    Soils—7.00-500.00 (average 13.70)
    Freshwater—0.015
    Seawater—0.40

2. **Organismal Concentrations (mg/g)**   4, 42, 47
    Plants—Marine: 10.00; land: 18.00

Animals—Marine: 1.50-20.00; land: 0.20-85.00 (260.00 bone, .20-.50 soft tissues)

Man—14.00

Special concentrators—Shellfish, vertebrates

3. **Dietary Sources (Variability due to Environment)**   5, 12, 26, 27, 36, 48, 52
   High (mg/100 g) 200-400
       Seafood—Sardines, pilchards, caviar, smelt
       Meat/Organs—Egg yolk
       Nuts/Seeds—Almonds, sesame seeds, filberts
       Vegetables—Kale, collards, mustard greens, turnip greens, soybeans
       Dairy products—Cheeses (blue, cheddar, swiss, brick, Limburger, American Parmesan)
       Miscellaneous—Milk chocolate, molasses (blackstrap), kelp, brewer's yeast, torula yeast
   Medium (mg/100 g) 100-200
       Seafood—Shrimp, salmon, mackerel, anchovy, scallops
       Nuts/Seeds—Brazil, pilinuts, pistachios, sunflower
       Grains—Oats, buckwheat, wheat bran
       Fruit—Figs (dry)
       Vegetables—Cabbage, chickpeas, horseradish, dandelion greens, chard, beet greens, mung beans, broccoli, watercress, parsley, onions, red kidney beans
       Dairy products—Buttermilk, ice cream, milk, yogurt
       Miscellaneous—Light molasses, cocoa, maple syrup, maple sugar
   Low (mg/100 g) 50-100
       Seafood—Clams, flounder, herring (kippered), crayfish, carp, lobster, oysters
       Meat/Organs—Eggs
       Nuts/Seeds—Peanuts, pecans, walnuts, pumpkin seeds
       Grains—Wheat germ
       Fruit—Dates (dry), prunes (dry), raisins, rhubarb, olives, oranges, lemons, black currants
       Vegetables—Romaine lettuce, lima beans, green beans, okra, artichokes, chives, lentils (dry), peas, parsnips, rutabagas, celery, endive, spinach, leeks
       Dairy Products—Cheeses (Camembert, cottage, cream), sherbet
       Miscellaneous—Chocolate, brown sugar

CHEMISTRY

1. **Atomic Properties (Element)**   6, 7, 9, 30, 49
   Periodic table group no.—II-A, period 4
   Category of element—Alkaline earth, metal
   Atomic weight—40.08
   Atomic number—20
   Atomic radius (metallic)—1.874 Å
   Electron shells—2, 8, 8, 2
   Orbital electrons—$1s^2$, $2s^2$, $2p^6$, $3s^2$, $3p^6$, $4s^2$
   Natural isotopes—Ca^{40} (97%), Ca^{42} (0.6%), Ca^{44} (2.1%)
   Long-lived radioactive isotopes—Ca^{41} (10^5 yr), Ca^{45} (164 days), Ca^{47} (4.9 days)

2. **Ionic Properties (Biological Forms)**   6, 7, 9, 30, 49
   Oxidation states (valences)—Ca^{2+}
   Ionic radius (Å)—0.94 Å
   Oxidation potentials—$Ca^0 \rightarrow Ca^{2+}$ (2.87 v)

3. **Molecular Properties (Biological Forms)**   6, 7, 9, 16, 25, 30, 43, 49
   Covalent radius (Å)—1.39 Å
   Coordination numbers—6, 8
   Stereochemistry—Hexahedral, octahedral
   Electron transfer compounds—None reported
   Typical molecular complexes—Ca (EDTA)

4. **Analytical Methods**   3, 30, 31, 40, 55
   Physical—Atomic absorption
   Chemical—Spectrophotometric: glyoxal-bis (2-hydroxyanil)
   Hair/Nail analysis—Hair feasible
   Comments—Precautions as for Mg^{2+}

5. **Chemical Properties of Compounds**   6, 7, 9, 49, 54
   See Table 2.1.

Table 2.1. Properties of Calcium Compounds

	REACTIONS			SOLUBILITY			
	Heat °C	Air	Water	g/100 cc H_2O	Alc.	Eth.	Acid
Ca lactate $Ca(C_3H_5O_3)_2 \cdot 5H_2O$	$-H_2O(100°)$	efflor.	neut., pH7	5.4^{15}	I	I	SS
Ca gluconate $Ca(C_6H_4O_7) \cdot H_2O$	$-H_2O(120°)$	stable	neut., pH7	3.3^{15}	I	I	NA
Ca chloride $CaCl_2 \cdot 2H_2O$	$-2H_2O(200°)$	deliq.	heat acidic	74.5^{20}	S	NA	NA
Ca phosphate monobasic $CaH_4(PO_4)_2 \cdot H_2O$	$-H_2O(100°)$	deliq.	acidic	1.8^{30}	I	NA	S
Ca phosphate dibasic $CaHPO_4 \cdot 2H_2O$	$-2H_2O(100°)$	deliq.	acidic	$.03^{18}$	I	NA	S
Ca phosphate tribasic $Ca_3(PO_4)_2$	stable	NA	basic	$.002^{20}$	I	NA	S
Ca carbonate $CaCO_3$	$-CO_2(825°)$	stable	NA	$.001^{20}$	I	NA	S

Table 2.1   Properties of Calcium Compounds (continued)

	Density	MW hyd./anh.	MP °C	XL Form	Color XL/Powd.	Appearance Commercial Form	% Element h./anh.	Odor	Taste	Synonyms
Ca lactate $Ca(C_3H_5O_3)_2 \cdot 5H_2O$	NA	308.3/ 218.2	d	need.	col./wh.	G, P	13.0/ 18.4	0	NA	NA
Ca gluconate $Ca(C_6H_4O_7) \cdot H_2O$	NA	448.4/ 430.4	d	need.	col./wh.	C, G, P	8.9/ 9.3	0	0	calciofon glucal ebucin
Ca chloride $CaCl_2 \cdot 2H_2O$	0.835	147.0/ 110.0	d	cubic	col./wh.	G, F, P	27.3/ 36.1	0	NA	NA
Ca phosphate monobasic $CaH_4(PO_4)_2 \cdot H_2O$	2.22	252.1/ 234.1	d	triclin.	col./wh.	G, P. C	15.9/ 17.1	NA	acidic	Ca biphos. Ca superphos.
Ca phosphate dibasic $CaHPO_4 \cdot 2H_2O$	2.31	172.1/ 136.1	d	triclin.	col./wh.	C	23.3/ 29.5	NA	0	NA
Ca phosphate tribasic $Ca_3(PO_4)_2$	3.14	-/310.2	1670°	amorph.	col./wh.	P	-/38.8	0	0	trical PO_4 tertcal PO_4
Ca carbonate $CaCO_3$	2.83/ 2.71	-/100.1	d	hex. rhomb.	col./wh.	P, C	-/40.0	0	chalky	limestone chalk

Abbreviations: efflor. = effloresces; neut. = neutral; need. = needles; hex. = hexagonal; F = flakes; C = crystals; h. = hydrated. Others as in Table 1.1.

MEDICINAL AND NUTRITIONAL ROLE

1. **Units of Measurement**
   Weight—μg (microgram); 1 mg (milligram) = 1000 μg = .001 g
   Concentration—ppm (parts per million) = μg/g; mg% = mg/100 ml

2. **Human Body Fluid Levels (Normal) (mg/100 ml)**   1, 2, 4, 12, 23, 35
   Blood—6.20-9.70 (8.00)
   Plasma, serum—8.80-10.40 (10.00)
   Urine—3.30-26.40 (15.40)

3. **Human Tissue Levels (mg/g)**   4, 12, 24, 46
   Hair—0.36-0.85
   Bone—110.00-260.00
   Muscle—0.07
   Nerve—0.12
   Liver—0.12

4. **Important Dietary Levels**   5, 21, 27, 30, 35, 39, 57
   Recommended dietary allowance—800 mg/day
   Deficiency limits—<200 mg/day
   Toxic limit—No data

5. **Estimated Human Daily Balance (average American diet, 70 kg ♂, 30 yr)**
   18, 21, 30, 53
   Average intake—1000 mg/day (977 food, 23 water)
   Average output—1000 mg/day (800 feces, 175 urine, 25 sweat)
   Net gain/loss—Balanced (accumulation in aorta, kidneys, prostate, thyroid,
   trachea, with age)

6. **Indications for Supplementation of Above Diet**   5, 21, 27, 30, 35, 57
   Healthy normal—None
   Special conditions—Pregnancy, lactation, senescence (osteoporosis)

7. **Factors Affecting Availability from Diet**   18, 21, 27, 51, 53
   Decreased (See absorption section, inhibitors)
       Low protein diet
       High Fat diet
       Excessive divalent metals and phosphates
       Alkali ingestion
   Increased (See absorption section, synergists)
       High protein diet
       Hypocalcemia
       Acidity in gut
       Vitamin D and PTH

8. **Deficiency Symptoms**   18, 21, 23, 30, 36, 51
    Man: Tetany, paresthesias, hyperirritability, laryngospasm, muscle cramps, convulsions (grand mal), bone demineralization, parathyroid hyperplasia, stunted growth

9. **Effects of Dietary Excess (Salts or Concentrates)**   18, 23, 36, 39, 51
    Acute—Ca salts practically nontoxic except for: Ca arsenate (arsenic toxicity), Ca molybdate (molybdenum toxicity), Ca chloride (gastric irritant); hypothyroid individuals (hypercalcemia), vitamin D overdosage
    Chronic—Practically nontoxic except for: Ca arsenate (arsenic toxicity), Ca molybdate (molybdenum toxicity), Ca chloride (gastric irritant), hypothyroid individuals (hypercalcemia), vitamin D overdosage

METABOLIC ROLE

1. **Intestinal Absorption**   3, 18, 30, 35, 39, 44, 51
    Chemical forms—Sulfates, phosphates, chlorides, protein complexes, phytates
    Preferred valence—Ca^{2+}
    Poorly absorbed—Phytates, complexes, multivalent salts
    Well absorbed—Lactates, chlorides, gluconates
    Sites—Duodenum, upper jejunum
    Efficiency—30-40%
    Active transport—Yes
    Synergizers—Vitamin D_3 (1.25 $(OH_2)D$), PTH, lysine, arginine, lactose, Ca-binding protein
    Antagonists—Calcitonin, glucocorticoids, phytates, oxalates, phosphates, Mg

2. **Blood carriers**   18, 30, 51
    Ca-protein complexes (35%) not physiologically active; ionic Ca^{2+} (65%) physiologically active

3. **Half-Life of Element in Blood**   20, 21, 51, 53
    Not available; est. 0.04% of plasma Ca excreted per minute at normal plasma levels

4. **Target (Initial) Sites**   30, 51, 53
    Tissues—All
    Cells—Mitochondria, endoplasmic reticulum

5. **Storage**   21, 30, 35, 51, 53
   Sites—Bone (accumulations with age in aorta, kidneys, prostate), mitochondria
   Forms—Bone crystal, (hydroxyapatite) $Ca_{10}(PO_4)_6(OH)_2$

6. **Homeostatic Mechanisms**   18, 21, 30, 35, 42, 51, 53
   Relative efficiency in element retention—80-100%
   Kidney participation—90% reabsorption ($\uparrow$ by PTH, vitamin D_3 $\downarrow$ by adrenal
      steroids, calcitonin)
   Intestinal participation—Secretion and reabsorption
   Liver (bile) participation—Secretion and reabsorption (the last two systems
      via the enterohepatic circulation)

7. **Specific Functions (via Cofactors/Metalloenzymes, Metalloproteins/Ions)**
      13, 18, 21, 25, 30, 32, 51, 53
   Molecular level
      Bone crystal structure component
      Regulation of certain enzymes—Cofactor
      Insolubilizing agent
      Intracellular electrolyte balance
   Cellular level
      Decreased membrane permeability to Na, K
      Maintenance of irritability of nerves, muscles
      Intercellular cement
      Inhibition of adenyl cyclase
      Activator of muscle contraction
      Enzyme catalyst—Mitochondrial granules
      Mitotic agent (stimulant)
      Universal regulator—calmodulin
   Organismal level
      Blood clotting mechanisms
      Maintenance of muscular contractility
      Release of hormones (TRH, ADH, calcitonin)
      Major bone structure component
      Maintenance of neural transmission (acetylcholine)
      Homeostasis of blood vessels and heart
      Maintenance of electrolyte balance
      Energy metabolism participation
      Phosphorus metabolism homeostasis

8. **Metalloenzymes Cofactors, Metalloproteins** 8, 10, 11, 15, 18, 25, 30, 32, 35, 50, 51, 53

System Type	Organ	Metallo-enzyme/Protein	Cofactors	System Function
Metallo-protein Cofactor	Muscle	Troponin	Ca^{2+}	Contraction of muscle
	Endocrine glands	Adenyl cyclase	Ca^{2+}	Inhibition of C-AMP
	Bone, Kidney	Kinases	Ca^{2+}	Stimulated (form PO_4-proteins)
	Nerves	Choline esterase	Ca^{2+}	Destruction of acetycholine
	Blood	Prothrombin	Ca^{2+}	Formation of thrombin, blood clotting
	Pancreas	Lipase	Ca^{2+}	Fat digestion
	Liver	Succinic deHase	Ca^{2+}	Krebs cycle
	Muscle	ATP-ase	Ca^{2+}	ATP → ADP (muscle energy)

9. **Excretion** 18, 20, 21, 30, 39, 51
Chemical forms—Urine (phosphate, citrate, Ca^{2+} ion, chlorides), feces (bile compounds, phytates, oxalates, PO_4, Ca soaps)
Organs—Kidney (urine): 15-20%; intestine (feces): 70-80%; liver (bile, intestine): some reabsorption; skin: 2-5%; other: 0

MISCELLANEOUS

1. **Relationship to Other Minerals** 18, 27, 30, 51, 53
Mg—Absorption antagonist, synergist in bone and metabolism
Na—Antagonist or synergist to Ca, depending on organ and concentration
K—Antagonist or synergist to Ca, depending on organ and concentration
PO_4—Absorption synergist (antagonist in excess Ca), synergist in bone
F—Absorption antagonist
Fe—Utilization stimulated by Ca (hematopoiesis)

2. **Relationship to Vitamins** 18, 27, 36, 37, 51, 53
Vitamin D—Synergist in absorption
Vitamin A—Synergist in absorption
Vitamin C—Synergist in bone growth

3. **Relationship to Hormones**   18, 20, 27, 50, 51, 53
   PTH—Regulates Ca in blood (increases blood Ca)
   TRH—Ca releases TRH
   Calcitonin—Regulates Ca in blood (decreases blood Ca)
   ADH—Ca releases ADH
   Cyclic AMP—Ca inhibits adenyl cyclase

4. **Unusual Features**   18, 21, 27, 30, 36, 50, 51, 53
   High protein diet increases Ca loss in urine
   Endocrine glands output depends on Ca concentration
   High reabsorption of Ca by kidney
   Accumulation in certain tissues with age
   Nontoxicity of Ca salts orally
   Mitochondrial concentration of Ca
   Increase in respiration rate of certain organs
   Mitotic stimulation
   Muscular contraction (Ca-binding protein—Calmodulin)
   Universal regulator—Calmodulin

5. **Possible Relationship of Deficiency Symptoms to Metabolic Action**   18, 21,
       27, 30, 35, 51, 53
   Bone demineralization—PTH action, to restore blood Ca
   Stunted growth—Lack of available Ca for bone growth
   Parathyroid hyperplasia—Overstimulation of parathyroid gland
   Tetany, convulsions, laryngospasm ⎫ Increased neuronal permeability to
                                     ⎬ Na + K
   Hyperirritability, death   ⎭ Decreased neuronal transmitters

Chapter 3. Magnesium (Mg)

Although about 60% of the body Mg is in structural form in the skeleton, the remainder of the Mg in the body is chiefly in the intracellular form, with three major metabolic functions:

1. Membrane effects, including permeability, muscular contraction, nerve impulse conduction, and antagonism to Ca
2. Intracellular fluid regulation, including viscosity, buffering, PO_4 transport, activation of enzyme systems, chelating agent, and antagonism to Ca
3. Regulation of protein synthesis

Magnesium is found in all animals and plants (except some insects) and is essential for their life, good health, and normal longevity. Its mode of action is chiefly due to its transport properties, alkalinity, hydration, conductivity, and chelating effects. Intracellular fluid containing high Mg (relative to Ca) is considered by some to represent the original fluid (pre-Cambrian seas) in which life evolved. Without Mg, chlorophyll might never have developed to be the efficient photon trap it has become, and life might never have survived without the products of photosynthesis—oxygen and plentiful carbohydrates. Also, protein synthesis cannot proceed without Mg. Magnesium plays a key role in many physiological functions (especially protein synthesis) and is associated with many key enzymes and a few hormones and vitamins. It is absorbed as the free ion, and its chief synergizer is potassium; its chief antagonist is Ca.

There is no evidence of a Mg deficiency in the average American diet. It may be beneficial to balance the Ca intake with Mg in cases of nephrocalcinosis, tissue repair, hyperirritability, and muscular weakness. High dietary Mg items include some nuts, some grains, soybeans, brewer's yeast, kelp, blackstrap molasses, and dolomite.

Deficiencies of Mg are found mainly in cases of hyperirritability, soft tissue calcification, muscular dysfunction, intestinal losses, and malnutrition. Body Mg is fairly well conserved by the kidney, although fecal losses do occur in the form of sequestered Mg compounds.

GENERAL INFORMATION

1. **Dietary and Medicinal Forms**   18, 49, 53, 54

   Element—Magnesium: metal; not used medicinally

   Inorganic salts—Sulfate (epsom salts), oxide (magnesia), hydroxide (milk of magnesia), magnesium calcium carbonate (dolomite)

   Chelated forms—Citrate, gluconate, palmitate

2. **History of Biological Significance**   18, 21, 35, 50, 53

   1905—Meltzer and Aver: first description of anesthetic action of Mg in animals

   1932—Kruse: first detailed Mg deficiency in animals

   1934—Hirschfelder: first human Mg deficiency reported

   1936—Fisher et al.: Mg a part of chlorophyll structure

   1951—Cotlove: Mg deficiency reduces K in cells

   1956—Flink: confirmed existence of Mg deficiency in man

   1959—Tissieres: ribosomal subunits require Mg for aggregation

   1963—MacIntyre: evidence for PTH control of plasma Mg

   1967—Durlach et al.: detailed description of human Mg deficiency

   1969—Shils: Mg essential for mobilization of Ca from bone

   1969—Barnes: Mg conserved by kidney in humans

3. **Physiological (Blood) Forms**   18, 21, 50, 51 53

   Mg^{2+} ion, "protein-bound-Mg," "complexed Mg"

4. **Synergistic Agents**   30, 35, 39

   Metabolic (some functions)—Na, K, Ca

   Absorption—Vitamin D (?), lactic acid, lactose

5. **Antagonistic Agents**   30, 35, 39
   Metabolic (some functions)—Ca, Na, K
   Absorption—Ca, phytates, $PO_4{}^{2-}$, F^-, Na^+, fats

6. **Physiological Functions (Maintenance of Systems/Components)**   18, 20, 21, 30, 50, 51
   Circulatory—Maintenance heart muscle and EKG; vasodilatation blood vessels
   Excretory—Prevention of nephrocalcinosis
   Respiratory—Maintenance of pulmonary activity
   Digestive—Laxative properties (Mg excess)
   Nervous—Maintenance of neuromuscular transmission
   Special sensory—Neuronal homeostasis
   Reproductive—Growth of fetus (protein synthesis)
   Endocrine—Synergizes the secretion of PTH, antagonizes T4
   Blood—Blood lipids homeostasis
   Muscular—Maintenance of irritability; prevention of soft tissue calcification
   Skeletal—Maintenance of bone structure
   Integument—Prevention of hyperemic skin (rats)
   Protective/Immune—Homeostasis of clotting mechanisms
   Metabolic—Glucose and fatty acid catabolism; interaction in protein synthesis, Na, Ca, K metabolism; body temperature maintenance
   Detoxification—Liver maintenance
   Growth—+
   Health—+
   Longevity—+

7. **Body Content**   12, 21, 35, 50
   g/70 kg = 20-28; μg/g = 300-420

8. **Relative Organ Concentrations**   12, 21, 35, 50
   Bone has 50-70% body Mg
   Bone > kidney > muscle > gut > heart > spleen > nerve > skin > liver > fat ≥ lungs

9. **Deficiencies**   18, 21, 23, 30, 36, 51
   Man—Hypomagnesemia
   Animals—Hyperemia (rats), hypomagnesemia (sheep)

10. **Excess Conditions**   18, 21, 23, 30, 36, 38, 39
    Man—Hypermagnesemia
    Animals—Hyperemia, convulsions, neutomuscular changes, grass tetany (cattle)

11. **Essentiality**   1, 38, 42
Man—Vital, good health, normal longevity
Other species—All: vertebrates, invertebrates, fungi, spermatophytes, protozoa, algae; some: insects, bacteria

12. **Major Commercial Uses (Biological Interface)**   6, 22, 30, 54
Element—Pyrotechnics, flares (metal); alloys (Mg-Al-Fe)
Compounds—Fertilizer ($MgSO_4$), cements (MgO), firebrick (MgO), glue (MgO), fireproofing ($MgSO_4$)

13. **Medicinal Applications**   18, 27, 30, 53, 54
Mineral waters ($MgSO_4$)
Cathartic (various Mg salts)
Antacid [$Mg(OH)_2$], (MgO)
Sedative ($MgBr_2$)
Muscular relaxant ($MgSO_4$)
Cholagogue ($MgSO_4$)

14. **Hazards and Toxicity**   18, 30, 46, 39, 54
Element
    Inhalation—Metal fume fever, irritation
    Contact—Blebs on skin
Compounds
    Inhalation—Leukocytosis, granulomas, fever
    Contact—Generally nontoxic
    Oral toxicity—See nutrition section, dietary excess
Carcinogenicity/Mutagenicity = —/—

DISTRIBUTION AND SOURCES

1. **Occurrence and Environmental Concentrations (mg/g)**   3, 4, 6, 42
Relative terrestrial abundance—#8
Chief minerals—kieserite ($MgSO_4$); periclase (MgO); brucite [$Mg(OH)_2$]; dolomite [$MgCa(CO_3)_2$]
Earth's crust—20.90
Rocks—2.70-23.30 (limestone-igneous)
Soils—5.00
Freshwater—0.004
Seawater—1.35

2. **Organismal Concentrations (mg/g)**   4, 42, 47
Plants—Marine: 5.20; land: 3.20

Animals—Marine: 5.00; land: 1.00

Man—0.29

Special concentrators—Calcareous red algae, Foraminifera, Bryozoa, Porifera

3. **Dietary Sources (Variability due to Environment)**   5, 12, 26, 27, 36, 48, 52
   High (mg/100 g) 200-400
       Nuts/Seeds—Almonds, brazils, cashews
       Vegetables—Soybeans, parsnips
       Grains—Buckwheat, wheat bran, germ
       Miscellaneous—Chocolate, cocoa, blackstrap molasses, brewer's yeast, kelp
   Medium (mg/100 g) 100-200
       Nuts/Seeds—Filberts, hickory, peanuts, pecans, pistachio, walnuts, sesame
       Grains—Barley, millet, oats, rye, wheat, wildrice
       Vegetables—Beet greens, corn, peas, carrots
       Miscellaneous—Salt, torula yeast, brown sugar, sugar cane
   Low (mg/100 g) 50-100
       Seafood—Shrimp, tuna, clams
       Grains—Brown rice
       Fruits—Apricots, dates, figs (dry)
       Vegetables—Lima beans, chard, parsley, collards, cowpeas, turnip greens,
          lentils (dry), spinach
       Miscellaneous—Molasses (medium), baker's yeast, coconut (dry), raw sugar

CHEMISTRY

1. **Atomic Properties (Element)**   6, 7, 9, 30, 49
   Periodic table group no.—II-A, period 3
   Category of element—Metal, alkaline earth
   Atomic weight—24.31
   Atomic number—12
   Atomic radius (metallic)—1.60 Å
   Electron shells—2, 8, 2
   Orbital electrons—$1s^2$, $2s^2$, $2p^6$, $3s^2$
   Natural isotopes—Mg^{24} (77.4%), Mg^{25} (11.5%), Mg^{26} (11.1%)
   Long-lived radioactive isotopes—Mg^{27} (9.5 min), Mg^{28} (21.4 hr)

2. **Ionic Properties (Biological Forms)**   6, 7, 9, 30, 49
   Oxidation states (valences)—Mg^{2+}

Ionic radius (Å)—0.65-0.75
Oxidation potentials—$Mg^0 \rightarrow Mg^{2+}$ (+2.375 v)

3. **Molecular Properties (Biological Forms)**   6, 7, 9, 16, 25, 30, 43, 49
Covalent radius (Å)—1.20
Coordination numbers—4, 5, 6, 8
Stereochemistry—4, tetrahedral; 5, planar; 6, hexahedral; 8, octahedral
Electron transfer compounds—Chlorophyll (?)
Typical molecular complexes—$[Mg(NH_3)_6]^{2+}$, $[Mg(H_2O)_6]^{2+}$

4. **Analytical Methods**   3, 30, 31, 40, 55
Physical—Atomic absorption (flameless)
Chemical—Spectrophotometric, titan yellow method
Hair/Nail analysis—Feasible, many reports of hair analysis
Comments—protein interferes with atomic absorption; lack of reference
    standards causes difficulty in comparison of methods

5. **Chemical Properties of Compounds**   6, 7, 9, 49, 54
See Table 3.1

MEDICINAL AND NUTRITIONAL ROLE

1. **Units of Measurement**
Weight—μg (microgram); 1 mg (milligram) = 1000 μg = .001 g
Concentration—ppm (parts per million) = $\mu g/g$; mg% = mg/100 ml

2. **Human Body Fluid Levels (Normal) (mg/100 ml)**   1, 2, 4, 12, 23, 35
Blood—4.24
Plasma/Serum—1.00-3.00 (2.00)
Urine—1.96-11.20 (6.30)

3. **Human Tissue Levels ($\mu g/g$)**   4, 12, 24, 46
Hair—53-135
Liver—22.0
Muscle—23.0
Nerve—16.0
Bone—105.0

4. **Important Dietary Levels**   5, 21, 27, 30, 35, 39, 57
Recommended dietary allowance—350 mg/day ♂ (300 ♀)

Table 3.1.   Properties of Magnesium Compounds

	REACTIONS			SOLUBILITY			
	Heat °C	Air	Water	g/100 cc H_2O	Alc.	Eth.	Acid
Mg sulfate $MgSO_4 \cdot 7H_2O$	$-7\ H_2O(250°)$	efflor.	neut. pH 6-7	71^{20}	SS	NA	NA
Mg citrate $Mg_3(C_6H_5O_7)_2 \cdot 14H_2O$	NA	NA	NA	SS	I	NA	S
Mg palmitate $MgC_{16}H_{31}O_{22}$	NA	NA	NA	$.008^{25}$	SS	SS	NA
Mg gluconate $Mg(C_6H_{11}O_7)_2 \cdot H_2O$	NA	NA	NA	NA	NA	NA	NA
MgCa carbonate $CaCO_3 \cdot MgCO_3$	d. 730°	NA	NA	$.032^{18}$	NA	NA	NA
Mg oxide MgO	BP 3600^c	adds CO_2 deliq.	alk. pH 10.3	$.0006^{15}$	I	NA	S
Mg hydroxide $Mg(OH)_2$	$-H_2O(350°)$	adds CO_2	alk.	$.0009^{15}$	NA	NA	NA

Table 3.1   Properties of Magnesium Compounds (continued)

	Density	MW hyd./anh.	MP °C	XL Form	Color XL/Powd.	Appearance Commercial Form	% Element h./anh.	Odor	Taste	Synonyms
Mg sulfate $MgSO_4 \cdot 7H_2O$	1.68	246.5/ 120.4	d	rhomb. monocl.	col./wh.	C, P	9.9/ 20.2	O	bitter saline	epsom salts
Mg citrate $Mg_3(C_6H_5O_7)_2 \cdot 14H_2O$	NA	703.4/ 451.1	NA	NA	co./wh.	P, G	10.4/ 16.2	O	pleasant	NA
Mg palmitate $MgC_{16}H_{31}O_{22}$	NA	$-$/535.2	121.5°	need.	col./wh.	L, need.	$-$/4.5	NA	NA	NA
Mg gluconate $Mg(C_6H_{11}O_7)_2 \cdot H_2O$	NA	NA	NA	NA	NA	NA	NA	NA	NA	NA
MgCa carbonate $CaCO_3 \cdot MgCO_3$	2.87	$-$/184.4	d	trig.	col./wh.	NA	$-$/13.2	NA	NA	dolomite
Mg oxide MgO	3.58	$-$/40.3	2852°	cubic	col./wh.	P	$-$/60.3	O	NA	NA
Mg hydroxide $Mg(OH)_2$	2.36	$-$/58.3	d	hex.	col./wh.	P, PL	$-$/41.7	NA	NA	milk of magnesia

Abbreviations: Pr = prisms; S = scales; PL = plates; alk. = alkaline; monocl. = monoclinic; hex. = hexagonal; trig. = trigonal. Others as in Tables 1.1 and 2.1.

Deficiency limits—< 0.85 mg/day
Toxic limit—> 15 g/day
Estimated daily intake range—180-480 (average 330) mg/day

5. **Estimated Human Daily Balance (average American diet, 70 kg ♂, 30 yr)**
    18, 21, 30, 53
    Average intake—330 mg/day (324 food, 6 water)
    Average output—330 mg/day (215 feces, 104 urine, 11 sweat)
    Net gain/loss—Balanced, no change

6. **Indications for Supplementation of Above Diet**   5, 21, 27, 30, 35, 57
    Healthy normal—None
    Special conditions—Deficiency, malnutrition, intestinal losses

7. **Factors Affecting Availability from Diet**   18, 21, 27, 51, 53
    Decreased
        Insolubility of Mg compounds
        See absorption section, antagonists
        Alcoholism, diarrhea, old age
        Cooking in water
        Low Mg content in food
        Low protein diet
    Increased
        Solubility of Mg compounds
        See absorption section, synergists
        Ca deficiency
        High protein diet

8. **Deficiency Symptons**   18, 21, 23, 30, 36, 51
    Man: Poor growth, hyperirritability, convulsions, tetany, death

9. **Effects of Dietary Excess (Salts or Concentrates)**   18, 23, 36, 39, 51
    Acute—Purgative; nausea; malaise; muscular weakness and paralysis; paralysis
        of respiratory, cardiovascular, and CNS
    Chronic—Muscle weakness, hypotension, ECG changes, sedation, confusion

METABOLIC ROLE

1. **Intestinal Absorption**   13, 18, 30, 35, 39, 44, 51
    Chemical forms—Chlorides, sulfates, phosphates, phytates, protein complexes
        Preferred valence—Mg^{2+}
        Poorly absorbed—Sulfates, oxides, phosphates, phytates, complexes

Well absorbed—Ionized forms, lactates, chlorides, gluconates
Sites—Duodenum, ileum
Efficiency—30-40%
Active transport—Yes, similar to Ca
Synergists—Lactic acid, lactose; vitamin D_3: 1,25 $(OH)_2D_3$
Antagonists—Phytates, Ca, PO_4, Na, fats, PTH (?), calcitonin (?)

2. **Blood Carriers**   18, 30, 51
Plasma protein complexes

3. **Half-Life of Element in Blood**   20, 21, 51, 53
(Not available; est. 0.19% of Mg in plasma excreted per minute at normal plasma levels

4. **Target (Initial) Sites**   30, 31, 53
Tissues—Connective, skin, liver, intestine
Cells—Mitochondria, cytosol

5. **Storage**   21, 30, 35, 51, 53
Sites—Skeleton, muscles, soft tissues, RBC
Forms—Bone crystal structure, protein complexes, ions

6. **Homeostatic Mechanisms**   18, 21, 30, 35, 42, 51, 53
Relative efficiency in element retention—80-100%
Kidney participation—Critical controller of reabsorption
    Reabsorption—↓ by Mg, ↑ by PTH
Intestinal participation   Enterohepatic circulation
Liver (bile) participation   All secreted Mg reabsorbed

7. **Specific Functions (via Cofactors/Metalloenzymes, Metalloproteins/Ions)** 13, 18, 21, 25, 30, 32, 51, 53
Molecular level
    Binding agent for ribosomes and mRNA
    Regulation of enzymatic activity—Cofactor
    Bone crystal structure
    Chelating agent
Cellular level
    Enzyme systems activator—Cofactor
    Binding of cellular organelles
    Regulation of neuronal irritability
    Participation in protein synthesis and DNA synthesis
    Participation in cyclic AMP formation
    ATP synthesis

Organismal level
    Maintenance of neuromuscular transmission
    Maintenance of heart muscle and blood vessels
    Maintenance of bone structure (with Ca)
    Maintenance of CNS
    Homeostasis of calcium

8. Metalloenzymes, Cofactors, Metalloproteins   8, 10, 11, 15, 18, 25, 30, 32, 35, 50, 51, 53

System Types	Organ	Metalloenzyme/Protein	Co-factors	System Function
Cofactors	Various tissues	Phosphokinases Carboxylase Pyruvate oxidase	Mg, B_1	Glucose metabolism
	Various tissues	Thiokinases Glucokinase Myokinase	Mg	Fatty acid degradation
	Various tissues	Phosphatases Alkaline Phosphatase Pyrophosphatase	Mg	Phosphate splitting off
	Various tissues	Enolase	Mg	Glucose metabolism
	Various tissues	Isocitric dehydrogenase	Mg	Glucose metabolism
	Various tissues	Peptidases	Mg	Split peptides

9. Excretion   18, 20, 21, 30, 39, 51

Chemical forms—Urine: ionic (Mg^{2+}), phosphates, chlorides; feces: oxalates, phytates, bile compounds

Organs—Kidney (urine): 30-40%; intestine (feces): 60-70%; liver (bile, intestine): reabsorbed; skin (sweat): 10-15%

MISCELLANEOUS

1. Relationship to Other Minerals   18, 27, 30, 51, 53

Ca—Antagonist or synergist to Mg, depending on system
Na—Antagonist or synergist to Mg, depending on system

K—Antagonist or synergist to Mg, depending on system
F—Absorption antagonist
PO_4—Absorption antagonist

2. **Relationship to Vitamins**   18, 27, 36, 37, 51, 53
   B_1—Cofactor in glucose metabolism
   D—Absorption synergist
   B_6—Mg acts as binding agent in enzyme reactions
   C—Synergist in collagen synthesis

3. **Relationship to Hormones**   18, 20, 27, 50, 51, 53
   PTH—Regulation of Ca + Mg in bone
   STH—Synergist in growth action
   T4—Increases intracellular Mg

4. **Unusual Features**   18, 21, 27, 30, 36, 50, 51, 53
   Radiation damage causes large losses of body Mg
   Radiation protective action of Mg
   Body-temperature-lowering effect of Mg
   Intracellular location
   Anesthetic action
   Central atom in chlorophyll
   Protein and DNA synthesis

5. **Possible Relationship of Deficiency Symptoms to Metabolic Action**   18, 21, 27, 30, 35, 51, 53
   Poor growth—Mg required for protein and DNA synthesis
   Hyperirritability ⎫
   Convulsions   ⎬ Maintenance of nervous system, ionic balance
   Tetany—Disturbed ionic balance in muscles

Chapter 4. Sodium (Na)

Sodium in the body is chiefly an extracellular ion with many functions:

1. Extracellular body fluid regulation including osmotic and blood pressure, buffering, viscosity, CO_2 transport, and solubilization of proteins and organic acids
2. Membrane effects including membrane permeability, sodium pump action, neuromuscular irritability, and nerve impulse conduction

Sodium is found in all animals but in very few plants. It is essential for animal life and normal growth, development, and life span in man as well as most vertebrates. Its mode of action is mainly by way of its transport properties, hydration, alkalinity, conductivity, and charge effects. Without the Na pump and consequent development of a nervous system, human life as we know it could not have evolved. Extracellular fluid containing high Na (relative to K) is considered by many to represent the environmental fluid in post-Cambrian seas in which animal organisms continued to develop before emerging on dry land. Sodium plays a key role in many physiological functions (especially blood pressure) but is not associated with many hormones or enzyme systems. It is absorbed as the free ion, and its chief synergist is K (certain functions), while its chief antagonists are also K (different functions) along with Ca.

There is some evidence the average American diet includes too much Na because of the increasing incidence of hypertension with consequent heart disease (note the association of Na with hypertension). An increased craving for salt has added extra Na to our body fluids and has become a national habit.

It may be necessary to screen American diets for removal of excessively high-Na items. High-Na dietary items include table salt, dairy products, meats, seafood, and many processed foods.

Deficiencies of Na are found mainly in cases of gastrointestinal fluid losses, heavy perspiration, and individuals with endocrine, renal, and adrenal defects. Body Na is very tightly conserved with an extremely efficient homeostatic mechanism; hence less Na is needed than K.

GENERAL INFORMATION

1. **Dietary and Medicinal Forms**   18, 49, 53, 54
   Element—Sodium metal; not used medicinally
   Inorganic salts—Chloride, phosphate, borate, bicarbonate, acetate, tartrate, citrate
   Organic forms—Gluconate

2. **History of Biological Significance**   18, 21, 35, 50, 53
   1871—Salkowski: first description of absorption and excretion of Na
   1874—Ringer: balance of ions in natural fluids, effects of Na on heart beat
   1895—Biedermann: skeletal muscle contracts rhythmically in Na solutions
   1926—St. John: dietary Na essential for normal growth and life
   1927—Clark: osmotic action of Na on heart described
   1939—Mathews: Na stimulates (sciatic) nerve
   1940—Wilbrandt: Na increases permeability of human cells (RBC)
   1952—Simpson and Tait: discovery of aldosterone regulation of body Na
   1966—Woodbury: electrogenic Na-K pump in cell membrane postulated
   1972—Coleman et al.: blood Na elevation a possible cause of hypertension

3. **Physiological (Blood) Forms**   18, 21, 50, 51, 53
   Ionic form—Na^+

4. **Synergistic Agents**   30, 35, 39
   Metabolic (some functions)—K, Mg, Ca
   Absorption—Glucose

5. **Antagonistic Agents**   30, 35, 39
   Metabolic (other functions)—K, Mg, Ca
   Absorption—Ca

6. **Physiological Functions (Maintenance of Systems/Components)**   18, 20, 21, 30, 50, 51

    Circulatory—Dilation of arterioles, ↓ heart rate; maintenance of blood pressure

    Excretory—↑ membrane permeability, tubular reabsorption and K, NH_4 exchange; maintenance of acid-base balance

    Respiratory—Lung homeostasis; CO_2 transport ($NaHCO_3$)

    Digestive—Glucose absorption; production of gastric HCl, digestive fluids

    Nervous—Maintenance of nerve irritability

    Special sensory—Taste sensations, homeostasis of eyes

    Reproductive—Homeostasis of testicles

    Endocrine—↓ aldosterone, ↑ ADH in blood

    Blood—Maintenance of viscosity, osmolarity, ionic balance, pH

    Muscular—Maintenance of muscle irritability

    Skeletal—Homeostasis of bone

    Integument—Absorption, excretion, storage of Na

    Immune—Solubilization of immune glubulins

    Metabolic—Protein, CHO metabolism, Na-K pump

    Detoxification—Homeostasis of liver, solubilization of organic compounds and acids

    Growth—+

    Health—+

    Longevity—+

7. **Body Content**   12, 21, 35, 50

    mg/70 kg = 105; μg/g = 1500

8. **Relative Organ Concentrations**   12, 21, 35, 50

    Serum > lungs > liver > heart > skeleton > kidney > brain > skin > uterus > pancreas > muscle > RBC

9. **Deficiencies**   18, 21, 23, 30, 36, 51

    Man

    Hyponatremia

    Water intoxication   } Na deficiency is a

    Adrenal insufficiency   component of other deficiencies

    Renal insufficiency

10. **Excess Conditions**   18, 21, 23, 30, 36, 38, 39

    Man—Hypernatremia, hypertension

11. **Essentiality**   1, 38, 42

    Man—Vital, needed for good health, normal life span

Other species—All: vertebrates, fungi; some: protozoans, bacteria, algae

12. **Major Commercial Uses (Biological Interface)**   6, 22, 30, 54
Element—Sodium lamps, heat transfer media, photoelectric cells, manufacture of tetraethyl Pb
Compounds—Preservative; curing of hides; soap; dyes; photography; mordant; heat trap

13. **Medicinal Applications**   18, 27, 30, 54, 53
Cathartic—Na_2HPO_4, Na Tartrate
Emetic—NaCl
Anti-inflammatory—NaCl
Antiseptic—Na borate
Expectorant—Na acetate
Acidifier—NaH_2PO_4
Electrolyte replenisher—NaCl
Alkalizer, antacid—$NaHCO_3$, Na acetate, Na citrate

14. **Hazards and Toxicity**   18, 30, 39, 46, 54
Element—Extremely caustic to all tissue
   Inhalation—No data
   Topical—Burns, extremely caustic to all tissue
Compounds—Not considered toxic except when toxic anions present
   Inhalation—No data
   Topical—Nontoxic except as above noted
   Oral toxicity—see nutrition section, dietary excess
Carcinogenicity/Mutagenicity = $-/-$

DISTRIBUTION AND SOURCES

1. **Occurrence and Environmental Concentrations (mg/g)**   3, 4, 6, 42
Relative terrestrial abundance—#6
Chief minerals—Halite (NaCl), saltpeter (KNO_3), kernite (Na borate), cryolite (Na_3AlF_6), borax ($Na_2B_4O_7$), soda ash (Na_2CO_3)
Earth's crust—28.10
Rock's—0.40-23.60 (limestone-igneous)
Soils—6.30
Freshwater—.0063
Seawater—10.50

2. **Organismal Concentrations (mg/g)**   4, 42, 47
Plants—Marine: 33.00; land: 1.20

Animals—Marine: 4.00-48.00 (fish—coelenterates); land: 4.00
Man—1.40
Special concentrators—Maritime and salt marsh plants
Indicator plants—No data

3. **Dietary Sources (Variability due to Environment)**   5, 12, 26, 27, 36, 48, 52
   High (100-700 mg/100 g)
       Seafood—Tuna, clams, caviar, lobster, sardines, scallops, shrimp
       Meat/Organs—Brains, eggs, beef kidneys, beef liver
       Vegetables—Beet greens, celery, swiss chard, olives, peas
       Dairy products—Butter, buttermilk, cheeses (cream, Parmesan, swiss, cheddar, cottage)
       Miscellaneous—Pickles, table salt, kelp, brewer's yeast
   Medium (50-100 mg/100 g)
       Seafood—Flounder, haddock, halibut, herring, lingcod, shad, perch, oysters, red snapper, salmon, sea bass, bluefish, carp, cod, croaker
       Meat/Organs—Goose, beef heart, lamb, beef, chicken, duck, chicken gizzard, pork, turkey, liver (chicken, lamb, turkey, pig), veal
       Nuts/Seeds—Sesame
       Vegetables—Beets, kale, spinach, turnips, watercress
       Dairy Products—Milk
   Low (1-50 mg/100g)
       Seafood—Albacore, clams
       Nuts/Seeds—Coconuts, filberts, peanuts, sunflower, walnuts, almonds, brazils, cashews, chestnuts
       Fruits—Berries (blackberries, blueberries, boysenberries, cranberries, gooseberries, loganberries, raspberries, strawberries), figs (dry), dates (dry), apples, apricots, avocados, bananas, cherries, currants, cantalopes, oranges, papayas, pineapples, plums, prunes, raisins, mangoes, grapefruit, grapes, guavas, kumquats, lemons, limes
       Vegetables—Green beans, broccoli, brussels sprouts, cabbage, carrots, artichokes, asparagus, lima beans, bean sprouts, garlic, cauliflower, cress, cucumbers, eggplant, endive, horseradish, kohlrabi, lentils, lettuce, mustard greens, okra, onions, parsley, peas, green peppers, potatoes, pumpkins, squash, turnips, tomatoes, sweet potatoes
       Grains—Barley, rice (brown), rye, wheat
       Miscellaneous—Chocolate, molasses, mushrooms, yeast

CHEMISTRY

1. **Atomic Properties (Element)**   6, 7, 9, 30, 49
   Periodic table group no.—I-A, period 3

Category of element—Alkali metal
Atomic weight—22.99
Atomic number—11
Atomic radius (metallic)—1.857 Å
Electron shells—2, 8, 1
Orbital electrons—$1s^2$, $2s^2$, $2p^6$, $3s^1$
Natural isotopes—Na^{23} (100%)
Long-lived radioactive isotopes—Na^{22} (2.6 yr), Na^{24} (15 hr)

2. **Ionic Properties (Biological Forms)**   6, 7, 9, 30, 49
   Oxidation states (valences)—+1
   Ionic radius (Å)—0.95-1.00 (2.76 Å hydrated)
   Oxidation potentials—$Na^0 \rightarrow Na^+$ (2.712 v)

3. **Molecular Properties (Biological Forms)**   6, 7, 9, 16, 25, 30, 43, 49
   Covalent radius (Å)—1.539
   Coordination numbers—6 (hydration number = 16.6)
   Stereochemistry—tetrahedral
   Electron transfer compounds—No data
   Typical molecular complexes—$[Na(NH_3)_4]^+$, Na pyrophosphate, Na EDTA

4. **Analytical Methods**   3, 30, 31, 40, 55
   Physical—Flame photometry, spark mass spectrometry, atomic absorption
   Chemical—Spectrophotometric, zinc uranylacetate and dithizone
   Hair/Nail analysis—Feasible, values reported
   Comments—Flame photometry and atomic absorption favored methods;
      interferences from other metals occur

5. **Chemical Properties of Compounds**   6, 7, 9, 49, 54
   See Table 4.1

MEDICINAL AND NUTRITIONAL ROLE

1. **Units of Measurement**
   Weight—μg (microgram); 1 mg (milligram) = 1000 μg = .001 g
   Concentration—ppm (parts per million) = μg/g; mg% = mg/100 ml

Table 4.1. Properties of Sodium Compounds

	REACTIONS			SOLUBILITY			
	Heat °C	Air	Water	g/100 cc H_2O	Alc.	Eth.	Acid
Na citrate, $Na_3C_6H_5O_7 \cdot 2H_2O$	$-2H_2O(150°)$	stable	alk, pH 8	72^{25}	I	NA	NA
Na bicarbonate, $NaHCO_3$	$-CO_2(270°)$	NA	alk, pH 8.3	$69°$	SS	NA	NA
Na borate, $Na_2B_4O_7 \cdot 10H_2O$	$-10H_2O(320°)$	efflor.	alk, pH 9.5	2^6	SS	NA	I
Na chloride, NaCl	BP 1413°	stable	neut. pH 6-7	35.7^{20}	SS	NA	SS
Na acetate, $CH_3COON_a \cdot 3H_2O$	$-3H_2O(120°)$	efflor.	alk. pH 8.9	$76.2°$	S	S	NA
Na tartrate, $Na_2C_4H_4O_6 \cdot 2H_2O$	$-2H_2O(120°)$	NA	alk. pH 7-9	29^6	I	NA	NA

Table 4.1. Properties of Sodium Compounds (continued)

	Density	MW hyd./anh.	MP °C	XL Form	Color XL/Powd.	Appearance Commercial Form	% Element h./anh.	Odor	Taste	Synonyms
Na citrate, Na₃C₆H₅O₇ · 2H₂O	NA	294.1/258.1	d.	NA	wh./wh.	C, G, P	23.5/26.7	NA	cool saline	trisodium citrate
Na bicarbonate, NaHCO₃	2.16	−/84.0	d.	monocl.	wh./wh.	P, G	−/27.4	NA	NA	baking soda
Na borate, Na₂B₄O₇ · 10H₂O	1.73	381.4/201.2	75°	monocl.	col./wh.	C, G, P	11.3/22.8	O	NA	borax
Na chloride, NaCl	2.17	−/58.4	801°	cubic	col./wh.	G, P	−/39.3	NA	saline	table salt
Na acetate, CH₃COONa · 3H₂O	1.45	136.1/82.0	58°	monocl.	col./wh.	C, P, PR	16.4/28.0	NA	NA	NA
Na tartrate, Na₂C₄H₄O₆ · 2H₂O	1.82	230.1/194.1	d.	rhomb.	col./wh.	C, G	55.7/23.7	NA	NA	NA

Abbreviations as in earlier tables.

2. **Human Body Fluid Levels (Normal) (mg/100 ml)**   1, 2, 3, 12, 23, 35
   Blood—182-209 (196.3 average)
   Plasma/Serum—306-331 (321.8 average)
   Urine—146-548 (350.0 average)

3. **Human Tissue Levels (mg/g)**   4, 12, 24, 46
   Hair—1.21
   Bone—180
   Muscle (skeletal)—72
   Nerve—170
   Liver—190

4. **Important Dietary Levels (mg/day)**   5, 21, 27, 30, 35, 39, 57
   Recommended dietary allowance—Not established; suggested ca. 1200
     (3000 NaCl)
   Deficiency limits—< ca. 500 (1270 NaCl)
   Toxic limit—> 18,000 (30,000 NaCl)
   Average daily intake—3000-9000 (5000-15,000 NaCl)

5. **Estimated Human Daily Balance (average American diet 70 kg ♂, 30 yr)**
     18, 21, 30, 53
   Average intake—1724 mg/day (food 1717, water 7)
   Average output—1724 mg/day (urine 1701, feces 12, sweat 11)
   Net gain/loss—Balanced normally

6. **Indications for Supplementation of Above Diet**   5, 21, 27, 30, 35, 57
   Healthy normal—Negative, possibly decrease
   Special conditions—Heavy sweating, vomiting, diarrhea, adrenal cortical
     insufficiency, excess water intake

7. **Factors Affecting Availability from Diet**   18, 21, 27, 51, 53
   Decreased
       See absorption section, antagonists
       Boiling food in cooking
       Increased water intake
       Vegetarian diets
       Diarrhea
   Increased
       See absorption section, synergizers
       Salting food in cooking
       Increased processing of foods and use of them
       Eating habits, craving for salt
       Meat diets

8. **Deficiency Symptons**   18, 21, 23, 30, 36, 51
   Man: Anorexia, nausea, muscle atrophy, retarded bond development, poor growth, weight loss, death

9. **Effects of Dietary Excess (Salts or Concentrates)**   18, 23, 36, 39, 51
   Acute—Animals: excessive water intake, diarrhea, stiff gait, salivation, muscular fibrillation, exhaustion, respiratory failure, encephalopathy, congestion of organs, death (terminally)
   Chronic—Animals: inhibition of growth, increased water intake, increased urinary volume, massive edema, hypertension, anemia, lipemia, hypoproteinemia, azotemia, death (terminally)

METABOLIC ROLE

1. **Intestinal Absorption**   13, 18, 30, 35, 39, 44
   Chemical forms—ionic (Na^+)
   Preferred valence—+1
   Poorly absorbed—No data
   Well absorbed—Ionic form
   Sites—Complete intestinal tract
   Efficiency—$> 98\%$
   Active transport—Yes $>$ intracellular to serosal fluid
   Synergizers—Cl^-, K^+, Mg^{2+}; deoxycorticosterone, 9-α-fluorocortisone; hexoses, animo acids
   Antagonists—Ca^{2+}, cardiac glycosides

2. **Blood Carriers**   18, 30, 51
   None, ionic form (Na^+)

3. **Half-Life of Element in Blood**   20, 21, 51, 53
   Not available; est. 0.03% of plasma Na excreted per minute at normal plasma levels

4. **Target (Initial) Sites**   30, 51, 53
   Tissues—All (extracellular fluids)
   Cells—Mainly extracellular fluid, very small amount intracellular fluid-cytosol

5. **Storage**   21, 30, 35, 51, 53
   Sites—Only in extracellular fluids, small amount in bone
   Forms—Na^+ ions

6. Homeostatic Mechanisms   18, 21, 30, 35, 42, 51, 53
Relative efficiency in element retention $> 98\%$
Kidney participation—Controlled by tubular reabosrption in proximal
tubules by anti-diuretic hormone (ADH), aldosterone, and body pH
Intestinal participation $\Big\}$ Very small
Liver (bile) participation

7. Specific Functions (via Cofactors/Metalloenzymes/Metalloprotein/Ions)
13, 18, 21, 25, 30, 32, 51, 53
Molecular level
Regulation of osmotic pressure, acid-base balance
CO_2 transport, hydration of proteins, solubilization of organic acids
Cellular level
Regulation of cell permeability
Neuromuscular irritability
Na pump action
Organismal level
Synergizer of bone and body growth weight gain
Muscle homeostasis, respiration of CO_2
Regulation of blood pressure and extracellular fluids as noted above
Homeostasis of digestive and nervous system
Homeostasis of protein, CHO metabolism

8. Metalloenzymes, Cofactors, Metalloproteins Systems   8, 10, 11, 15, 18,
25, 30, 32, 35, 50, 51, 53

System Type	Organ	Metalloenzyme/Protein	Cofactors	System Function
Cofactors	All	Na-K-ATPase	Na, K	Na pump

9. Excretion
Chemical forms—Ionic Na^+
Organs
Kidney (urine): 98% (glomecular filtration and reabsorption)
Intestine (feces) $\Big\}$ 2%
Liver (bile, intestine)

MISCELLANEOUS

1. Relationship to Other Minerals   18, 27, 30, 51, 53
K—Synergist in Na-K pump, antagonist in intracellular reactions

Ca—Antagonist in absorption, synergist in bone metabolism
Mg—Antagonist in absorption, synergist in bone metabolism
PO_4—Synergist in pH maintenance
HCO_3—Synergist in CO_2 transport (as $NaHCO_3$)

2. **Relationship to Vitamins**   18, 27, 36, 37, 51, 53
B_6—Involved in electrolyte balance
D—Possible synergist in bone metabolism with Na

3. **Relationship to Hormones**   18, 20, 27, 50, 51, 53
Aldosterone—Na decreases aldosterone output
ADH—Na increases ADH output

4. **Unusual Features**   18, 21, 27, 30, 36, 50, 51, 53
Na is major ion involved in osmotic pressure of body fluids and blood pressure
Na causes gelation of intracellular fluid
Pure Na salt solutions are toxic to cells
Nerves are stimulated in pure Na salt solutions
Na causes increase in membrane permeability
Na is absent in most plants

5. **Possible Relationship of Deficiency Symptoms to Metabolic Action**   18, 21
    27, 30, 35, 51, 53
Anorexia ⎫
Nausea ⎭ Loss of gastric HCl and digestive fluids
Muscle atrophy—Loss of neuromuscular irritability
Retarded bone development—Loss of synergism with Ca
Poor growth—Loss of synergism with Mg
Weight loss—Decreased protein and CHO metabolism

Chapter 5. Potassium (K)

Potassium in the body is chiefly intracellular with many functions:

1. Intracellular body fluid regulation including osmotic pressure, buffering, viscosity, CO_2 transport (RBC), and solubilization of proteins
2. Membrane effects including membrane permeability, sodium pump action, muscular contraction, and nerve impulse conduction

Potassium is found in all plants and animals. It is essential for all life and normal growth, development, and life span in man as well as all life forms with the possible exception of some bacteria. Its mode of action is chiefly due to its transport properties, hydration, alkalinity, conductivity, and charge effects. Intracellular fluid containing high K (relative to Na) is considered by many to represent the original fluid (pre-Cambrian seas) in which life evolved. The Na pump (actually the Na-K pump) could not have evolved without the presence of K, and thus no development of a nervous system (and hence of human life) could have occurred. Potassium plays a key role in many physiological functions (especially the heart beat) and is associated with several key hormones and enzyme systems. It is absorbed as the free ion, and its chief synergizer is Na (certain functions), which is also its chief antagonist (alternate functions) along with Mg.

There is no evidence that the average American diet includes too much K. Indeed, since K antagonizes excess Na (e.g., in hypertension), it is likely that increased K (relative to Na) in our diet would be beneficial. This would mean a return to vegetable-based diets (as opposed to the increasing trend to carnivorous diets), and use of NaCl/KCl mixtures in place of table salt. High-K dietary items include unsalted nuts, seeds, yeasts, grains, mushrooms, molasses, chocolate, dried fruits, and many fresh fruits and vegetables.

Deficiencies of K are found mainly in cases of gastrointestinal losses, starvation, diuresis, and adrenal or renal malfunction. Body K is not very tightly conserved under a system of partial homeostasis—losses are appreciable; hence the need for replenishment, more than for Na.

GENERAL INFORMATION

1. **Dietary and Medicinal Forms**   18, 49, 53, 54
   Element—Potassium metal; not used medicinally
   Inorganic salts—Chloride, bicarbonate, nitrate, phosphate, acetate, citrate, tartrate
   Organic forms—Gluconate

2. **History of Biological Significance**   18, 21, 35, 50, 53
   1871—Salkowski: first description of absorption and excretion of K (animals)
   1874—Ringer: balance of ions in natural fluids, effects of K on heart beat
   1894—Von Bunge: relations between dietary Na and K described
   1925—Serenyi: discovery that skeletal muscle loses excitability in K solutions
   1926—Miller: dietary K essential for normal growth and life
   1939—Mathews: discovery that K causes loss of irritability in muscle
   1940—Wilbrandt: discovery that K increases permeability of human RBC
   1942—Orent-Keiles et al.: low K found to cause sterility, heart and kidney damage in rats
   1955—Ruegamer and Elvehjem: low-K diets found to cause paralysis in dogs
   1966—Woodbury: electrogenic Na-K pump in cell membrane postulated

3. **Physiological (Blood) Forms**   18, 21, 50, 51, 53
   Ionic—K^+

4. **Synergistic Agents**   30, 35, 39
   Metabolic (certain functions)—Ca, Mg, Na; insulin
   Absorption—Ionophores

5. **Antagonistic Agents**   30, 35, 39
   Metabolic (some functions)—Ca, Mg, Na
   Absorption—Ca

6. **Physiological Functions (Maintenance of Systems/Components)**   18, 20, 21, 30, 50, 51

   Circulatory—Dilation of arterioles, ↓ heart rate; regulation of blood pressure

   Excretory—↑ membrane permeability, tubular reabsorption or Na, NH_4 exchange; maintenance of acid-base balance

   Respiratory—CO_2 transport (RBC), $KHCO_3$

   Digestive—Motility of gastrointestinal tract

   Nervous—Maintenance of irritability

   Special sensory—Homeostasis of eyes

   Reproductive—Homeostasis of gametogenesis

   Endocrine—↑ FSH, ↑ ADH, ↑ aldosterone in blood; insulin synergism

   Blood—Viscosity, osmolarity, volume, pH maintenance

   Muscular—Maintenance of irritability

   Skeletal—Synergizer of bone growth

   Integument—Excretion, absorption K

   Immune—Solubilization of globulins

   Metabolic—Na-K pump; protein, CHO metabolism

   Detoxification—Liver homeostasis

   Growth—+

   Health—+

   Longevity—+

7. **Body Content**   12, 21, 35, 50

   mg/70 kg = 250.0; μg/g = 3600

8. **Relative Organ Concentrations**   12, 21, 35, 50

   RBC > muscle > brain > intestine > heart > pancreas > liver > kidney > lungs > uterus > skin > adrenal > skeleton > serum

9. **Deficiencies**   18, 21, 23, 30, 36, 51

   Man—Hypokalemia; potassium depletion; metabolic alkalosis (K deficiency is a component of other deficiency)

10. **Excess Conditions**   18, 21, 23, 30, 36, 38, 39

    Man—Hyperkalemia; renal insufficiency (K excess is a component of other disorder)

11. **Essentiality**   1, 38, 42

    Man—Vital, needed for good health, normal life span

    Other species—All: vertebrates, invertebrates, insects, protozoa, algae, fungi, spermatophytes; some: bacteria

12. Major Commercial Uses (Biological Interface)   6, 22, 30, 54
Element—Heat transfer medium; organic syntheses
Compounds—Photography; buffer solutions; electrode cells; fertilizer

13. Medicinal Applications   18, 27, 30, 53, 54
Electrolyte replenisher—KCl, $KHCO_3$, K gluconate
Table salt substitute—KCl
Dietary supplement—K gluconate
Antacid—$KHCO_3$, K citrate
Diuretic—KNO_3
Cathartic—K_2HPO_4, K tartrate

14. Hazards and Toxicity   18, 30, 46, 39, 54
Element—Extremely caustic to all tissue
    Inhalation—No data
    Topical—Burns, extremely caustic to all tissue
Compounds—Not considered toxic except when toxic anions present
    Inhalation—No data
    Topical—Nontoxic except as above noted
    Oral toxicity—See nutrition section, dietary excess
Carcinogenicity/Mutagenicity = $-/-$ (except for natural radioactive iso-
    tope—K^{40})

DISTRIBUTION AND SOURCES

1. Occurrence and Environmental Concentrations (mg/g)   3, 4, 6, 42
Relative terrestrial abundance—#7
Chief minterals—Sylyite (KCl), kainite ($KCl\text{-}MgSO_4$), carnallite (KCl-
    $MgCl$), sylvinite (KCl-NaCl), polyhalite (K, Mg, $CaSO_4$), orthoclase
    ($K_2O \cdot Al_2O_3$)
Rocks—0.270-26.60 (limestones-shales)
Soils—14.00
Freshwater—0.0023
Seawater—0.380

2. Organismal Concentrations (mg/g)   4, 42, 47
Plants—Marine: 52.00; land: 14.00
Animals—Marine: 5.00-30.00; land: 7.40
Man—2.00
Special concentrators—No data
Indicator plants—No data

3. Dietary Sources (Variability due to Environment)   5, 12, 26, 27, 36, 48, 52
  High (400-1000 mg/100 g)
    Seafood—Halibut, herring, lingcod, sardines
    Meat/Organs—Goose
    Nuts/Seeds—Pecans, sesame, sunflower, walnuts, almonds, brazils, cashews, chestnuts, filberts, peanuts
    Fruits—Avocados, dates (dry), figs (dry), prunes (dry, raisins (dry)
    Vegetables—Cress, garlic, horseradish, lentils (dry), parsley, potatoes, spinach, artichokes, lima beans, beet greens, swiss chard, collards
    Grains—Buckwheat, rye, wheat bran
    Miscellaneous—Chocolate, molasses, mushrooms, kelp, yeast (bakers', brewer's)
  Medium (200-400 mg/100 g)
    Seafood—Haddock, perch, red snapper, salmon, scallops, shad, shrimp, tuna, albacore, sea bass, carp, clams, cod, croaker, flounder, sole
    Meat/Organs—Liver (beef, pig, lamb), pork, turkey, beef, beef brains, chicken, duck, chicken gizzard, beef kidneys, lamb
    Nuts/Seeds—Coconut, macadamia
    Grains—Brown, rice, wheat
    Fruits—Kumquats, cantaloupes, papayas, plums, rhubarb, apricots, bananas, currants, elderberries, guavas
    Vegetables—Carrots, cauliflower, celery, chives, eggplant, endive, kale, kohlrabi, asparagus, green beans, beets, broccoli, brussels sprouts, cabbages, lettuce, mustard greens, okra, onions, peas, green peppers, pumpkins, squash, sweet potatoes, tomatoes, turnips
  Low (50-200 mg/100 g)
    Seafood—Caviar, lobster, oysters
    Meat/Organs—Eggs, beef heart, (turkey, chicken) liver, beef tongue
    Grains—Barley
    Fruits—Persimmons, pears, tangerines, mangos, pineapples, (cran-, goose-, rasp-, logan-, straw-, black-, blue-, boysen-) berries, cherries, apples, oranges, grapes, lemons, grapefruit, limes
    Vegetables—Bean sprouts, corn, cucumbers, onions, peas
    Dairy products—Cream, milk, buttermilk, cheeses (cheddar, cottage, cream, Parmesan, Swiss)
    Miscellaneous—Pickles, vinegar, maple syrup

CHEMISTRY

1. Atomic Properties (Element)   6, 7, 9, 30, 49
  Periodic table group no.—I-A, period 4

Category of element—Alkali metal
Atomic weight—39.10
Atomic number—19
Atomic radius (metallic)—2.272 Å
Electron shells—2, 8, 8, 1
Orbital electrons—$1s^2$, $2s^2$, $2p^6$, $3s^2$, $3p^6$, $4s^1$
Natural isotopes—K^{39} (93.1%), K^{40} (<.01%), K^{41} (<6.9%)
Long-lived radioactive isotopes—K^{40} (1.3×10^9 yr), K^{42} (12.5 hr), K^{43}
   (22.4 hr)

2. **Ionic Properties (Biological Forms)**   6, 7, 9, 30, 49
   Oxidation states (valences)—+1
   Ionic radius (Å)—1.33 (2.32 hydrated)
   Oxidation potentials—$K^0 \rightarrow K^+$ (2.924 v)

3. **Molecular Properties (Biological Forms)**   6, 7, 9, 16, 25, 30, 43, 49
   Covalent radius (Å)—1.962
   Coordination numbers—6, 8 (hydration number = 10.5)
   Stereochemistry—Tetrahedral (?)
   Electron transfer compounds—No data
   Typical molecular complexes—KSCN, KOCN, KHF_2

4. **Analytical Methods**   3, 30, 31, 40, 55
   Physical—Flame photometry, spark mass spectrometry, atomic absorption
   Chemical—Spectrophotometric, dipicrylamine
   Hair/Nail analysis—Feasible, values reported
   Comments—Flame photometry and atomic absorption are favored methods;
      interferences from other metals occur

5. **Chemical Properties of Compounds**   6, 7, 9, 49, 54
   See Table 5.1

MEDICINAL AND NUTRITIONAL ROLE

1. **Units of Measurement**
   Weight—μg (microgram); 1 mg (milligram) = 1000 μg = .001 g
   Concentration—ppm (parts per million) = μg/g; mg% = mg/100 ml

2. **Human Body Fluid Levels (Normal) (mg/100 ml)**   1, 2, 4, 12, 23, 25
   Blood—(177.9 average)
   Plasma/Serum—13.7-21.5 (17.2 average)
   Urine—93.3-326.6 (110.8 average)

Table 5.1.   Properties of Potassium Compounds

	REACTIONS			SOLUBILITY			
	Heat °C	Air	Water	g/100 cc H_2O	Alc.	Eth.	Acid
K chloride, KCl	sublimes 1500°	stable	neut. pH 7	34.7^{20}	SS	S	SS
K gluconate, $KC_6H_{11}O_7$	d. 180°	stable	alk. pH 7.5-8.5	S	I	I	NA
K bicarbonate, $KHCO_3$	d. 100-200°	NA	alk. pH 8.2	36.1^{25}	I	NA	NA
K acetate, CH_3COOK	MP 292°	deliq.	alk. pH 9.7	253^{20}	S	I	S
K phosphate dibasic, K_2HPO_4	d.	deliq.	alk. pH 8.5-9.0	167^{20}	S	NA	NA

Table 5.1.   Properties of Potassium Compounds (continued)

	Density	MW hyd./anh.	MP °C	XL Form	Color XL/Powd.	Appearance Commercial Form	% Element h./anh.	Odor	Taste	Synonyms
K chloride, KCl	1.98	−/74.6	776°	cubic	col./wh.	C, P	−/52.4	NA	saline	NA
K gluconate, $KC_6H_{11}O_7$	NA	−/234.2	d.	NA	wh.-y/−	C, P, G	−/16.7	O	saline	NA
K bicarbonate, $KHCO_3$	2.17	−/100.1	d.	monocl.	col./wh.	C, G, P	−/39.0	NA	NA	NA
K acetate, CH_3COOK	1.57	−/98.2	292°	NA	col./wh.	P, F	−/39.6	NA	NA	NA
K phosphate dibasic, K_2HPO_4	NA	−/174.2	d.	amorph.	wh.	G	−/44.9	O	NA	dipotassium phosphate

3. **Human Tissue Levels (mg/g)**   4, 12, 24, 46
   Hair—.0723
   Bone—61
   Muscle (skeletal)—360
   Nerve—330
   Liver—215

4. **Important Dietary Levels (mg/day)**   5, 21, 27, 30, 35, 39, 57
   Recommended dietary allowance—Not established; suggested ca. 2500
      (4760 KCl)
   Deficiency limits—< 585-1170 (1110-2220 KCl)
   Toxic limit—> 12,000 (25,000 KCl)
   Average daily intake—960-2880 (2000-6000 KCl)

5. **Estimated Human Daily Balance (average American diet, 70 kg ♂, 30 yr)**
      18, 21, 30, 53
   Average intake—1955 mg/day (food 1952, water 3)
   Average output—1955 mg/day (urine 1760, feces 195, sweat 0)
   Net gain/loss—Balanced normally

6. **Indications for Supplementation of Above Diet**   5, 21, 27, 30, 35, 57
   Healthy normal—Negative
   Special conditions—Diarrhea, renal disease, diabetic acidosis

7. **Factors Affecting Availability from Diet**   18, 21, 27, 51, 53
   Decreased
      See absorption section, antagonists
      Boiling food in cooking
      Excessive use of salt
      Meat diets
      Increased processing of foods and use of them
      Diarrhea
   Increased
      See absorption section, synergizers
      Vegetarian diets
      Use of salt substitutes

8. **Deficiency Symptoms**   18, 21, 23, 30, 36, 51
   Man: Muscle weakness, cardiac arrhythmia, paralysis, bone fragility, sterility,
      adrenal hypertrophy, decreased growth rate, loss of weight, death

9. **Effects of Dietary Excess (Salts or Concentrates)**   18, 23, 36, 39, 51
   Acute—Animals: tonoclonic convulsions, CNS paralysis, asphyxial con-

vulsions, diarrhea, gastroenteritis, polydipsia, diuresis, dehydration, renal necrosis, fever, prostration, dialation of heart, cardiac arrhythmia, collapse of lungs, respiratory failure

Chronic—Man: cardiac and central nervous system depression, mental confusion, weakness, vomiting, numbness, tingling, flaccid paralysis of extremeties

METABOLIC ROLE

1. **Intestinal Absorption**   13, 18, 30, 35, 39, 44, 54
   Chemical forms—Ionic K^+
      Preferred valence—+1
      Poorly absorbed—No data
      Well absorbed—Ionic form
   Sites—Small intestine
   Efficiency—ca. 90%
   Active transport—Passive diffusion and/or facilitation
   Synergizers—Na^+, Mg^{2+}, ionophores
   Antagonists—Cardiac glycosides, Ca^{2+}; aldosterone (reverse secretion in gut)

2. **Blood Carriers**   18, 30, 51
   None, ionic form K^+

3. **Half-Life of Element in Blood**   20, 21, 51, 53
   Not available; est. 0.39% of K in plasma excreted per minute at normal plasma levels

4. **Target (Initial) Sites**   30, 51, 53
   Tissues—All (mainly intracellular)
   Cells—Cytosol, small amount extracellular fluid

5. **Storage**   21, 30, 35, 51, 53
   Sites—No storage as such, RBCs and muscles contain more than average
   Forms—K^+ ions

6. **Homeostatic Mechanisms**   18, 21, 30, 35, 42, 51, 53
   Relative efficiency in element retention—ca. 90%
   Kidney participation—Major controller, via ADH, aldosterone, and body pH
   Intestinal participation—Small but have K^+ secretion into colon
   Liver (bile) participation—Very small

7. **Specific Functions (via Cofactors/Metalloenzymes, Metalloproteins/Ions)**
   13, 18, 21, 25, 30, 32, 51, 53
   Molecular level
       Regulation of pH, osmotic pressure, protein hydration
       Cellular level
       Irritability of muscles and nerves
       Regulation of cell permeability, pH, and osmotic pressure
       K-Na pump action
   Organismal level
       Homeostasis of muscles and heart
       Homeostasis of CNS and heart rhythms
       Homeostasis of bones, sex organs, adrenals
       Synergizer of body growth and weight gain
       Homeostasis of protein, CHO metabolism
       Homeostasis of body fluids

8. **Metalloenzymes, Cofactors, Metalloproteins Systems**   8, 10, 11, 15, 18, 25, 30, 32, 35, 50, 51, 53

System Type	Organ	Metalloenzyme/Protein	Cofactors	System Function
Cofactors	All	Na-K-ATPase	Na, K	Na-K pump
	All	Some glycolytic enzymes	K	Anaerobic metabolism
	All	Some oxidative phosphorylation enzymes	K	Cell { oxidation respiration

9. **Excretion**   18, 20, 21, 30, 39, 51
   Chemical forms—Ionic K^+
   Organs
       Kidney (urine): ca. 84% (glomerular filtration and reabsorption)
       Intestine (feces)   } 15%
       Liver (bile, intestine) }
       Skin: small amounts

MISCELLANEOUS

1. **Relationship to Other Minerals**   18, 27, 30, 51, 53
   Na—Synergistic in Na-K pump, antagonistic in intracellular reactions
   Ca—Antagonist in absorption, synergist in effects on smooth muscle
   Mg—Antagonist in absorption, synergist in anesthetic actions
   PO_4—Synergist in pH maintenance (intracellular)
   HCO_3—Synergist in CO_2 transport in RBCs

2. **Relationship to Vitamins**   18, 27, 36, 37, 51, 53
   B_6—Involved in electrolyte balance
   D—Involved in Ca-K antagonisms in absorption (?)

3. **Relationship to Hormones**   18, 20, 27, 50, 51, 53
   FSH—K increases secretion of FSH
   ADH—K increases ADH output
   Aldosterone—K increases aldosterone output
   Insulin—K is synergistic to insulin
   STH—is synergistic to K in growth

4. **Unusual Features**   18, 21, 27, 30, 36, 50, 51, 53
   K is major ion involved in heart action
   Absorption mechanisms for K remain a mystery
   K causes liquefaction of intracellular fluid
   Pure K salt solutions are toxic to cells, cause nerves to lose irritability
   K causes increase in cell permeability
   Ionophore transport of K

5. **Possible Relationship of Deficiency Symptoms to Metabolic Action**   18, 21, 27, 30, 35, 51, 53
   Muscle weakness—Loss of nerve irritability
   Cardiac arrhythmia—Heart regulation lost
   Paralysis—High Na/K paralyzes nerves
   Bone fragility—Loss of Ca synergism
   Sterility—Loss of FSH action
   Adrenal hypertrophy—Stress reactions
   Decreased bone growth—Loss of growth
   Loss of weight—Loss of synergism with protein, CHO metabolism

Chapter 6.   Zinc (Zn)

Zinc is found in all plants and animals. It is essential for normal growth, development and life span in humans, although life may continue for a while without it. Its mode of action is mainly by way of its enzyme action as activator and constituent of many key enzymes of the body, especially the nucleic acid polymerases which affect protein synthesis. It is very important for the maintenance of the sex glands, especially the prostate, as well as the metabolism of carbohydrates by virtue of its synergism with insulin. It also is very important in preventing and reversing Cd toxicity symptoms such as in hypertension, testicular damage, and prostate involvement. It appears that Zn is optimally absorbed as a chelated complex made in the intestines, but its chemical nature is not yet known; the existence of a vitamin-like form of Zn (as with other trace elements) is a possibility.

There is some evidence that the average American diet does not include sufficient amounts of Zn for replacement of losses; so a readjustment of the diet to include high-Zn foods may be considered. Dietary Zn can be obtained from liver, muscle, cheeses, yeasts, oysters, herring, sunflower seeds, wheat germ, and bran.

GENERAL INFORMATION

1. **Dietary and Medicinal Forms**   37, 49, 53, 54
   Element—Metallic zinc; not used medicinally

Inorganic salts—Carbonate, chloride, oxide, sulfate
Metallovitamin—Zinc-histidine peptide complex (?)
Chelated forms—Gluconate, glycinate, citrate

2. **History of Biological Significance**   8, 21, 37, 46, 50, 53
    1869—Raulin: Zn is required by a mould (A-Niger) for growth
    1905—Mendel and Bradley: Zn is a component of snail respiratory pigment
    1926—Somner and Lipman: higher plants require Zn
    1934—Todd: Zn is essential in rat diet
    1939—Keilin and Mann: carbonic anhydrase in red cells contains Zn
    1961—Prasad et al.: demonstrated human deficiency of Zn
    1964—Fujioka and Lieberman: DNA synthesis in rat liver requires Zn
    1974—Vallee et al.: reverse transcriptase contains Zn

3. **Physiological (Blood) Forms**   17, 21, 37, 46, 50, 53
    α_2-macroglobulin, Zn-albumin complex, metallothionin, insulin, alkaline
        phosphatase, glutamic/lactic/malic dehydrogenases

4. **Synergistic Agents**   30, 35, 37, 39, 46
    Metabolic—Vitamins A, D, E, B_6; Mn, STH, insulin testosterone
    Absorption—Pancreatic ligands, chelating agts, amino acids, peptides

5. **Antagonistic Agents**   30, 35, 37, 39, 46
    Metabolic—Cu, Fe, Cd, 6-mercaptopurine
    Absorption—Cu, Cd, Fe, Cr, Co, Mn, Se

6. **Physiological Functions (Maintenance of Systems/Components)**   17, 21, 30,
        37, 46, 50, 53
    Circulatory—Arterial walls homeostasis
    Excretory—Kidney peptidase, acid-base balance
    Respiratory—Carbonic anhydrase (CO_2 removal), a Zn enzyme
    Digestive—Liver functions, proteolysis, pancreatic enzymes cofactor
    Nervous—Brain development
    Special sensory—Appetite, taste, smell
    Reproductive—Testes, ovary, prostate, fertility maintenance
    Endocrine—↑ pituitary gonadotrophins, insulin, glucagon, peptide hormone
        synthesis
    Blood—RBCs, serum proteins maintenance
    Muscular—Muscle homeostasis

Skeletal—Bone structure homeostasis
Integument—Skin, hair, nails maintenance
Protective/Inmune—Lymphocytes, wound healing homeostasis
Metabolic—Protein, nucleic acids, carbohydrates, metabolism; aerobic and
   phosphate metabolism
Detoxification—Cd, pentobarbital, ethanol
Growth—+
Health—+
Longevity—+

7. **Body Content**   8, 12, 21, 35, 42, 46
   mg/70 kg = 1400-2300; μg/g = 20-33

8. **Relative Organ Concentrations**   12, 21, 42, 46, 53
   Choroid $>$ prostate $>$ muscle, kidney, liver $>$ heart, pancreas $>$ spleen,
   testes $>$ lung, brain, adrenals

9. **Deficiencies**   21, 30, 36, 37, 46
   Man—Dwarfism, sexual infantilism, dermatitis, hyposmia, hypogeusia,
   koilonychia
   Pigs—Parakeratosis
   Rats—Alopecia, birth defects

10. **Excess Conditions**   21, 30, 36, 37, 39, 38, 46
    Man—Metal fume fever, other Zn salt fume fevers
    Animals—Zinc tremor

11. **Essentiality**   1, 17, 37, 38, 46
    Man—Vital; needed for good health, normal longevity
    Other species—All: vertebrates, fungi, spermatophytes; some protozoans,
    algae, insects, bacteria

12. **Major Commercial Uses (Biological Interface)**   6, 22, 30, 54
    Element—Alloys: bronze (Cu, Zn, Sn), brass, (Zn, Cu), Babbitt metal (Sn,
    As, Sb, Pb), German silver (Cn, Zn, Ni); galvanizing: Zn, Cd
    Compounds—Pigments, disinfectants, preservatives, deodorants, embalming
    agents, mordants, fungicide, rodenticide

13. **Medicinal Applications**   18, 27, 30, 37, 53, 54
    Emetics ($ZnSO_4$)
    Astringents (Zn salts)
    Antiseptics ($ZnCl_2$)
    Hormones (insulin)

Dentin desensitizers (ZnCl$_2$)
Ointments (Zn stearate)
Dental cement [Zn$_3$(PO$_4$)$_2$]

14. **Hazards and Toxicity—Symptoms**   19, 30, 37, 39, 41, 46, 54
Element—Low toxicity
   Topical—Irritation
   Inhalation—Respiratory problems, chills, fever, nausea, vomiting
Compounds
   Topical—Irritation
   Inhalation—Respiratory problems, chills, fever, nausea, vomiting
   Oral toxicity—See nutrition section, dietary excess
Carcinogenicity/Mutagenicity = +/+ (rats) cocarcinogenic (?)

DISTRIBUTION AND SOURCES

1. **Occurrence and Environmental Concentrations** (μg/g)   3, 4, 6, 29, 42, 47
Relative terrestrial abundance—#23
Chief minerals—Sphalerite (ZnS), smithsonite (ZnCO$_3$), calamine (ZnSiO$_4$),
   franklinite (Fe, ZnMnO)
Earth's crust—65
Rocks—16-95 (sandstones—shales)
Soils—10-300 (50 average)
Freshwater—.0002-1.0 (.01 average)
Seawater—.01-.015

2. **Organismal Concentrations** (μg/g)   4, 42, 46, 47
Plants—Marine: 150; land: 25-100
Animals—Marine: 6-1500; land: 160
Man—33
Special concentrators—Plankton, radiolaria, coelenterates, mollusc, snakes
   (venom)
Indicator plants—Oranges, apples (deficiency)

3. **Dietary Sources (Variability due to Environment)**   5, 8, 26, 32a, 37, 36, 42,
   46, 52
High (mg/100 g) 4-10
   Seafood—Oysters, herring
   Meat/Organs—Beef, lamb, liver (beef, pork)
   Nuts/Seeds—Sunflower, pumpkin
   Diary products/fats—Cheese (American, Swiss, Cheddar, Colby, Parmesan,
      Provolone, Edam, Gouda)

Grains—Wheat (germ, bran)

Miscellaneous—Yeast (brewers', torula), maple syrup, bone meal, gluten, tea (dry)

Medium (mg/100 g) 0.4-4

Seafood—Lobster, crab, shrimp, tuna, perch, clams, anchovies, kippers

Meat/Organs—Chicken, turkey, mutton, pork, veal; chicken and turkey: liver, gizzard, heart; eggs

Nuts/Seeds—Peanuts, cashews

Grains—Oats, barley, wheat, brown rice, rye, buckwheat

Fruits—Avocados

Vegetables—Corn, lentils (dry), peas, spinach, beets, watercress, parsely, okra, carrots, asparagus

Dairy products—Cheese (Camembert, Limburger, Mozzarella, Munster, Roquefort, Monterey), yogurt

Miscellaneous—Raw sugar, molasses, coffee (dry)

Low (mg/100 g) 0-0.4

Fruits—Apples, grapes, grapefruit, oranges, pears, pineapples, bananas, peaches, cherries, watermelon, strawberries, apricots, red currants, lemons, cantaloupes, raisins

Vegetables—Beans (green, soy), cabbage, lettuce, onions, potatoes, tomatoes, radishes, yams, cauliflower, brussels sprouts, cucumber, eggplant, pumpkin, turnips, rutabagas, polished rice

Dairy products—Butter, cream, milk, margarine, lard, oil (olive, corn)

Miscellaneous—White sugar, sugar cane, honey, dates, mushrooms

CHEMISTRY

1. **Atomic Properties (Element)**   6, 7, 9, 30, 49

   Periodic table group no.—II-B, period 4

   Category of element—Metal, transition element

   Atomic weight—65.38

   Atomic number—30

   Atomic radius (metallic)—1.33, 1.45 Å

   Electron shells—2, 8, 18, 2

   Orbital electrons—$3s^2$, $3p^6$, $3d^{10}$, $4s^2$

   Natural isotopes—Zn^{64} (49%), Zn^{66} (28%), Zn^{67} (4%), Zn^{68} (19%)

   Long-lived radioactive isotopes—Zn^{62} (9 hr), Zn^{65} (244 days), Zn^{69} (14 hr), Zn^{72} (47 hr)

2. **Ionic Properties (Biological Forms)**   6, 7, 9, 30, 49
   Oxidation states (valences)—Zn^{2+}
   Ionic radius (Å)—0.75
   Oxidation potentials—$Zn^0 \rightarrow Zn^{2+}$ (0.762 v)
   Reducing/Oxidizing forms—None
   Unstable in aqueous solutions—None

3. **Molecular Properties (Biological Forms)**   6, 7, 9, 16, 25, 30, 43, 49
   Covalent radius (Å)—1.34
   Coordination numbers—4, 6
   Stereochemistry—Tetra-, octahedral
   Electron transfer compounds—None
   Typical molecular complexes—$[Zn(CN)_4]^{2-}$, $[Zn(NH_3)_6]^{2+}$, $[Zn(OH)_4]^{2-}$

4. **Analytical Methods**   3, 30, 31, 40, 47, 55
   Physical—Electrothermal atomic absorption; neutron activation
   Chemical—Spectrophotometric color, dithizone
   Hair/Nail analysis—Feasible, widely used
   Comments—Proteins interfere in atomic absorption; lack of standard procedures and reference materials to compare methods; blood Zn analysis problems from high Zn in RBC, WBC, platelets

5. **Chemical Properties of Compounds**   6, 7, 9, 49, 54
   See Table 6.1

MEDICINAL AND NUTRITIONAL ROLE

1. **Units of Measurement**
   Weight—μg (microgram); 1 mg (milligram) = 1000 μg
   Concentration—ppm (parts per million) = $\mu g/g$; $\mu g\%$ = $\mu g/100$ ml;

2. **Human Body Fluid Levels (Normal) ($\mu g/100$ ml)**   1, 2, 12, 37, 46
   Blood—509-650 (580) (RBC—1300; WBC—8000)
   Plasma/Serum—100-120 (11); circadian rhythm
   Urine—51.3-154.0 (84.0)
   Decreased serum levels in pregnancy, hepatitis, cirrhosis, tissue injury, myocardial infarction, renal insufficiency, tuberculosis, steroid therapy, increased age, women

3. **Human Organ Levels ($\mu g/g$)**   4, 8, 24, 46, 47
   Hair—150-190
   Liver—55

Table 6.1.   Properties of Zinc Compounds

	REACTIONS			SOLUBILITY				Taste	Synonyms
	Heat °C	Air	Water	g/100 cc H_2O	Alc.	Eth.	Acid		
Zn sulfate, $ZnSO_4 \cdot H_2O$	$-H_2O(238°)$	efflor.	acid pH 4.5	S	SS	NA	NA		zinc vitriol
Zn chloride, $ZnCl_2$	BP 732°	deliq.	acid pH 4	432^{25}	S	S	S	astringent	butter of zinc
Zn carbonate, $ZnCO_3$	$-CO_2 (300°)$	NA	NA	$.001^{15}$	I	S	S	NA	NA_1
Zn oxide, ZnO	stable	adds CO_2	NA	$.0002^{29}$	I	NA	S	NA	flowers of zinc

	Density	MW hyd./anh.	MP °C	XL Form	Color XL/Powd.	Appearance Commercial Form	% Element h./anh.	Odor
Zn sulfate, $ZnSO_4 \cdot H_2O$	1.97	179.4/161.4	d.	rhomb.	col./wh.	G, P	36.4/40.5	O
Zn chloride, $ZnCl_2$	2.91	−/136.3	290°	hex.	col./wh.	G	−/48.0	O
Zn carbonate, $ZnCO_3$	4.40	−/125.4	d.	trig. rhomb.	col./wh.	NA	−/52.1	O
Zn oxide, ZnO	5.61	−/81.4	1975°	hex.	y.-wh./−	P	−/80.3	O

Abbreviations as in earlier tables. y. = yellow.

Muscle—54
Brain—14
Bone—110

4. **Important Dietary Levels (mg/day)**   5, 21, 27, 30, 37, 39, 46
   Recommended dietary allowance—15 (15,000 μg/day)
   Deficiency limits—< 2
   Toxic limit—> 1000

5. **Estimated Human Daily Balance (average American diet, 70 kg ♂, 30 yr)**
   (μg/day)   27, 30, 42, 46
   Average intake—14,000 (13,000 food, 1000 water)
   Average output—14,000 (13,170 feces, 50 urine, 780 sweat)
   Net gain/loss—Balance, normally

6. **Indications for Supplementation of Above Diet**   5, 27, 30, 42, 46
   Healthy normal—Possible deficit (15,000 RDA − 14,000 average = 1000 μg/
   day)
   Special conditions—Related to body size, sex, age, stress, pregnancy, lactation

7. **Factors Affecting Availability from Diet**   17, 21, 27, 37, 46, 53
   Decreased
       Phytic acid in diet (vegetarian, soybean, cereals)
       Bulk in diet
       Absorption inhibitors (see absorption section)
       Zn-poor soils for vegetables
       Boiling vegetables
   Increased
       High-protein (casein, liver extract, etc.) diet
       Zn deficiency
       Absorption synergizers (see absorption section)
       Chelated complexes of Zn
       High-Zn content of water for drinking
       Zn-enriched or acid soils for vegetables

8. **Deficiency Symptoms**   21, 30, 36, 37, 46
   Man: Growth failure, anorexia, hypogonadism, hypogeusia, hyposmia,
       dermatitis, koilonychia, impaired wound healing
   Animals: Alopecia, skin lesions, hyperkeratosis, dermatitis, hypogonadism,
       skeletal abnormalities, impaired wound healing, growth failure, impaired
       brain development, increased developmental abnormalities

9. **Effects of Dietary Excess (Salts or Concentrates)** 19, 33, 36, 39, 46

   Acute—Lassitude, slow tendon reflexes, bloody enteritis, diarrhea, leukopenia, CNS depression, tremors, paralysis of extremities

   Chronic—Poor growth, microcytic hypochromic anemia, anorexia, symptoms of Ca and Fe deficiency

METABOLIC ROLE

1. **Intestinal Absorption** 17, 30, 35, 37, 39, 46

   Chemical forms

       Preferred valence—Zn^{2+}

       Poorly Absorbed—Oxides, metal

       Well absorbed—Chelates, salts.

   Sites—Duodenum, ileum, jejunum

   Efficiency—15-51% (increased in deficiency)

   Active transport—Present, not exclusive for Zn

   Synergizers—Amino acids, peptides, chelating agents, pancreatic ligands, histidine, cysteine

   Antagonists

       Competitors—Cu, Cd, Fe, Cr, Ca

       Sequestrants—Phytate, PO_4, Se, mucosal proteins

2. **Blood Carriers** 17, 30, 37, 46

   Serum (12-20%)—Macroglobulin, albumin-Zn, amino acid-Zn complexes

   RBC (80%)—Carbonic anhydrase

   WBC (3%)—Alkaline phosphatase

3. **Half-Life of Element in Blood** 8, 17, 37, 46

   < 3 hr

4. **Target (Initial) Sites** 17, 30, 37, 46

   Tissues—Liver, choroid, prostate, skin, bones, spleen, kidney

   Cells—Nuclei, cytosol, endoplasmic reticulum

5. **Storage** 17, 30, 37, 46

   Sites—Bones, spleen, kidney, liver, muscle (small amount), RBC

   Forms—Metallothionin (complexes)

6. **Homeostatic Mechanisms** 17, 30, 37, 42, 46

   Relative efficiency in element retention—80-97%

   Kidney participation—No controls reported

   Intestinal participation—Mucosal absorption controls; enteropheatic circulation

   Liver (bile) participation—secretion of Zn in bile and pancreatic juice

7. Specific Functions (via Cofactors/Metalloenzymes/Metalloproteins/Ions)
17, 21, 25, 30, 37, 46, 58

Molecular level
- Ligand; participant in catalysis
- Stabilizer/regulator of enzymes
- Stabilizer of DNA

Cellular level
- (Via enzyme action) Synthesis of nucleic acids, proteins, and porphyrins; activation of adenyl cyclase; mitogenic action on lymphocytes; stabilizing of ribosomes

Organismal level
- Synergism with hormones: growth (STH), CHO metabolism (insulin)
- Sex development (sex hormones)
- Maintenance: sensory functions, immune functions, respiration; brain development

8. Metalloenzymes, Cofactors, Metalloproteins   8, 10, 11, 15, 25, 30, 35, 37, 46

System Type	Organ	Metalloenzyme/Protein	Cofactors	System Function
Metallo-enzymes	Pancreas	Carboxypeptidases A+B	O	Digestion of peptides
	RBC	Carbonic anhydrase	O	CO_2 transfer
	Kidney	Renal dipeptidase	O	Digestion of peptides
	Liver	Glutamate de-Hase	NAD	Deaminations
	Heart	Malate de-Hase	NAD	Citric acid cycle
	Kidney	Alkaline phosphatase	O	Metabolism of organic PO_4
	Liver	Alcohol de-Hase	NAD	Metabolism of alcohol
	Muscle	Glyceraldehyde-3-P de-Hase	NAD	Glucose metabolism
	Kidney	Leucine amino peptidase/dipeptidase	O	Hydrolysis of peptides
	Muscle	AMP aminohydrolase	O	Conversion AMP → IMP
	Liver	Delta-Aminolevulinic acid dehydrogenase	O	Porphyrin synthesis
	Sea urchin	DNA polymerase	Mg	DNA synthesis
Metallo-protein	Liver	Metallothionin	Cd, Hg, Cu	Storage form
Co-factors	Various	Peptidases, enolase, arginase, deaminase, lecithinase, aldolase, decarbosylase	Zn, Mn, Mg, Co	Degredative

9. Excretion   21, 30, 37, 39, 42, 46
Chemical forms—Zn-amino acid complexes, fecal complexes

Organs
- Kidney (urine): 0.5-10% (increased by cortisol)
- Intestine (feces) ⎫
- Liver (bile, intestine) ⎬ 80-94%

Skin: ca. 6%
Other: hair—negligible

MISCELLANEOUS

1. **Relationship to Other Minerals**   27, 30, 37, 46, 53
   Cu—Absorption and metabolic antagonist to Zn
   Cd—Absorption and metabolic antagonist to Zn; major toxin
   Fe—Absorption and metabolic antagonist to Zn
   Cr—Absorption antagonist (competitive)
   Ca—Absorption antagonist (competitive)
   Mn—Absorption antagonist (competitive)
   P—Absorption antagonist (sequestrant)

2. **Relationship to Vitamins**   27, 36, 37, 46, 53
   A—Mobilized from liver by Zn
   D—Affects Zn intestinal absorption in some animals
   E—Synergist with Zn
   B_6—Synergist with Zn
   Niacin—NAD a cofactor with many Zn metalloenzymes

3. **Relationship to Hormones**   37, 46, 53
   Insulin—Zn complex with insulin; synergism with Zn (CHO metabolism)
   STH
   Testosterone   } Synergism with Zn in growth
   Cortisol—Increased urinary excretion of Zn, lowered serum Zn levels
   Progesterone—Lowered serum Zn levels

4. **Unusual Features**   21, 30, 36, 37, 46, 50, 53
   Zn reverses Cd-induced hypertension
   Zn inhibits ribonuclease
   Increased developmental abnormalities in Zn-deficient rats
   Presence of Zn in snake venoms and toxins
   Zn depletion by oral administration of histidine
   High serum Zn/Cu ratios show correlations with high serum cholesterol
   Circadian rhythm in Zn levels in blood serum
   Deposits of Zn in bones on high-Ca diet
   Rapid movement of serum Zn to liver during stress

5. **Possible relationship of Deficiency Symptoms to Metabolic Action of Zn**
   21, 30, 27, 36, 37, 46, 53
   Growth failure—DNA synthesis impaired

Hypogonadism—Maintenance germinal epithelium decreased
Dermatitis—Mucopolysaccharide synthesis decreased
Hyposmia   ⎫
Hypogeusia   ⎬   No data
Anorexia   ⎭
Impaired wound healing—Mucopolysaccharide synthesis decreased

Chapter 7. Iron (Fe)

Iron in the body has three major functions: oxygen transport, cellular respiration, and peroxide scavenging. Iron is found in all cells in plants and animals. It is essential for normal growth, development, and life span in humans. Its mode of action is mainly by way of oxygen transport by hemoglobin and myoglobin as well as by Fe enzymic roles in energy transformations in the cell, plus its role in the deactivators of deadly peroxides in the cells. Thus it plays a key role in many facets of respiration. It appears that Fe is optimally absorbed in the heme form, a chelated porphyrin complex made in the bone marrow. We thus have a vitamin-like form of Fe as is the case of most trace minerals. Iron's major mineral synergizer is Cu, and a major vitamin synergizer is folic acid. A major antagonist is Zn.

There is some evidence that the average American diet includes too much Fe for the human male but perhaps insufficient Fe for the human female. The effects of excess Fe in human male diets is exacerbated by vitamin plus Fe pill intake, lack of Fe excretion mechanisms, and may be related to the elevated cardiovascular disease rates in human males. Excess Fe also causes an antagonism and replacement of valuable zinc so important for the male prostate gland. Therefore human male diets should be examined for high-Fe items, while premenopausal human female diets should be increased in high-Fe items because of Fe losses from menstruation. High-Fe dietary items include liver, kidneys, clams, oysters, blackstrap molasses, brewer's and torula yeast, bone meal, soybeans, sunflower and pumpkin seeds, and soybeans.

Deficiencies are mainly found in children and menstruating females.

GENERAL INFORMAION

1. **Dietary and Medicinal Forms**   37, 49, 53, 54
   Element—Iron metal; not used medicinally at present
   Inorganic salts—Ferrous carbonate, sulfate
   Metallovitamin—Heme (porphyrin)
   Chelated forms—Ferrous citrate, lactate, fumarate, gluconate, succinate, glycinate

2. **History of Biological Significance**   8, 21, 37, 46, 50, 53
   1681—Sydenham: made first use of iron in medicine
   1713—Lemery and Geoffy: demonstrated that iron is present in blood
   1746—Menghini: iron-rich foods elevate blood iron
   1832—Blaud: cured chlorosis (anemia) with large doses of FE
   1832—Fodisch: blood of anemics is low in iron
   1842—Andral: Fe therapy increases RBCs in anemia
   1936—Reiman et al.: inorganic Fe is incorporated into hemoglobin
   1947—Holmberg and Laurell: transferrin in blood plasma contains Fe
   1953—Schoden et al.: ferritin is primary storage form of Fe
   1974—Siimes et al.: transferrin is primary blood carrier of Fe

3. **Physiological (Blood) Forms**   17, 21, 37, 46, 50, 53
   Transferrin, serum ferritin, hemoglobin (Hb) (RBC), catalase (RBC)

4. **Synergistic Agents**   30, 35, 37, 39, 46
   Metabolic—Porphyrin, Cu, Se, Mo, B_{12}, folic acid, ceruloplasmin
   Absorption—Alcohol, histidine, lysine, gastroferrin, vitamin C, citric, lactic, pyruvic, succinic acid, lactose, fructose, glucose, sucrose, sorbitol, porphyrin

5. **Antagonistic Agents**   30, 35, 37, 39, 46
   Metabolic—Zn, Co
   Absorption—Phytate, phosphate, egg proteins, long-chain fatty acids, Mn, Co, Ni, Cr, Zn, Ca, Mg, Cd, Cu, desferrioxamine

6. **Physiological Functions (Maintenance of System/Components)**   17, 21, 30, 37, 46, 50
   Circulatory—Heart muscle homeostasis (myoglobin)
   Execretory—Xanthine oxidase (purines catabolism)
   Respiratory—Hemoglobin, O_2 transport
   Digestive—Gastrointestinal tract homeostasis (Fe enzymes)
   Nervous—Oxygen for brain cells; ATP from cell oxidations (cytochromes)
   Special sensory—Retina metabolism (highest); ATP via cytochromes

Reproductive—Fetal Hb loss; replacement of pregnancy losses of Fe
Endocrine—Catecholamine synthesis (Fe enzymes)
Blood—Hemoglobin transferrin, ferritin, catalase component, hemopoiesis
Muscular—Myoglobin (skeletal muscle)
Skeletal—Bone marrow homeostasis, hemopoiesis
Integument—Skin and nails homeostasis; ATP via cytochromes (energy)
Protective/Immune—Resistance to infection; ATP via cytochromes (energy)
Metabolic—TCA cycle enzymes; cell oxidations, Krebs cycle (peroxidases)
Detoxification—Peroxides by peroxidases (heme enzyme); organic hydro-
    carbons by catalase (P-450)
Growth—+
Health—+
Longevity—+

7. **Body Content**   8, 12, 21, 35, 42, 46
   mg/70 kg = 4000-5000; μg/g = 57-70

8. **Relative Organ Concentrations**   12, 21, 42, 46
   Liver, spleen > bone marrow > kidney > heart > muscle > brain

9. **Deficiencies**   21, 30, 36, 37, 46, 39
   Man—Hypochromic microcytic anemia, polycythemia
   Pigs—Thumps

10. **Excess Conditions**   21, 30, 36, 37, 38, 46
    Man—Hemochromatosis, hemosiderosis

11. **Essentiality**   1, 17, 37, 38, 46
    Man—Vital; needed for good health, normal life span
    Other species—All: vertebrates, protozoa, algae, fungi, spermatophytes;
        some: invertebrates, insects

12. **Major Commercial Uses (Biological Interface)**   6, 22, 30, 54
    Element—Alloys steels [stainless (Cr, Ni, Cu, No, C); Mn; Cr-V; W; Ni],
        irons [duriron (Si); cast (C, Si, S, Mn, P); malleable (C, S, Si, P)]
    Compounds—Fertilizers, electroplating, feed supplements, reducing agents,
        wood preservative, weed killer, pesticide, ink, dye, lithography, water
        treatment, catalyst

13. **Medicinal Applications**   18, 27, 30, 37, 53, 54
    Hematinic ($FeSO_4$)
    Dietary supplement ($FeSO_4$, chelated forms)
    Tracer studies (Fe^{55}, Fe^{59})

14. **Hazards and Toxicity**   19, 30, 37, 39, 41, 46, 54
    Element—Low toxicity of metal
      Inhalation—No data
      Topical—No data
    Compounds
      Inhalation—Siderosis, mottling of lungs
      Topical—No data
      Oral toxicity—See nutrition section, dietary excess
    Carcinogenicity/Mutagenicity = ±/±   (cocarcinogenic?);   only   Fe-dextron
      carcinogenic

DISTRIBUTION AND SOURCES

1. **Occurrence and Environmental Concentrations** ($\mu g/g$)   3, 4, 6, 29, 42, 47
   Relative terrestrial abundance—#4
   Chief minerals—Magnetite (Fe_3O_4), hematite (Fe_2O_3), limonite (FeO_2),
      siderite ($FeCO_3$), pyrite (FeS_2), melanterrite ($FeSO_4$)
   Earth's crust—50,000
   Rocks—3800-56,300 (limestone-igneous)
   Soils—7000-550,000
   Freshwater—.01-1.4 (0.67 average)
   Seawater—.003-4.0 (0.01 average)

2. **Organismal Concentrations** ($\mu g/g$)   4, 42, 46, 47
   Plants—Marine: 700; land: 140
   Animals—Marine: 400; land: 160
   Man—60
   Special concentrators—Blue-green algae, horsetails, bryophytes, sponges,
      corals
   Indicator plants—In South America

3. **Dietary Sources (Variability due to Environment)**   8, 26, 36, 42, 46, 52
   High (mg/100 g) 5-18
      Seafood—Clams, oysters, caviar
      Meat/Organs—Liver and kidneys (beef, calf, pork, chicken, lamb), rein-
         deer
      Nuts/Seeds—Pistachio, pinon nuts, black walnuts, sesame, sunflower,
         pumpkin seeds
      Vegetables—Iris moss, chives, parsley, soybeans (dry)
      Grains—Wheat germ and bran, rice bran

Miscellaneous—Red wine, blackstrap molasses, sorghum syrup, bone meal, yeast (brewers', torula)

Medium (mg/100 g) 1-5

Seafood—Herring, mackerel, sardines, tuna, swordfish, scallops, shrimp, abalone

Meat/Organs—Chicken, duck, goose, turkey, eggs, lamb, pork, veal, beef tongue and heart

Nuts/Seeds—Almonds, brazils, cashews, chestnuts, peanuts, coconut, pecans, walnuts

Grains—Barley, brown rice, rye, wheat, oats, buckwheat

Fruits—Gooseberries, dates, figs, raisins, prunes, olives

Vegetables—Beets, radishes, beet greens, brussels sprouts, chard, endive, kale, spinach, watercress, artichokes, lima beans, green beans, broccoli, cauliflower, peas, brussel sprouts, lentils, red kidney beans, garbanzos

Dairy products—Cheese (cheddar)

Miscellaneous—Maple sugar, brown sugar, bakers' yeast, mushrooms

Low (mg/100 g) 0.1-1.10

Seafood—Carp, shad, salmon, halibut haddock, flounder, cod, blue fish, lobster, crab

Grains—White rice

Fruits—Lemons, limes, apricots, bananas, grapes, guavas, peaches, rhubarb, avocados, grapefruit, oranges, tangerines, cantaloupe, honeydew, watermelon, apples, cherries, papayas, pears, currants, berries (black-, blue-, cran-, logan-, rasp-, straw-)

Vegetables—Corn, cucumbers, eggplant, okra, green peppers, pumpkin, squash, tomatoes, carrots, parsnips, potatoes, sweet potatoes, rutabagas, turnips, asparagus, cabbage, celery, kohlrabi, lettuce, onion

Dairy products—Butter, buttermilk, cheeses (cream, cottage, swiss, blue), cream, milk

Miscellaneous—Oils, honey, white sugar, kelp

CHEMISTRY

1. **Atomic Properties (Element)**   6, 7, 9, 30, 49
   Periodic table group no.—VIII, period 4
   Category of element—Metallic transition element
   Atomic weight—55.85
   Atomic number—26
   Atomic radius (metallic)—1.24 Å
   Electron shells—2, 8, 8, 6, 2

Orbital electrons—$3s^2$, $3p^6$, $3d^6$, $4s^2$
Natural isotopes—Fe^{54} (5.8%), Fe^{56} (91.7%), Fe^{57} (2.2%), Fe^{58} (0.3%)
Long-lived radioactive isotopes—Fe^{52} (8.2 hr), Fe^{55} (2.6 yr), Fe^{59} (45 days), Fe^{60} (3×10^5 yr)

2. **Ionic Properties (Biological Forms)**   6, 7, 9, 30, 49
   Oxidation states (valences)—Fe^{2+}, Fe^{3+}
   Ionic radius (Å)—Fe^{2+}: 0.82; Fe^{3+}: 0.67
   Oxidation potentials—$Fe^0 \rightarrow Fe^{2+}$ (0.441 v); $Fe^0 \rightarrow Fe^{3+}$ (0.036 v); $Fe^{2+} \rightarrow Fe^{3+}$ (−0.771 v)
   Reducing/Oxidizing forms—Fe^{2+}/Fe^{3+}
   Unstable in aqueous solutions—Fe^{2+}

3. **Molecular Properties (Biological Forms)**   6, 7, 9, 16, 25, 30, 43, 49
   Covalent radius (Å)—Fe^{2+}: 1.165; Fe^{3+}: 1.39
   Coordination numbers—Fe^{2+} (6); Fe^{3+} (6)
   Stereochemistry—Fe^{2+} (octahedral); Fe^{3+} (octahedral)
   Electron transfer compounds—Heme enzymes, nonheme Fe proteins
   Typical molecular complexes—$Fe(CN)_6{}^{3-}$, $Fe(CN)_6{}^{4-}$, $Fe(H_2O)_4 (NH_3)_2{}^{2+}$

4. **Analytical Methods**   3, 30, 31, 40, 47, 55
   Physical—Packed cell volume; atomic absorption; emission spectroscopy
   Chemical—Spectrophotometric, bathophenanthroline sulfonate
   Hair/Nail analysis—Feasible, widely used
   Comments—Lack of standard procedures and reference materials to compare methods gives uncertainty

5. **Chemical Properties of Compounds**   6, 7, 9, 49, 54
   See Table 7.1

MEDICINAL AND NUTRITIONAL ROLE

1. **Units of Measurement**
   Weight—μg (microgram); 1 mg (milligram) = 1000 μg
   Concentration—ppm (parts per million) = μg/g; μg% = μg/100 ml

2. **Human Body Fluid Levels (Normal) (μg/100 ml)**   1, 2, 12, 37, 46
   Whole blood—38,000-45,000 (41,500)
   Plasma/serum—♀ 63-202 (average 113); ♂ 67-191 (average 127); circadian rhythm
   Urine—32.7
   Decreased serum levels—Caused by malignant tumors, uremia, leukemia,

Table 7.1.   Properties of Iron Compounds

$Fe = 2+$ (ferrous)	REACTIONS			SOLUBILITY			
	Heat °C	Air	Water	$g/100\ cc$ H_2O	Alc.	Eth.	Acid
Fe carbonate, $FeCO_3$	d.	NA	NA	$.007^{25}$	NA	NA	S
Fe citrate, $FeC_6H_6O_7 \cdot H_2O$	d. 350°	NA	NA	SS	i	i	NA
Fe sulfate, $FeSO_4 \cdot 7H_2O$	$-7\ H_2O$ (300°)	oxidizes efflor.	NA	15.7^{20}	SS	NA	NA
Fe lactate, $FeC_6H_2O_6 \cdot 3H_2O$	d.	darkens deliq.	NA	2.1^{10}	SS	NA	NA
Fe fumarate, $FeC_4H_2O_4$	NA	NA	NA	$.14^{25}$	SS	NA	NA
Fe gluconate, $FeC_{12}H_2O_{14} \cdot 2H_2O$	NA	NA	acid	S	i	NA	NA
Fe succinate, $FeC_4H_4O_4 \cdot 4H_2O$	NA	NA	NA	SS	NA	NA	NA

Table 7.1.   Properties of Iron Compounds (continued)

Fe = 2+ (ferrous)	Density	MW hyd./anh.	MP °C	XL Form	Color XL/Powd.	Appearance Commercial Form	% Element h./anh.	Odor	Taste	Synonyms
Fe carbonate, $FeCO_3$	3.8	−/115.9	d.	trig.	gr.-gray/br.	NA	−/48.2	O	NA	siderite
Fe citrate, $FeC_6H_6O_7 \cdot H_2O$	NA	264.0/246.0	d.	rhomb.	col./wh.	P, S	20.8/22.3	O	NA	NA
Fe sulfate, $FeSO_4 \cdot 7H_2O$	1.9	278.1/151.9	64°	monocl.	bl.-gr./?	C, G	20.1/36.8	O	saline	melan-terite
Fe lactate, $FeC_6H_2O_6 \cdot 3H_2O$	NA	288.0/234.0	d.	NA	gr.-wh./?	C, P	19.4/23.9	charact.	sweet	NA
Fe fumarate, $FeC_4H_2O_4$	NA	−/169.9	280°	NA	r.-gr.-r. br./?	G, P	−/32.9	O	O	NA
Fe gluconate, $FeC_{12}H_{22}O_{14} \cdot 2H_2O$	NA	482.2/446.2	NA	NA	y.-gray/gr.-y.	NA	11.6/12.5	caramel	NA	NA
Fe succinate, $FeC_4H_4O_4 \cdot 4H_2O$	NA	171.9/99.2	NA	NA	NA	NA	32.5/55.9	NA	NA	NA

Abbreviations: gr = green; br. = brown; bl. = blue; r. = red; charact. = characteristic; others as in earlier tables.

liver cirrhosis, myelomatosis in pregnancy, polycythemia, chronic Fe deficiency, infections

Increased serum levels—Caused by anemias (hemolytic, pernicious, aplastic),
hemochromatosis, hepatitis

3. **Human Tissue Levels (μg/g)**   4, 8, 24, 46, 47
   Hair—26-32
   Bone—111
   Muscle—28
   Liver—104
   Nerve—20

4. **Important Dietary Levels (mg/day)**   5, 21, 27, 30, 37, 39, 46
   Recommended dietary allowance—♀ 18, ♂ 10
   Deficiency limits—< 2
   Toxic limit—> 100

5. **Estimated Human Daily Balance (average American diet, 70 kg ♂, 30 yr)**   27,
   30, 42, 46
   Average intake—13,000 mg/day (12,833 food, 140 water, 27 air)
   Average output—13,000 mg/day (12,250 feces, 250 urine, 500 sweat)
   Net gain/loss—Balance normally

6. **Indications for Supplementation of Above Diet**   5, 27, 30, 42, 46
   Healthy normal—Males, none; females, need
   Special conditions—Needed for infants, adolescents, pregnancy, lactation

7. **Factors Affecting Availability from Diet**   17, 21, 27, 37, 46, 53
   Decreased
       Senescence
       Cu deficiency
       Achlorhydria
       Antacids
       Plant (vegetarian) diet
       Boiling of food
       Inhibitors (see absorption section)
   Increased
       Animal foods
       Acidic foods
       Hypoxia
       Accelerated erythropoiesis
       Iron cooking utensils
       Synergizers (see absorption section)

Alcohol
Anemia
FE deficiency
Hemochromatosis
B_6 deficiency
Gastroferrin

8. **Deficiency Symptoms**   21, 30, 36, 37, 46
Man: (Hypochromic microcytic anemia), listlessness, fatigue, palpitation on exertion, sore tongue, angular stomatitis, dysphagia, koilonychia, depressed growth, decreased resistance to infection

9. **Effects of Dietary Excess (Salts or Concentrates)**   19, 33, 36, 39, 46
Acute—Biphasic shock, rapid increase in respiration, and pulse rates, congestion of blood vessels, hypotension, pallor, drowsiness in 6-8 hr, prostration, coma, death from cardiac failure in 36 hr
Chronic—Hemorrhagic necrosis of gastrointestinal tract, hepatotoxicity, metabolic acidosis, prolonged clotting time, increased plasma levels of serotonin and histamine

METABOLIC ROLE

1. **Intestinal Absorption**   17, 30, 35, 37, 39, 46
Chemical forms—Fe^{2+}, Fe^{3+} salts; heme (independently absorbed)
Preferred valence—Fe^{2+} (Fe^{3+} reduced to Fe^{2+})
Poorly absorbed—Phytates, SO_4, PO_4
Well absorbed—Amino acids, chelates, gluconates, citrates, ascorbates
Sites—Duodenum, stomach, upper jejunum
Efficiency—5-15% (varies with deficiency and disease); heme absorbed very efficiently
Active transport—At higher intake levels
Synergizers—Ascorbic acid; citric, lactic, pyruvic, succinic acids; lactose, fructose, glucose, sucrose; histidine, lysine, valine, gastroferrin, alcohol, sorbitol
Antagonists (not for heme)
Competitors—Desferrioxamine, Co, Zn, Cd, Cu, Mn
Sequestrants—Phytate (?), PO_4, egg proteins

2. **Blood Carriers**   17, 30, 37, 46
Transferrin (siderophilin), long-chain fatty acids, serum ferritin

3. **Half-Life of Element in Blood**   8, 17, 37, 46
   90-100 min

4. **Target (Initial) Sites**   17, 30, 37, 46
   Tissues—Liver, spleen, bone marrow
   Cells—Mitochondria (heme synthesis)

5. **Storage**   17, 30, 37, 46
   Sites—Liver, spleen, intestinal mucosa, bone marrow, muscle
   Forms—Ferritin, hemosiderin

6. **Homeostatic Mechanisms**   17, 30, 37, 42, 46
   Relative efficiency in element retention—95-100%
   Kidney participation—Negligible
   Intestinal participation—Epithelial cells concentrate Fe
   Liver (bile) participation—Excreted in bile but reabsorbed in enterohepatic
      circulation

7. **Specific Functions (via Cofactors/Metalloenzymes/Metalloproteins/Ions)**
      17, 21, 25, 30, 37, 46, 58
   Molecular level
      Ligand; enzyme stabilizer or regulator
      Catalyst; electron transfer agent
   Cellular level
      Cellular respiration and energy production (ATP) via Krebs cycle; main-
         tenance cell membranes
      Detoxification of peroxides; electron transfer
   Organismal level
      Maintenance of all systems
      Preservation of membranes
      Key element in respiration

8. **Metalloenzymes, Cofactors, Metalloproteins**   8, 10, 11, 15, 25, 30, 35,
      37, 46

System Types	Organ	Metalloenzyme/Protein	Cofactors	System Function
Metallo-enzymes	Heart	Cytochrome oxidase (heme)	Fe^{2+}/Cu^{2+}	Electron transport
	Heart	Cytochrome C (heme)	Fe^{2+}/Fe^{2+}	Electron transport
	RBC	Catalase (heme)	Fe^{2+}/Fe^{2+}	Peroxide detoxication
	RBC	Glutathione peroxidase (heme)	Fe^{2+}/Se	Peroxide detoxication
	Liver	Peroxidase (heme)	Fe^{2+}/Fe^{2+}	Peroxide detoxication
	Heart	Succinic dehydrogenase	Fe^{2+}/FAD	Electron transport
	Heart	NAD dehydrogenase	Fe^{2+}/FAD	Electron transport
	Mammary gland	Xanthine oxidase	Fe^{2+}/Mo	Electron transport

System Types	Organ	Metalloenzyme/Protein	Cofactors	System Function
Metallo-proteins	RBC	Hemoglobin (heme)	Fe^{2+}	Oxygen transport
	Skeletal muscle	Myoglobin (heme)	Fe^{2+}	Oxygen transport
	Liver	Ferritin	Fe^{3+}	Iron storage
	Liver	Hemosiderin	Fe^{3+}	Iron storage
	Blood	Transferrin	Fe^{31}	Iron transport
	Egg white	Conalbumin	Fe^{3+}	Iron transport
	Egg yolk	Phosvitin	Fe^{3+}	Iron transport

9. **Excretion**   21, 30, 37, 39, 42, 46
   Chemical forms—Ferritin, food iron
   Organs—Kidney (urine): ca. 2%; intestine (feces): ca. 94%; liver (bile, intestine): trace, resorption via enterophepatic circulation; skin: ca. 4%; other: menstrual losses (blood)

MISCELLANEOUS

1. **Relationship to Other Minerals**   27, 30, 37, 46, 53
   Co, Zn, Cd, Cu, Ni, Mn—Competitive absorption inhibitors
   Mo—With Fe in xanthine oxidase
   Cu—As ceruloplasmin acts as ferroxidase
   Cu—With Fe in cytochrome oxidase
   Pb—Inhibits heme synthesis
   Zn—Deficiency mimics Fe deficiency anemia
   Se—With Fe in glutathione peroxidase
   Co—As B_{12} synergizes hemoglobin production

2. **Relationship to Vitamins**   27, 36, 37, 46, 53
   B_2—Cofactor with iron for succinic and NAD dehydrogenase (FAD)
   B_6—Deficiency increases Fe absorption
   B_{12}, folic acid—Synergize Fe, control pernicious anemia

3. **Relationship to Hormones**   37, 46, 53
   Cortisol—Diurnal variation of serum Fe (via Cu)
   Epinephrine, norepinephrine—Synthesis requires Fe enzyme
   Erythropoietin—Stimulates RBC formation

4. **Unusual Features**   21, 30, 36, 37, 46, 50, 53
   Low efficiency of FE absorption

High efficiency of body conservation of Fe

Multiple valence changes in Fe during Fe metabolism

No excretion mechanisms for excess Fe in body

Diurnal plasma Fe variation

Unavailability of egg yolk Fe

Low levels of Fe in milk

Excessive deposits of Fe from self-medication in males (cardiovascular problems)

5. **Possible Relationship of Deficiency Symptoms to Metabolic Action**   21, 30, 27, 36, 37, 46, 53

Listlessness, fatigue, palpitation on exertion—Lacks synergism of Fe with B-complex

Sore tongue, angular stomatitis—Lacks synergism of Fe enzymes with FAD (B_2)

Dysphagia, koilonychia—Exposure of Cd/Zn antogonism

Depressed growth and infection resistance—Synergism of Fe with B-complex

Chapter 8. Cobalt (Co)

Cobalt salts are effective only in satisfying ruminant and microorganismal nutritional requirements. Soil and gut microorganisms convert the salts to the needed form of vitamin B_{12}. All vertebrates including man require their cobalt in the form of vitamin B_{12}. For further information about the vitamin please consult the vitamin B_{12} chapter.

Cobalt salts themselves have some biological effects, mostly deleterious, such as polycythemia, hyperlipemia, thyroid and heart damage, and insulin inhibition. They are also found to be mutagenic or carcinogenic. Any cobalt assimilated in the human diet that is not in the vitamin form is not used, but is promptly excreted in the urine or feces. Cobalt salts also exert a competitive effect on absorption of iron and manganese. Therefore, supplementation with cobalt salts should be avoided in favor of the vitamin B_{12} form, which is required. Values of dietary contents of cobalt are highly variable, depending on soil, location, climate, and methodology. Very few species of microorganisms can incorporate cobalt into vitamin B_{12}, the main ones that can are the nitrogen-fixing bacteria (legumes) and the rumen bacteria in ruminants. There may be no direct relationship between cobalt content and vitamin B_{12} content of the diet.

There is no evidence available to justify dietary supplementation of cobalt salts in the human diet, but cobalt as vitamin B_{12} is definitely needed (see the vitamin B_{12} chapter). Ruminants do require Co salts in the diet.

GENERAL INFORMATION

1. **Dietary and Medicinal Forms**   37, 49, 53, 54

   Element—Cobalt, metal; not used medicinally except as Co^{60} radiation source

   Inorganic salts—Cobaltous chloride, acetate

   Chelated forms—Cobalamins (see vitamin B_{12})

   Metallovitamin—Vitamin B_{12} and cobalamins

2. **History of Biological Significance**   8, 21, 37, 46, 50, 53

   1926—Bertrand et al.: first demonstration of Co in animals

   1929—Waltner et al.: discovery that polycythemia develops in rats ingesting Co

   1935—Underwood et al.: discovery of Co requirement in animals

   1948—Smith and Parker: Co an essential part of vitamin B_{12}

   1951—Keener: Co alone effective in restoring B_{12} microflora (ruminants)

   1955—Hodgkin et al.: structure of B_{12} determined

   1967—Morin et al.: myopathy caused by Co in beer

3. **Physiological (Blood) Forms**   17, 21, 37, 46, 50, 53

   Hydroxocabalamin, aquocobalamin, transferrin

4. **Synergistic Agents (see also vitamin B_{12})**   30, 35, 37, 39, 46

   Metabolic—I^-, Mn^{2+}, penicillin, Cu^{2+}, Zn^{2+}

   Absorption—See iron, synergists

5. **Antagonistic Agents (see also vitamin B_{12})**   30, 35, 37, 39, 46

   Metabolic—I^- (excess)

   Absorption—Fe^{2+}, EDTA; see iron, antagonists

6. **Physiological Functions (Maintenance of Systems/Components) (via B_{12} or Co^{2+})**   17, 21, 30, 37, 46, 50

   Circulatory—Increase cardiac glycogen (via Co^{2+})

   Excretory—Stimulates erythropoietin in kidney (via Co^{2+})

   Respiratory—Maintenance erythropoiesis; maintenance bone marrow (via B_{12})

   Digestive—Maintenance mucosa of gastrointestinal tract (via B_{12})

   Nervous—Maintenance myelin sheath (via B_{12})

   Special sensory—Maintenance vision, coordination (via B_{12})

   Reproductive—Prevention congenital anomalies; maintenance gametogenesis (via B_{12})

   Endocrine—Release of erythropoietin (via Co^{2+}); release of glucagon, T4; inhibition of insulin release (via B_{12})

   Blood—Hyperlipemia (via Co^{2+})

   Muscular—Muscle homeostasis and control (via B_{12})

   Skeletal—Maintenance bone marrow (via B_{12})

Integument—Maintenance of skin (via B_{12})
Immune—Maintenance of leukopoiesis (via B_{12})
Metabolic—Nucleic acid, protein, lipid synthesis (via B_{12})
Detoxification—Methylation and sulfhydryl reactions (via B_{12})
Growth—+ (via B_{12})
Health—+ (via B_{12})
Longevity—+ (via B_{12})

7. **Body Content Total Co**   8, 12, 21, 35, 42, 46
mg/70 kg = 1.0-1.5; μg/g = 14-21

8. **Relative Organ Concentrations (as Co^{2+})**   12, 21, 42, 46
Muscle > bones > kidney > liver > heart > spleen > pancreas

9. **Deficiencies**   21, 30, 36, 37, 46
Man (as vitamin B_{12})—Glossitis, sprue, anemias (pernicious, megaloblastic, macrocytic-hyperchromic)
Animals—Bush sickness, phalaris staggers (ruminants) (as Co^{2+})

10. **Excess Conditions**   21, 30, 36, 37, 39, 38, 46
Man—Polycythemia, cardiomyopathy, goiter (as Co^{2+})
Animals—Polycythemia, thyroid hyperplasia (rats); anemia (sheep) (as Co^{2+})

11. **Essentiality**   1, 17, 37, 38, 46
Man—Vital, normal helath and longevity (only as B_{12})
Other species—All: vertebrates, insects (as B_{12} except ruminants), blue-green algae, N-fixing bacteria (as Co^{2+})
   some: spermatophytes, protozoa, bacteria (except N-fixing), fungi, algae (except blue-green) as B_{12}

12. **Major Commercial Uses (Biological Interface)**   6, 22, 30, 54
Element—Alloys [stellite (Cr, W, Mo, Fe, Ni); Alnico (Al, Ni)], nuclear technology
Compounds—Catalyst, electroplating, fertilizer and feed additive, poison gas adsorbent, bleaching agent, foam stabilizer, paints and indicators

13. **Medicinal Applications**   27, 30, 37, 53, 54
Vitamin B_{12} manufacture ($CoNO_3$)
Trace mineral (veterinary use) ($CoCl_2$, $CoCO_3$)
Radiation source (Co^{60}) (Co metal)
Hematinic—Refractory anemias ($CoCl_2$)

14. **Hazards and Toxicity**   19, 30, 37, 39, 41, 46, 54
Element

Inhalation—Pulmonary symptoms, bone marrow hyperplasia, peritoneal and pericardial effusion

Contact—Dermatitis

Compounds

Inhalation—Pulmonary edema

Contact—Dermatitis (contact)

Oral toxicity—See nutrition section, dietary excess

Carcinogenicity/Mutagenicity = +/+ (carcinogenic only by injection)

DISTRIBUTION AND SOURCES

1. **Occurence and Environmental Concentrations (μg/g) (as Co^{2+})**   3, 4, 6, 29, 42, 47

   Relative terrestrial abundance—#34

   Chief minerals—Cobaltite (CoAsS); smaltite ($CoAs_2$); erythrite [$CO_3(AsO_4)$ · $8H_2O$]

   Earth's crust—23.0

   Rocks—0.1-25.0 (limestones-igneous)

   Soils—1.0-40.0

   Freshwater—.00090

   Seawater—.00027

2. **Organismal Concentrations (μg/g) (as Co^{2+})**   4, 42, 46, 47

   Plants—Marine: 0.7; land: 0.5

   Animals—Marine: 0.5-5.0; land: 0.03

   Man—0.02

   Special concentrators (land plants)—*Nyssa Sylvatica, Clethra Barbinervis*

3. **Dietary Sources (Variability due to Environment) as Total Cobalt (B_{12} Co plus Co^{2+})**   8, 26, 36, 42, 46, 52

   High (μg/100 g) 22-100

   Seafood—Sardines, salmon, herring

   Meat/Organs—Liver (pig, lamb), kidney (lamb, beef)

   Nuts/Seeds—Peanuts

   Vegetables—Peas, okra

   Dairy products/fats—Butter

   Grains—Buckwheat, wheat bran, wheat germ

   Miscellaneous—Molasses, raw sugar, cornstarch, corn meal

   Medium (μg/100 g) 10-22

   Seaford—Oysters, clams, crabs

   Meat/Organs—Pork, lamb, sheep, beef, chicken

   Grains—Brown rice, wheat

   Fruits—Pears, figs

Vegetables—Onion, cassava tuber, spinach, corn, cucumber, cauliflower, beans, cabbage, yams

Miscellaneous—Corn oil

Low (µg/100 g) 1-10

Meat/Organs—Eggs, beef liver, egg yolk

Nuts/Seeds—Walnuts, sunflower seeds

Grains—Polished rice, barley

Fruits—Bananas, apples, cherries, apricots, raisins

Vegetables—Carrots, beans, beets, chard, lettuce, tomatoes, eggplant, brussels sprouts, radishes, potatoes

Dairy products—Milk

Miscellaneous—Wine, white sugar, sugar cane

CHEMISTRY

1. **Atomic Properties (Element)**   6, 7, 9, 30, 49

   Periodic table group no.—VIII, period 4

   Category of element—Transition element, metallic

   Atomic weight—58.93

   Atomic number—27

   Atomic radius (metallic)—1.253 Å

   Electron shells—2, 8, 15, 2

   Orbital electrons—$3s^2$, $3p^6$, $3d^7$, $4s^2$

   Natural isotopes—Co^{59} (100%)

   Long-lived radioactive isotopes—Co^{55} (18.21 hr), Co^{56} (77 days), Co^{57} (270 days), Co^{58} (71.3 days), Co^{60} (5.3 yr), Co^{61} (1.7 hr)

2. **Ionic Properties (Biological Forms) (as Co^{2+})**   6, 7, 9, 30, 49

   Oxidation States (Valences)—Co^{2+}, Co^{3+} (vitamin B_{12})

   Ionic radius (Å)—Co^{2+}: 0.74; Co^{3+}: 0.63

   Oxidation potentials—$Co^0 \rightarrow Co^{2+}$ (+0.277 v); $Co^{2+} \rightarrow Co^{3+}$ (−1.84 v)

3. **Molecular Properties (Biological Forms) (as Co^{2+})**   6, 7, 9, 16, 25, 30, 43, 49

   Covalent radius (Å)—Co^{2+}: 1.55; Co^{3+}: 1.35

   Coordination numbers—4, 6 (Co^{2+}); 6 (Co^{3+})

   Stereochemistry—4, tetrahedral; 6, octahedral

   Electron transfer compounds—Aquocobalamine, coenzyme B_{12}

   Typical molecular complexes—$[Co(NH_3)_6]^{3+}$, $[Co(CN)_6]^{3-}$

4. **Analytical Methods**   3, 30, 31, 40, 47, 55
   Physical—Atomic absorption (flameless), neutron activation
   Chemical—Spectrophotometric color, 1-nitroso-2-naphthol
   Hair/Nail analysis—Hair feasible, values reported
   Comments—Co determination not an indicator of B_{12}; high variability
   among methods—no reference standards

5. **Chemical Properties of Compounds**   6, 7, 9, 49, 54
   See Table 8.1

MEDICINAL AND NUTRITIONAL ROLE

1. **Units of Measurement**
   Weight—μg (microgram); 1 mg (milligram) = 1000 μg
   Concentration—ppm (parts per million) = μg/g; μg% = μg/100 ml

2. **Human Body Fluid Levels (Normal) (μg/100 ml) (as Total Cobalt)**   1, 2,
   12, 37, 46
   Blood—0.35-1.70 (1.02)
   Plasma/Serum—0.01-0.12 (0.03)
   Urine—0.23-0.56 (0.33)

3. **Human Organ Levels** μg/g (as Total Cobalt)   4, 8, 24, 46, 47
   Hair—.03-.24
   Liver—0.095
   Nerve—0.015
   Muscle (skeletal)—0.007
   Bone—0.028

4. **Important Dietary Levels (as Total Cobalt)**   5, 21, 27, 30, 37, 39, 46
   Estimated dietary level—100-1000 μg/day (need only 40 μg/day as B_{12})
   Toxic limit—490 μg/day

5. **Estimated Human Daily Balance (average American diet, 70 kg ♂, 30 yr)**
   (as Total Cobalt)   27, 30, 42, 46
   Average intake—300 μg/day (food 290, water 10)
   Average output—300 μg/day (urine 200, feces 94, sweat 4)
   Net gain/loss—Balanced

6. **Indications for Supplementation of Above Diet**   5, 21, 27, 30, 42, 46
   Healthy normal—None
   Special conditions (as B_{12} only—Anemia, deficiencies, growth, pregnancy

Table 8.1.   Properties of Cobalt Compounds

Co = 2+ (cobaltous)	REACTIONS			SOLUBILITY			
	Heat °C	Air	Water	g/100 cc H_2O	Alc.	Eth.	Acid
Co chloride, $CoCl_2 \cdot 6H_2O$	$-6H_2O(120°)$	deliq.	acid pH 4.6	76.7°	VS	S	S
Co acetate, $CoC_4H_6O_4 \cdot 4H_2O$	$-4H_2O(140°)$	deliq.	neut.	S	S	NA	S

Co = 2+ (cobaltous)	Density	MW hyd./anh.	MP °C	XL Form	Color XL/Powd.	Appearance Commercial Form	% Element h./anh.
Co chloride, $CoCl_2 \cdot 6H_2O$	1.92	257.9/ 129.9	87	monocl. prisms	red-pink/ ?	C	24.8/ 45.4
Co acetate, $CoC_4H_6O_4 \cdot 4H_2O$	1.71	249.1/ 177.0	NA	monocl. prisms	red-violet/?	C, need.	23.7/ 33.3

Abbreviations as in earlier tables. VS = very soluble.

7. **Factors Affecting Availability from Diet (as Co^{2+})**   17, 21, 27, 37, 46, 53
Decreased
    Food in stomach
    Protein in diet
    Absorption inhibitors (see absorption section)
    See also vitamin B$_{12}$
Increased
    Iron deficiency
    Hemochromatosis
    Absorption synergizers (see absorption section)
    See also vitamin B$_{12}$

8. **Deficiency Symptoms (see vitamin B$_{12}$)**   21, 30, 36, 37, 46
Man—See vitamin B$_{12}$
Animals—Ruminants (as Co^{2+}): weakness, emaciation, anemia, high mortality, tachycardia, incoordination
    Nonruminants: see vitamin B$_{12}$

9. **Effects of Dietary Excess (Salts or Concentrates (as Co^{2+})**   19, 33, 36, 39, 46
Acute—Nausea, vomiting, diarrhea, paralysis, low blood pressure, low body temperature, death
Chronic—Thyroid dysfunction, myxodema, goiter, congestive heart failure, polycythemia, pericardial effusion, damage to α cells in pancreas, cancer

METABOLIC ROLE

1. **Intestinal Absorption**   17, 30, 35, 37, 39, 46
Chemical forms—Cobalt salts and cobamides (including B$_{12}$)
    Preferred valence—Co^{2+} for salts; Co^{3+} for B$_{12}$
    Poorly absorbed—Large doses Co^{2+}, B$_{12}$ without intrinsic factor
    Well absorbed—Small doses of cobalt salts and cobamides, B$_{12}$ with intrinsic factor
Sites—Ileum (B$_{12}$), lower small intestine (Co^{2+})
Efficiency—20-95% (Co^{2+})
Active transport—Co^{2+} uses Fe transport system; B$_{12}$ uses intrinsic factor
Synergizers—See Fe synergizers
Antagonists—See Fe antagonists; Fe^{2+}, EDTA

2. **Blood Carriers**   17, 30, 37, 46
Transferrin (?), aquocobalamin, α globulin complexes, hydroxocobalamin; see vitamin B$_{12}$

3. **Half-Life of Element in Blood**   8, 17, 37, 46
   3 days (rabbit) (as Co^{2+}); also see vitamin B_{12}

4. **Target (Initial) Sites**   17, 30, 37, 46
   Tissues—All (see vitamin B_{12})
   Cells—Mitochondria, nucleus (?)

5. **Storage**   17, 30, 37, 46
   Sites—Kidney, liver, bone marrow, pancreas, spleen, heart; see also vitamin B_{12}
   Forms—Coenzyme B_{12}

6. **Homeostatic Mechanisms**   17, 30, 37, 42, 46
   Relative efficiency in element retention—0-20% (?) (as Co^{2+})
   Kidney participation—Major excretion organ; passive excretion of Co^{2+}
   Intestinal participation—Major controller for Co^{2+} absorption
   Liver (bile) participation—Yes, enterohepatic circulation of Co^{2+}

7. **Specific Functions (via Cofactors/Metalloenzymes/Metalloproteins/Ions)**
   17, 21, 25, 30, 37, 46
   Molecular level
     Redox agent
     Stabilizing agent
     Enzyme activator
   Cellular level
     See vitamin B_{12}
   Organismal level
     See vitamin B_{12}

8. **Metalloenzymes, Cofactors, Metalloproteins**   8, 10, 11, 15, 25, 30, 35, 37, 46

System Types	Organ	Enzyme/Protein	Co-factors	System Function
Metallo-enzyme	Animal tissues	Glycylglycine dipeptidase	—	Hydrolyzes dipeptides
Cofactor	Bacteria	Catalase	Co^{2+}	Destroys H_2O_2
Cofactor	Bacteria	Pyrophosphatase	Co^{2+}	Converts pyro- to ortho-PO_4

9. **Excretion**   21, 30, 37, 39, 42, 46
   Chemical forms—Co^{2+}, B_{12}, Co-histamine complex
   Organs
       Kidney (urine)—66%
       Intestine (feces)   ⎫
                         ⎬ 33%
       Liver (bile, intestine) ⎭
       Skin—1%

MISCELLANEOUS

1. **Relationship to Other Minerals**   27, 30, 37, 46, 53
   I—Co^{2+} antagonizes thyroid absorption of I
   Mo—Synergist with Co^{2+} in N-fixing bacteria
   Cu—Synergist with Co^{2+} in RBC production (as B_{12})
   Zn—Synergist with Co^{2+} in RBC production (as B_{12})
   Fe—Antagonist in absorption of Co^{2+}; synergist in RBC production (as B_{12})
   Mn—Antagonist in absorption of Co^{2+}

2. **Relationship to Vitamins (see also vitamin B_{12})**   27, 36, 37, 46, 53
   B_{12}—Co is central atom
   C—Increases Co^{2+} absorption in gut (chicks)
   Folic acid—cofactor with B_{12} in prevention of anemia

3. **Relationship to Hormones (see also vitamin B_{12})**   37, 46, 53
   T4—Co^{2+} antagonizes release of T4
   Cyclic AMP—Co^{2+} increases levels in kidney
   Glucagon—Release stimulated by Co^{2+}
   Insulin—Release inhibited by Co^{2+}
   Erythropoietin—Release stimulated by Co^{2+}
   Testosterone—Synergizes erythropoietin and B_{12}

4. **Unusual Features (see also vitamin B_{12})**   21, 30, 36, 37, 46, 50, 53
   Co^{2+} present in plants, not as B_{12}, not required
   Ruminants require Co as Co salts; convert to B_{12}
   Co^{2+} causes vasodilatation and flushing on injection
   Co absorbed as Co^{2+}; incorporated into B_{12} as Co^{3+}
   Humans require Co only as B_{12}
   Co^{2+} produces epileptic seizures on brain application
   Co^{2+} produces tumors on injection into skeletal muscles but exerts protective
       action against methylcholanthrene carcinogenesis
   N-fixing bacteria require Co^{2+} for B_{12} production and N-fixation

5. **Possible Relationship of Deficiency Symptoms to Metabolic Action**
   See vitamin B_{12}

Chapter 9. Copper (Cu)

Copper is a mineral essential to many key functions in the body. However, because it is richly present in practically all foods, there is a real possibility of a dietary excess of Cu in the American diet, which would antagonize Fe and Zn by replacement. Practically all soft water supplies have an excessive amount of Cu, due largely to dissolution of copper piping. Deficiencies in man have mainly been found in infancy. Some genetic defects have been found in Cu absorption. A major role of Cu in metabolism is in oxidation (both in ionic and enzyme form); thus its role in respiration, atherosclerosis (peroxidation), and anemias is important. Copper is optimally absorbed as a protein (metallothionin?) or an amino acid complex. A major synergist is Fe.

There is no evidence of need for supplementation of the average adult American diet with Cu. In fact, there may be an excess due to the Cu in water supplies. Also, Cu from cooking utensils and beverage containers adds to the Cu burden. Acute toxicity of ingested Cu is limited by its emetic action, and chronic toxicity is limited at higher values by regulated absorption in the intestine. However, sufficient data are not yet available for us to state that intermediate Cu intakes do not add to the body burden.

GENERAL INFORMATION

1. **Dietary and Medicinal Forms**   37, 49, 53, 54
   Element—Copper (metallic); sometimes used medicinally
   Inorganic salts—Carbonate, acetate, sulfate (blue vitriol)
   Metallovitamin—Cu-duodenal-protein complex (?)
   Chelated forms—Gluconate, glycinate, citrate

2. **History of Biological Significance**   8, 21, 37, 46, 50, 53
   1830—Buchholz: first identified Cu in plants
   1847—Harless: demonstrated Cu in snail blood
   1878—Frederick: identified Cu in hemocyanin
   1921—Bodansky: identified Cu in human brain
   1928—Hart: established essentiality of Cu for animals
   1931—Josephs: obtained first evidence of Cu deficiency in humans (infants)
   1935—Elvehjem: reversed Cu deficiency symptoms in animals with Cu
   1948—Holmberg: identified Cu in ceruloplasmin, blue serum protein
   1966—Osaki et al.: demonstrated ceruloplasmin involved in Fe metabolism
   1974—Dunlap: reported first adult human Cu deficiency

3. **Physiological (Blood) forms**   17, 21, 37, 46, 50, 53
   Hemocuprein, ceruloplasmin, erythrocuprein (RBC), hemocyanin (molluscs)
   Plasma amine oxidase, Cu-albumin, Cu-threonine, Cu-histidine

4. **Synergistic Agents**   30, 35, 37, 39, 46
   Metabolic—Fe (respiration)
   Absorption—Amino acids, duodenal proteins

5. **Antagonistic Agents**   30, 35, 37, 39, 46
   Metabolic—Zn, Fe, Mo, Cd, Ag
   Absorption—Fe, Cd, Hg, Ag, Mo, Zn, Ca, SO_4, S^{2-}, porphyrins, bile proteins,
   Vitamin C

6. **Physiological Functions (Maintenance of Systems/Components)**   17, 21,
   30, 37, 46, 50
   Circulatory—Aorta, myocardium, blood vessel structure, homeostasis
   Excretory—Purine excretion via Cu enzymes
   Respiratory—Stabilization Hb content (RBC)
   Digestive—Digestive tract homeostasis
   Nervous—Myelination of spinal cord maintenance
   Special sensory—Iris, choroid homeostasis
   Reproductive—Fertility, fetal nonresorption (homeostasis)
   Endocrine—Catecholamine synthesis

Blood—Hemoglobin synthesis
Muscular—Connective tissue, myoglobin maintenance
Skeletal—Bone structure homeostasis
Integument—Skin, nails, hair pigment, wool keratin maintenance
Protective/Immune—Infection resistance (reticuloendothelial system activa-
    tion); leukocyte factor (LEM) → ↑ ceruloplasmin synthesis in liver;
    neutrophils (homeostasis)
Metabolic—Elastin synthesis, Fe metabolism (synergism)
Detoxification—Aryl compounds, singlet oxygen (peroxidases)
Growth—+
Health—+
Longevity—+

7. **Body Content**   8, 12, 21, 35, 42, 46
mg/70 kg = 75-150; μg/g = 1.1-2.2

8. **Relative Organ Concentrations**   12, 21, 42, 46
Liver > brain > lung > kidney > ovary, testes > lymph node > muscle

9. **Deficiencies**   21, 30, 36, 37, 46
Man—Anemia (hypochromic), hypocupremia, neutropenia, Menke's syn-
    drome (defective absorption)
Cattle—Anemia (hypochromic macrocytic), falling disease, achromotrichia
Pigs—Anemia (hypochromic microcytic)
Sheep—Anemia (hypochromic), neonatal ataxia, achromotrichia
Rats—Anemia (hypochromic, microcytic), infertility

10. **Excess Conditions, Other Disorders**   21, 30, 36, 37, 39, 38, 46
Man—Wilson's disease (defective liver excretion and metabolism), metal
    fume fevers, icterus, hemoglobinuria, schizophrenia (?)

11. **Essentiality**   1, 17, 37, 38, 46
Man—Vital, needed for good health, normal life span
Other species—All: vertebrates, fungi, algae, spermatophytes; some: in-
    vertebrates, insects, protozoa

12. **Major Commercial Uses (Biological Interface)**   6, 22, 30, 54
Element—Alloys [bronze (Cu, Zn, Sn), brass (Cu, Zn), monel (Cu, Ni),
    German silver (Cu, Zn, Ni)] ; conductors: Cu metal
Compounds—Fungicides, herbicides, algicides, insecticides, bactericides,
    preservatives, mordants, pigments, pyrotechnics, food, feed additives

13. **Medicinal Applications**   18, 27, 30, 37, 53, 54
    Emetic ($CuSO_4$)
    Intrauterine device (Cu metal)
    Antifungal topical ($CuSO_4$)
    P-antidote ($CuSO_4$)
    Diet supplement—Cu gluconate, glycinate
    Oral deodorant—Cu gluconate

14. **Hazards and Toxicity—Symptoms**   19, 30, 37, 39, 41, 46, 54
    Element—Low toxicity
        Inhalation—Fume fever
        Topical—Irritation
    Compounds
        Inhalation—Fume fever
        Topical—Irritation
        Oral toxicity—See nutrition section, dietary excess
    Carcinogenicity/Mutagenicity = $-/\pm$ [cocarcinogenic (?)]

DISTRIBUTION AND SOURCES

1. **Occurrence and Environmental Concentrations** ($\mu g/g$)   3, 4, 6, 29, 42, 47
    Relative terrestrial abundance—#25
    Chief minerals—Malachite, $Cu_2(OH)_2CO_3$; azurite (basic carbonate), $Cu_3(OH)_2(CO_3)_2$; cuprite, Cu_2O; chalococite, Cu_2S
    Earth's crust—45
    Rocks—4-55 (limestones-shales)
    Soils—2-100
    Freshwater—.01-5.60
    Seawater—.003-.010

2. **Organismal Concentrations** ($\mu g/g$)   4, 42, 46, 47
    Plants—Marine: 11; land: 14
    Animals—Marine: 4-50; land: 2-4
    Man—1.2
    Special concentrators—Sponges, molluscs (blood), arthropods, annelids
    Indicator plants—Some bryophytes

3. **Dietary Sources (Variability due to Environment)**   8, 26, 36, 42, 46, 52
    High (mg/100 g) 1-10
        Seafood—Oysters, crabs, bluefish, perch, lobster
        Meat/Organs—Calf, duck, lamb, pork, beef (liver and kidney)
        Nuts/Seeds—Almonds, pecans, walnuts, filberts, brazils, sesame, sun-
            flower, pistachio

Vegetables—Soybeans

Grains—Wheat germ and bran

Miscellaneous—Yeast, gelatin, bone meal, corn oil, margarine, mushrooms

Medium (mg/100 g) 0.1-1.0

Seafood—Halibut, flounder, cod, tuna, mackerel, shrimp, crayfish, rainbow trout

Meat/Organs—Chicken, turkey, pork liver, mutton, beef heart

Nuts/Seeds—Peanuts

Grains—Barley, wheat, oats, rye, rice

Fruits—Apples, bananas, lemons, dates, apricots, raspberries, strawberries, avocados

Vegetables—Asparagus, artichokes, corn, kale, onion, potatoes, spinach, eggplant, lentils, sweet potatoes, lima beans, olives, celery, leeks, okra, horseradish

Dairy products—Cream, cheeses (American, Swiss, cheddar)

Miscellaneous—Eggs, honey, salt, black pepper

Low (mg/100 g) 0-0.1

Seafood—Sardines, salmon

Meat/Organs—Beef

Fruits—Grapes, oranges, apples, tangerines, cherries, grapefruit, pears, pineapples, watermelon, papaya, peach

Vegetables—Carrots, cabbage, cassava, radish, yam, brussels sprouts, cauliflower, lettuce

Dairy products—Milk, cheeses (cottage, Parmesan, Edam)

Miscellaneous—White sugar

CHEMISTRY

1. **Atomic Properties (Element)**   6, 7, 9, 30, 49

Periodic table group no.—I, period 4

Category of element—Metal, transition element

Atomic weight—63.66

Atomic number—29

Atomic radius (metallic)—1.278 Å

Electron shells—2, 8, 18, 1

Orbital electrons—$3s^2$, $3p^6$, $3d^{10}$, $4s^1$

Natural isotopes—Cu^{63} (69.1%), Cu^{65} (30.9%)

Long-lived radioactive isotopes—Cu^{61} (3.3 hr), Cu^{64} (12.8 hr), Cu^{67} (59 hr)

2. **Ionic Properties (Biological Forms)** 6, 7, 9, 30, 49
   Oxidation states (valences)—Cu^+, Cu^{2+}
   Ionic radius (Å)—0.96 (Cu^+), 0.72 (Cu^{2+})
   Oxidation potentials—$Cu^0 \rightarrow Cu^+$ (−.522 v); $Cu^+ \rightarrow Cu^{2+}$ (−.153 v)
   Reducing/Oxidizing forms—Cu^+/Cu^{2+}
   Unstable in aqueous solutions—Cu^+

3. **Molecular Properties (Biological Forms)** 6, 7, 9, 16, 25, 30, 43, 49
   Covalent radius (Å)—Cu^{2+}: 1.29, 1.43
   Coordination numbers—Cu^{2+}: 4, 6; Cu^+: 4
   Stereochemistry—Cu^{2+}: square/distorted octahedral; Cu^+: tetrahedral
   Electron transfer compounds—Various Cu metalloenzymes
   Typical molecular complexes—$[Cu(H_2O)_6]^{2+}$, $[CuCl_4]^{2-}$, $[Cu\ EDTA]^{2-}$.
      $[CuF_4]^{2-}$, $[Cu(NH_3)_4]^{2+}$

4. **Analytical Methods** 3, 30, 31, 40, 47, 55
   Physical—Electrothermal atomic absorption
   Chemical—Spectrophotometric: dithizone, bathocuproine
   Hair/Nail analysis—Feasible
   Comments—Proteins interfere; lack of reference standards

5. **Chemical Properties of Compounds** 6, 7, 9, 49, 54
   See Table 9.1

MEDICINAL AND NUTRITIONAL ROLE

1. **Units of Measurement**
   Weight—μg (microgram); 1 mg (milligram) = 1000 μg
   Concentration—ppm (parts per million) = μg/g; μg% = μg/100 ml

2. **Human Body Fluid Levels (Normal) (μg/100 ml)** 1, 2, 12, 37, 46
   Blood—89-98 (93.5)
   Plasma/Serum—81-147 (114)
   Urine—1.4-3.3 (2.3)
   Elevated serum Cu in: multiple sclerosis, infection, myocardial infarction,
      liver disease, old age, schizophrenia, estrogen, thyroid, pituitary hormone,
      surgery

3. **Human Tissue Levels (μg/gm)** 4, 8, 24, 46, 47
   Hair—12-21
   Bone—11.9
   Liver—7.1
   Muscle—1.25
   Brain—4.0

Table 9.1.   Properties of Copper Compounds

Cu = 2+ (cupric)	REACTIONS			SOLUBILITY			
	Heat °C	Air	Water	gm/100 cc H_2O	Alc.	Eth.	Acid
Cu acetate, $Cu(CH_3COO)_2 \cdot H_2O$	d. 240	NA	NA	7.2^{20}	S	SS	NA
Cu sulfate, $CuSO_4 \cdot 5H_2O$	$-5H_2O(250°)$	efflor.	acid pH 4.0	$32°$	I	NA	NA
Cu carbonate basic, $CuCO_3 \cdot Cu(OH)_2$	$-CO_2(200°)$	NA	NA	I	I	NA	S
Cu gluconate, $CuC_6H_4O_7 \cdot H_2O$	NA	NA	NA	30^{25}	SS	I	NA
Cu glycinate, $Cu(H_2NCH_2COO)_2 \cdot H_2O$	$-H_2O(123°)$	NA	NA	0.57^{16}	SS	NA	NA
$2Cu_2C_6H_4O_7 \cdot 5H_2O$ Cu citrate	$-H_2O(100°)$	NA	NA	I	NA	NA	S

Table 9.1.   Properties of Copper Compounds (continued)

Cu = 2+ (cupric)	Density	MW hyd./anh.	MP °C	XL Form	Color XL/Powd.	Appearance Commercial Form	% Element h./anh.	Odor	Taste	Synonyms
Cu acetate, $Cu(CH_3COO)_2 \cdot H_2O$	1.88	199.6/181.6	115	NA	dk. gr./?	P	-/35.0	NA	NA	NA
Cu sulfate, $CuSO_4 \cdot 5H_2O$	2.29	249.7/159.6	d.	triclin.	blue/?	C, G, P	25.4/39.8	NA	NA	blue vitriol
Cu carbonate basic, $CuCO_3 \cdot Cu(OH)_2$	4.0	-/222.1	d.	monocl.	green/?	C, amorph.	-/57.5	NA	NA	malachite
Cu gluconate, $CuC_6H_4O_7 \cdot H_2O$	NA	471.9/453.9	NA	NA	blue/?	C, P	13.5/14.0	O	astring.	NA
Cu glycinate, $Cu(H_2NCH_2COO)_2 \cdot H_2O$	NA	229.7/211.7	d.	rhomb.	blue/?	need.	27.7/30.0	NA	NA	bisglyci-nato copper
Cu citrate, $2Cu_2C_6H_4O_7 \cdot 5H_2O$	NA	720.4/630.4	NA	NA	bl. gr./?	P	-/40.3	NA	NA	NA

Abbreviations: dk = dark; astring. = astringent; others as in earlier tables. NA = not available

4. **Important Dietary Levels**   5, 21, 27, 30, 37, 39, 46
   Recommended dietary allowance—2 mg/day (2000 μg/day)
   Deficiency limits—$<$ 2 mg/day
   Toxic limit—mg/day $>$ 250

5. **Estimated Human Daily Balance (average American diet, 70 kg δ, 30 yr)**
   27, 30, 42, 46
   Average intake—4000 μg/day (3500 food, 60-500 water, 20 air)
   Average output—4000 μg/day (3500 feces, 50 urine, 40-400 sweat)
   Net gain/loss—Balance or excess of Cu

6. **Indications for Supplementation of Above Diet**   5, 27, 30, 42, 46
   Healthy normal—None; reduction may be desirable
   Special conditions—Certain infancy conditions

7. **Factors Affecting Availability from Diet**   17, 21, 27, 37, 46, 53
   Decreased
       High pH in gut
       Increased age
       Boiling foods
       Uncooked protein
       Absorption inhibitors (see absorption section)
   Increased
       Cu deficiency
       Cu cooking utensils
       Divalent Cu forms
       Cooking meat
       Raw vegetables
       Absorption synergizers (see absorption section)

8. **Deficiency Symptoms**   21, 30, 36, 37, 46
   Man—Neutropenia; anemia; bone disease
   Animals—Demyelination of nerves, degeneration, defective pigmentation,
       hair, wool, reproductive failure, cardiovascular lesions

9. **Effects of Dietary Excess of Supplements, Salts and Concentrates**   19, 33,
   36, 39, 46
   Acute—Sporadic fever, tachycardia, hypotension, hemolytic anemia, oliguria,
       uremia, coma, cardiovascular collapse, death
   Chronic—Nausea, vomiting, epigastric pain, yellow watery diarrhea, dizzi-
       ness, general debility, jaundice, green (stools, saliva, vomitus), antagonism
       to zinc

METABOLIC ROLE

1. **Intestinal Absorption**   17, 30, 35, 37, 39, 46
   Chemical forms
       Preferred valence—Cu^{2+}
       Poorly absorbed—Cu salts, Cu metal
       Well absorbed—Cu chelated compounds
   Sites—Stomach, small intestine
   Efficiency—32-60%
   Active transport—Some; not exclusive
   Synergizers—Amino acids, duodenal proteins
   Antagonists
       Competitors—Fe, Cd, Hg, Ag, Zn
       Sequestrants—Bile proteins, porphyrins, sulfides, SO_4, MoO_4, phytates
       Absorption inhibitor—Vitamin C

2. **Blood Carriers**   17, 30, 37, 46
   Albumin, ceruloplasmin (95%), histidine, threonine, glutamine

3. **Half-Life of Element in Blood**   8, 17, 37, 46
   3-7 days (ceruloplasmin-Cu)

4. **Target (Initial) Sites**   17, 30, 37, 46
   Tissues—Liver, kidney, gastrointestinal tract, brain, heart
   Cells—Cytosol, lysosomes, mitochondria

5. **Storage**   17, 30, 37, 46
   Sites—Liver, kidney, gastrointestinal tract
   Forms—Metallothionin (liver)

6. **Homeostatic Mechanisms**   17, 30, 37, 42, 46
   Relative efficiency in element retention—60-80%
   Kidney participation—No significant function
   Intestinal participation—Regulates Cu uptake and release
   Liver (bile) participation—Excretion in bile, no enterohepatic circulation

7. **Specific Functions (via Cofactors/Metalloenzymes/Metalloproteins/Ions)**
       17, 21, 25, 30, 37, 46, 58
   Molecular level
       Electron-transfer agent, crosslinking agent for collagen and elastin,
           catalyst (protein conformation), ligand to substrate, oxygen transport
           (hemocyanin)

Cellular level

Catecholamine synthesis, antioxidant (dismutases) cellular oxidations, phospholipid synthesis, iron metabolism, unsaturated fatty acid metabolism, mitochondrial energy production dependent on Cu enzymes

Organismal level

See physiological functions; mostly maintenance functions plus iron metabolism and mobilization, cellular oxidations, lipid and amine metabolism

8. Metalloenzymes, Cofactors, Metalloproteins   18, 10, 11, 15, 25, 30, 35, 37, 46

System Type	Organ	Metalloenzyme/Protein	Cofactors	System Function
Metallo-enzyme	Heart (mito-chondria)	Cytochrome c oxidase	Fe^{2+}	Myelin, catecho-lamine synthesis
	Heart, RBC, brain, liver, mitochondria	Superoxide dismutases, cerebrocuprein, hepa-tocuprein, hemocu-prein, erythrocuprein, mitochondrocuprein	Zn^{2+}, Mn^{2+}, Fe^{2+}	Superoxide degradation
	Plasma, liver	Ceruloplasmin (ferroxidase)	Fe^{2+}	Fe oxidation, mobilization
	Skin, melanomas	Tyrosinase	?	Melanin formation
	Liver, kidney	Uricase	?	Allantoin formation
	Adrenal	Dopamine β-hydroxylase	?	Norepinephrine synthesis
	Aorta, cartilage	Lysyl oxidase	B_6	Elastin, collagen crosslinking
	Plasma (beef)	Spermine oxidase	B_6	Oxidative deamination
	Plasma (pig)	Benzylamine oxidase	B_6	Oxidative deamination
	Kidney	Diamine oxidase	FAD, B_6	Oxidative deamination
Metallo-protein	Blood (mollusc)	Hemocyanin		Oxygen transport

9. Excretion   21, 30, 37, 39, 42, 46

Chemical forms—Bile: protein Cu complexes in feces

Organs

Kidney (urine)—Negligible (1%)

Intestine (feces) ⎫
Liver (bile, intestine) ⎭ Major (Cu 90%)

Skin—Negligible
Other (sweat)—Small (1-10%)

MISCELLANEOUS

1. **Relationship to Other Minerals**   27, 30, 37, 46, 53
   Fe, Cd, Hg, Ag, Zn—Competitive absorption inhibitors for Cu
   SO_4, Mo—Intestinal sequestrants for Cu
   Fe—Synergistic with Cu in heme synthesis
   Zn, Cd—Present with Cu in metallothionin

2. **Relationship to Vitamins**   27, 36, 37, 46, 53
   B_6—Cofactor for various Cu metalloenzymes
   B_2—FAD a cofactor for diamine oxidase (Cu enzyme)
   C—Inhibits absorption of Cu
   C, folic acid, B_{12}—Partially compensate for Cu deficiency anemia

3. **Relationship to Hormones**   37, 46, 53
   Estradiol, progesterone—Increase serum Cu (ceruloplasmin)
   Cortisol, ACTH—Decrease serum Cu
   Testosterone—Inceases serum Cu
   Epinephrine, norepinephrine—Synthesis is by Cu metalloenzymes
   Cortisol, progesterone—Synthesis involves Cu-dependent enzyme

4. **Unusual Features**   21, 30, 36, 37, 46, 50, 53
   Possible relationship of aging to Cu in tissues (peroxidation)
   Psychoses reported with high serum Cu
   Fetus accumulates Cu in liver
   Ceruloplasmin absent in turkeys, chickens
   Causes swelling of mitochondria
   Soft-water supplies usually high in Cu
   Cu-phytates soluble in alkaline intestine
   Zn/Cu ratios (rats) implicated in vascular disease
   Possible danger of excessive Cu intake in adults (self-medication)
   Cu deficiencies common in infants on cow's milk (low Cu)
   Increasing brain content of Cu during maturation
   Increased serum Cu correlated with atherosclerosis and peroxidation

5. **Possible Relationship of Deficiency Symptoms to Metabolic Action**   21,
   30, 27, 36, 37, 46, 53
   Neutropenia—Zinc toxicity symptom exposed; activation of reticuloendo-
      thelial system by Cu blocked
   Anemia—Formation of Fe-transferrin; Fe transport blocked
   Bone disease—Crosslinking of collagen stopped
   Demyelination—Phospholipid synthesis halted
   Defective pigmentation—Melanin synthesis blocked

Chapter 10. Chromium (Cr)

Chromium in the inorganic form shows only a small amount of biological activity. The biologically active form (i.e., vitamin form of Cr metallovitamin) is the GTF (glucose tolerance factor). Chromium has been shown to be effective in the GTF form to alleviate impaired glucose tolerance, and mild diabetes and to decrease serum cholesterol *in animals*. Presumably these results will be demonstrated in humans as well. The unique condition of a steady loss of Cr found in Americans with age may be related to the steady rise in atherosclerosis observed in Americans, and may trigger an interest in finding additional sources of biologically available organic Cr in unprocessed foods. The amount of Cr (which is obtainanle from high-Cr foods such as brewer's yeast, molasses, wheat germ, and kidney) needed to offset the daily losses is estimated at 50-200 μg/day. Some inorganic Cr salts are toxic, especially in the hexavalent form. The high content of Cr in RNA may indicate a more important function of Cr in human metabolism.

If supplementation of Cr in the human diet is proven beneficial, it should only be used in the food form (organic Cr), since Cr salts are usually toxic.

GENERAL INFORMATION

1. **Dietary and medicinal Forms**   37, 49, 53, 54
   Element—Chromium (metal); not used medicinally

Inorganic salts—Chromic trichloride, acetate
Metallovitamin—Clucose tolerance factor (GTF)
Chelated forms—Chromic glycinate, oxalate, perchlorate, salicylate

2. **History of Biological Significance**   8, 21, 37, 46, 50, 53
1929—Glaser and Halpern: yeast extracts potentiate insulin action
1955—Mertz and Schwarz: impaired glucose tolerance is refractory to known dietary factors
1957—Schwarz and Mertz: postulated new dietary glucose tolerance factor (GTF)
1959—Schwarz and Mertz: identified Cr as active ingredient of GTF in animal diets
1959—Wacker and Vallee: found high Cr levels in nucleic acids
1962—Schroeder: tissue levels of Cr decrease with age in man
1968—Hopkins and Price: Cr supplements improve glucose tolerance in humans
1969—Mertz: GTF facilitates action of insulin
1974—Polansky: active principle of GTF is a Cr-niacin complex
1975—Jeejeebhoy: made first report of human Cr deficiency

3. **Physiological (Blood) Forms**   17, 21, 37, 46, 50, 53
Glucose tolerance factor (GTF), Cr-transferrin, albumins, and globulins

4. **Synergistic Agents**   30, 35, 37, 39, 46
Metabolic—Insulin, glucose, Mg, B_6, Zn
Absorption—Oxalates, perchlorates, salicylates

5. **Antagonistic Agents**   30, 35, 37, 39, 46
Metabolic—Glucagon
Absorption—Zn, V, Fe, Mn, phytates

6. **Possible or Demonstrated Physiological Functions (Maintenance of Systems/ Components)**   17, 21, 30, 37, 46, 50

Circulatory—Serum cholesterol homeostasis (via insulin)
Excretory—Urinary sugar homeostasis (via insulin)
Respiratory—Increased cellular CO_2 output (via insulin)
Digestive—Glucose, amino acid absorption (via insulin)
Nervous—Neuronal homeostasis (via insulin)
Special sensory—corneal clarity
Reproductive—Homeostasis of fetal carbohydrate metabolism

Blood—Serum cholesterol homeostasis
Muscular—Energy for contraction (via insulin)
Skeletal—Component of bones ⎤
Integument—Component of hair ⎦ function unknown
Protective/Immune—Infection resistance of lung (via insulin)
Metabolic—Glucose, lipid, protein metabolism (via insulin)
Detoxification—Liver detoxification functions (via insulin, and liver homeostasis)
Growth—+ (?)
Health—+ (?)
Longevity—+ (?)

7. **Body Content**   8, 12, 21, 35, 42, 46
mg/70 kg = 0.6-1.4; μg/g = .009-.020

8. **Relative Organ Concentrations**   12, 21, 42, 46
Placenta > lung > stomach, muscle, kidney > spleen and liver

9. **Deficiencies**   21, 30, 36, 37, 46
Man—Impaired glucose tolerance, atherosclerosis (?)
Lab animals—Corneal opacity (rats), hyperglycemia (rats)

10. **Excess Conditions**   21, 30, 36, 39, 37, 38, 46
Man—Lung cancer (chromates—Cr^{6+})
Animals—Liver and kidney damage (Chromates—Cr^{6+})

11. **Essentiality**   1, 17, 37, 38, 46
Man—Not vital; may be needed for good health, normal life span
Other species—Some: vertebrates, fungi

12. **Major Commercial Uses (Biological Interface)**   6, 22, 30, 54
Element—Alloys (stainless steel, nichrome, stellite, chrome steel), chrome-plating
Compounds—Chromizing, catalyst, mordant, tanning, corrosion inhibitor, waterproofing, pigments

13. **Medicinal Applications**   27, 30, 37, 53, 54
Dietary supplement (Cr acetate, Cr glycinate, GTF)
Radioactive labeling of erythrocytes (Cr^{51})

14. **Hazards and Toxicity**   19, 30, 37, 39, 41, 46, 54
Element—Low toxicity of metal
Inhalation—Lung cancer (low incidence)

Compounds—Hexavalent (Cr^{6+}): dichromates and chromates, highly toxic; trivalent (Cr^{3+}): chromic salts, nontoxic

hexavalent Cr^{6+} only

    Inhalation—Lung cancer

    Topical—Primary irritation, ulceration, allergic exzema, dermatitis

    Oral toxicity—See nutrition section, (dietary excess)

    Carcinogenicity/Mutagenicity = +/+ (lungs) (hexavalent salts only)

DISTRIBUTION AND SOURCES

1. **Occurrence and Environmental Concentrations (μg/g) (or ppm)**   3, 4, 5, 29, 42, 47

   Relative terrestrial abundance—#25

   Chief minerals—Chromite (FeO · Cr_2O_3), lead chromate ($PbCrO_4$)

   Earth's crust—200 (average)

   Rocks—11-100 (limestones-igneous)

   Soils—5-3000 (100 average)

   Freshwater (.0000072-.00084)—0.00018 average

   Seawater—0.00005-.0020

2. **Organismal Concentrations (μg/g) (or ppm)**

   Plants—Marine: 1.0 (average); land: .02-.23

   Animals—Marine: 0.2-1.0; land: .11-.48

   Man—0.2 (average)

   Special concentrators—Ferns, ascidians

3. **Dietary Sources (Variability due to Environment)**   8, 26, 36, 42, 45, 46, 52

   High (mg/100 g) (30-200)

       Seafood—Oysters

       Meat/Organs—Calves' liver, egg yolk

       Nuts/Seeds—Peanuts

       Fruits—Grape juice

       Dairy products and fats—Cheese (American)

       Grains—Wheat, wheat germ

       Miscellaneous—Final molasses, brewer's yeast, sugar beet molasses, black pepper

   Medium (mg/100 g) (12-30)

       Seafood—Shrimp

       Meat/Organs—Beef and lamb (liver, heart, kidney), eggs

Grains—Brown rice
Fruits—Orange juice
Vegetables—Potato
Dairy products—Butter, margarine
Miscellaneous—Corn syrup, maple syrup, honey, blackstrap molasses, dark brown sugar, raw sugar
Low (mg/100 g) (0-12)
  Seafood—Haddock, lobster
  Meat/Organs—Pork, lamb, beef, chicken, ham
  Grains—Polished rice, barley
  Fruits—Raisins, apples, pears, rhubarb, bananas, blueberries, oranges, strawberries
  Vegetables—Parsnips, tomatoes, beans, carrots, spinach, corn
  Dairy products—Butter, corn oil, milk
  Miscellaneous—White sugar, light brown sugar, sugar cane, molasses, torula yeast, mushrooms

CHEMISTRY

1. Atomic Properties (Element)   6, 7, 9, 30, 49
Periodic table group No.—VI-B, period 4
Category of element—Transition element, metal
Atomic weight—51.99
Atomic number—24
Atomic radius (metallic)—1.249, 1.305 Å
Electron shells—2, 8, 13, 1
Orbital electrons—$3s^2$, $3p^6$, $3d^5$, $4s^1$
Natural isotopes—Cr^{50} (4.3%), Cr^{52} (83.8%), Cr^{53} (9.6%), Cr^{54} (2.4%)
Long-lived radioactive isotopes—Cr^{48} (23 hr), Cr^{51} (27.8 days), Cr^{49} (42 min)

2. Ionic Properties (Biological Forms)   6, 7, 9, 30, 49
Oxidation states (valences)—Cr^{2+}, Cr^{3+}, Cr^{6+}
Ionic radius (Å)—Cr^{2+}, 0.84; Cr^{3+}, 0.64; Cr^{6+}, 0.52
Oxidation potentials—$Cr^0 \rightarrow Cr^{2+}$ (0.56 v); $Cr^{2+} \rightarrow Cr^{3+}$ (0.41 v); $Cr^{3+} \rightarrow Cr^{6+}$ (−1.195 v)
Reducing/Oxidizing forms—Cr^{2+}/Cr^{6+}
Unstable in aqueous solution—Cr^{3+}

3. **Molecular Properties (Biological Forms)**   6, 7, 9, 16, 25, 30, 43, 49
   Covalent radius (Å)—Cr^{3+}, 1.45; Cr^{6+}, 1.16
   Coordination numbers—Cr^{3+}, 6; Cr^{6+}, 4, 6, 8
   Stereochemistry—Cr^{3+}, octahedral; Cr^{6+}, tetrahedral
   Typical molecular complexes—$[Cr(NH_3)_6]^{3+}$, $[Cr(H_2O)_6]^{3+}$, $[Cr(C_2O_4)_3]^{3+}$

4. **Analytical Methods**   3, 30, 31, 40, 47, 55
   Physical—Flameless atomic absorption, neutron activation
   Chemical—Spectrophotometric, diphenylthiocarbazone
   Hair/Nail analysis—Feasible, used
   Comments—*Volatilization* and contamination cause divergent results

5. **Chemical Properties of Compounds**   6, 7, 9, 49, 54
   See Table 10.1

MEDICINAL AND NUTRITIONAL ROLE

1. **Units of Measurement**
   Weight—μg (microgram); 1 mg (milligram) = 1000 μg
   Concentration—ppm (parts per million) = μg/g; μg% = μg/100 ml

2. **Human Body Fluid Levels (Normal) (μg/100 ml)**   1, 2, 12, 37, 46
   Blood—1.0-5.5 (2.8)
   Plasma/Serum—2.8
   Urine—.05-5.0 (2.5)

3. **Human Tissue Levels (μg/g)**   4, 8, 24, 46, 47
   Hair—0.65
   Bone—< 0.85
   Liver—0.02
   Muscle—0.03
   Brain—0.012

4. **Important Dietary Levels**   5, 21, 27, 30, 37, 39, 46
   Recommended dietary allowance—50-200 μg/day tentative
   Deficiency limits—< 50 μg/day
   Toxic limit—> 500 mg/day

Table 10.1.   Properties of Chromium Compounds

Cr = 3 + (chromic)	REACTIONS			SOLUBILITY			
	Heat °C	Air	Water	g/100 cc H₂O	Alc.	Eth.	Acid
Cr trichloride, CrCl₃	subl. 950°	deliq.	acid pH 2.4	SS	I	I	SS
Cr acetate, Cr (CH₃COO)₂	NA	NA	NA	SS	NA	NA	NA

Cr = 3 + (chromic)	Density	MW hyd./anh.	MP °C	XL Form	Color XL/Powd.	Appearance Commercial Form	% Element h./anh.
Cr trichloride, CrCl₃	2.87	-/158.4	1152	trig. monoclin.	violet/?	S	-/32.8
Cr acetate, Cr (CH₃COO)₂	NA	-/170.1	NA	NA	red/?	C	-/22.7

Abbreviations: subl. = sublimes; others as in earlier tables. NA = not available

5. **Estimated Human Daily Balance (average American diet, 70 kg ♂, 30 yr)** 27, 30, 42, 46
   Average intake—110.0 μg/day (food 100, water 10)
   Average output—110.6 μg/day (feces 98, urine 10, sweat 1, hair 0.6)
   Net gain/loss—0.6 μg/day loss

6. **Indications for Supplementation of Above Diet**   5, 21, 27, 30, 42, 46
   Healthy normal—Possibly needs supplementation
   Special conditions—Diabetes, sugar metabolism disorders

7. **Factors Affecting Availability from Diet**   17, 21, 27, 37, 46, 53
   Decreased
       See antagonists, absorption
       Refining of foods
       Soil quality
       Aging of humans
       Hexavalent form
       Inorganic form
   Increased
       See synergizers, absorption
       Organic complex form
       Chelating agents

8. **Deficiency Symptoms**   21, 30, 36, 37, 46
   Man—Impaired glucose tolerance
   Animals—Increased mortality, increased atherosclerosis, increased blood cholesterol levels, glycosuria, hyperglycemia, impaired glucose tolerance, inability to deal with stress

9. **Effects of Dietary Excess (Salts or Concentrates)**   19, 23, 33, 36, 39, 46
   Acute—(humans) Cr^{6+}: gastrointestinal ulceration, central nervous system symptoms; Cr^{3+}: little or no effect
   Chronic—(animals) Cr^{6+}: depressed growth, damaged liver and kidney; Cr^{3+}: vomiting and diarrhea; (humans): no reports of toxicity

METABOLIC ROLE

1. **Intestinal Absorption**   17, 30, 35, 37, 39, 46
   Chemical forms—Cr^{6+} and Cr^{3+} (salts), GTF, chelates
   Preferred valence—Cr^{3+}
   Poorly absorbed—Inorganic salts
   Well absorbed—Organic amino acid chelates, glucose tolerance factor, brewer's yeast extract

Sites—Small intestine, midsection
Efficiency—1.3% inorganic, 10-25% amino acid chelated
Active transport—Probably GTF, amino acid chelated forms
Synergizers—Oxalates, amino acids, perchlorates, salicylates
Antagonists—Phytates, alkalies, Zn, V

2. **Blood Carriers**   17, 30, 37, 46
   β Globulins (transferrin), GTF, albumins, globulins

3. **Half-Life of Element in Blood**   8, 17, 37, 46
   Few days

4. **Target (Initial) Sites**   17, 30, 37, 46
   Tissues—Heart, pancreas, lungs, brain, liver, bones, spleen, testes, epididymis
   Cells—Nuclei > cytosol > mitochondria, microsomes

5. **Storage**   17, 30, 37, 46
   Sites—Bones, spleen, testes, epididymis, liver (small amounts)
   Forms—Amino acid/niacin complexes, unknown forms

6. **Homeostatic Mechanisms**   17, 30, 37, 46, 42
   Relative efficiency in element retention—1-3% (?)
   Kidney participation—No evidence of controls
   Intestinal participation—Small amount
   Liver (bile) participation—Small amount

7. **Specific Functions (via Cofactors/Metalloenzymes/Metalloproteins/Ions)**
       17, 21, 25, 30, 37, 46
   Molecular level
       Enzyme activator, component of GTF
       Ligand to cell membrane receptors
   Cellular level
       Potentiates insulin in glucose and amino acid transport
       Involved in protein synthesis (via nucleic acids) (?)
       Increases swelling of mitochondria
       Participates in glucose, lipid, nucleic acid metabolism
   Organismal level (lab animals)
       Decreases serum cholesterol
       Improves growth and longevity
       Improves glucose tolerance
       Maintenance (see physiological functions)

8. Metalloenzymes, Cofactors, Metalloproteins 8, 10, 11, 15, 25, 30, 35, 37, 46

System Types	Organ	Metalloenzyme/Protein	Co-factors	System Function
Nonspecific enzyme	Liver	Phosphoglucomutase	Cr, Mg	Glucose metabolism

9. Excretion 21, 30, 37, 39, 42, 46
Chemical forms—Volatile compounds, inorganic, chelates
Organs
  Kidney (urine)—80%
  Intestine (feces) ⎱
  Liver (bile, intestine) ⎰ 20%
  Skin—Small amounts (hair)
  Other—Small amounts (sweat)

MISCELLANEOUS

1. Relationship to Other Minerals 27, 30, 37, 46, 53
  Zn ⎫
  V ⎬ Absorption inhibitors or competitors
  Mn ⎪
  Fe ⎭
  Mg—Synergist with Cr in enzyme action
  Zn—Synergist with insulin and Cr

2. Relationship to Vitamins 27, 36, 37, 46, 53
  Niacin—Part of GTF
  B_6—Synergist with Zn and Cr
  Pantothenic acid—Synergist in stress response

3. Relationship to Hormones 37, 46, 53
  Insulin—Synergist to GTF
  Glucagon—Antagonist to insulin and GTF
  Cortisol—antagonism to insulin and GTF

4. Unusual Features 21, 30, 36, 37, 46, 50, 53
  Lung accumulates Cr in nonmetabolic form
  Males more affected by deficiency of Cr than females
  High content of Cr in RNA

Tissue uptake of Cr decreases with age
Loss of Cr gradually with age (no other trace metal)
Organic Cr in egg yolk mostly unavailable
Hexavalent Cr carcinogenic, not biologically active
Trivalent Cr biologically active, not carcinogenic

5. **Possible Relationship of Deficiency Symptoms to Metabolic Action**   21, 30
    27, 36, 37, 46, 53
    Increased mortality—Impairment of protein synthesis (via insulin)
    Increased atherosclerosis and blood cholesterol—Mild diabetes, loss of
        insulin and Cr synergism
    Inpaired glucose tolerance—Loss of synergism of Cr with Zn and insulin
    Impaired stress response—Impairment of glucose metabolism with loss of GTF
    Corneal opacity—Cr^{3+} probably involved since cornea concentrates Cr
    Glycosuria, Hyperglycemia—Loss of synergism of Cr with insulin

Chapter 11. Manganese (Mn)

Manganese is found in all plants and animals. The biologically active form is Mn^{3+} (converted from Mn^{2+}), a basic ion, not involved in electron exchange reaction. It is a potential carcinogen. No Mn deficiency is known in man, although it is essential for many animals. Presumably it will be demonstrated essential for man in the future.

Manganese is poorly absorbed in the inorganic form as Mn^{2+}, but in the chelate form as Mn glycinate or gluconate it is very well absorbed. It is not known if a special vitamin-like form of Mn exists similar to that of Cr. In the oxidized form (MnO_4^-) it is very toxic, whereas the Mn^{2+} form is relatively nontoxic. Like Cr, it improves glucose tolerance; but in contrast to Cr, it seems to increase serum cholesterol. Manganese is conserved by homeostasis and is not lost with age as Cr is. The daily intake is estimated to be much larger than that of Cr, about 3800 μg. Similarly to Cr, Mn combines with RNA in the nucleus with an unknown function. Concentrated sources of Mn include tea, nuts, grains, bran, wheat germ, corn, and parsley.

There is no evidence that manganese supplements are needed in the average human diet, over and above the usual sources of intake.

GENERAL INFORMATION

1. **Dietary and Medicinal Forms**   37, 49, 53, 54
   Element—Manganese metal; not used medicinally
   Inorganic salts—Manganous sulfate, acetate
   Metallovitamin—Unknown
   Chelated forms—Manganous gluconate, glycinate, citrate

2. History of Biological Significance   8, 21, 37, 50, 46
1931—Kemmerer et al.: first evidence of Mn requirement (rats, mice)
1936—Wilgus et al.: Mn prevents perosis in chickens
1958—Cotzias: first inference of human need for Mn
1959—Bertinchamps: transmanganin is plasma protein carrier for Mn
1961—Curren and Azarnoff: Mn stimulates cholesterol synthesis in rat liver
1962—Leach and Munster: Mn active in bone formation in chicks
1968—Everson and Shrader: glucose intolerance caused by Mn deficiency
    (guinea pig)
1973—Doisy: first report of Mn deficiency in man

3. Physiological (Blood) Forms   17, 21, 37, 46
Transmanganin, transferrin, α_2 macroglobulin, corticoid complexes

4. Synergistic Agents   30, 37, 39, 46
Metabolic—Vitamin K, choline, Zn
Absorption—Ethanol

5. Antagonistic Agents   30, 37, 39, 46
Metabolic—Mg, Cu, V, Fe
Absorption—Ca, PO_4, Fe, Co, soy protein

**6. Possible or Demonstrated Physiological Functions (Maintenance of Systems/
    Components)**   17, 21, 30, 37, 46
Circulatory—Heart cell membranes (structure)
Excretory—Kidney cell membranes (structure)
Respiratory—Cellular O_2 uptake (mice)
Digestive—Food absorption, pancreatic cell membranes, liver cell membranes
    maintenance (guinea pig)
Nervous—Neurotransmitter synthesis
Special sensory—Conjunctival pigmentation, vestibular functions
Reproductive—Fertility, gonadal homeostatis (rabbit)
Endocrine—T4, acetylcholine, insulin, catecholamine synthesis (guinea pig)
Blood—↑ serum cholesterol
Muscular
    Glucose uptake
    Muscle glycogen (via insulin) } homeostasis
    Neuromuscular transmission
Skeletal—Mucopolysaccharide synthesis; chondrogenesis (chicks)
Integument—Coat color (mice); skin, connective tissues
Protective/Immune—Blood clotting mechanisms homeostasis
Metabolic—Lipid and CHO metabolism; glucose tolerance improved; muco-
    polysaccharide synthesis

Detoxification—Peroxides (superoxide dismutase)
Growth—+ ?
Health—+ ?
Longevity—+ ?

7. **Body Content** 21, 42, 46
mg/70 kg = 12-20; μg/g = 0.17.030

8. **Relative Organ Concentrations** 8, 21, 42, 46
Bone > pituitary, mammary gland > liver > pancreas > kidney > brain, lung
> prostate, spleen, heart > muscle

9. **Deficiencies** 21, 46, 30, 36, 37
Man—Glucose intolerance
Rats/Mice—Neonatal ataxia
Birds—Perosis, neonatal ataxia, parrot beak
Guinea pigs—Pancreatic hypoplasia

10. **Excess Conditions, Disorders** 21, 37, 30, 36, 38, 46, 39
Mice—Pallid mice congenital ataxia (genetic defects)
Man—Manganism, metal fume fever, locura manganica

11. **Essentiality** 1, 17, 38, 37, 46
Man—Vital (?); not clearly demonstrated
Other species—All: algae, fungi, spermatophytes; some: vertebrates, inverte-
brates, insects, protozoans

12. **Major Commercial Uses (Biological Interface)** 6, 22, 30, 54
Element—Alloys [ferromanganese (Fe, Mn), Mn bronze (Cu, Mn), manganin
(Cu, Mn, Ni), silicomanganese (Si, Mn)]
Compounds—Fertilizers, feeds, dyes, glazes, disinfectants, driers, pigments,
batteries, antiknock compounds (MMT, MCT), oxidizers

13. **Medicinal Applications** 27, 30, 37, 54
Nutritional supplement ($MnSO_4$, Mn glycinate, Mn gluconate)
Hematinic ($MnCO_3$)

14. **Hazards and Toxicity (Toxicity: $MnO_4^- > Mn^{2+} > Mn^{3+}$) (Varies with Species)**
19, 30, 37, 39, 46, 41, 54
Element (least toxic of essential trace minerals)
Inhalation—Fume metal fever: fatigue, anorexia, impotence, anemia, weakness, emotional disturbance, spastic gait, paralysis
Topical—Manganism: psychic and neurological disorders, nephritis, pneu-
monia, dyspnea, fever, lung hemorrhage, liver cirrhosis, muscle fatigue,
leukopenia, monocytosis, anemia, impotence

Compounds—Moderately toxic (neurotoxin)
  Inhalation—Similar to above
  Topical—Skin irritation from manganates, permanganates
  Oral toxicity—See nutrition section, dietary excess
Carcinogenicity/Mutagenicity = ±/+

DISTRIBUTION AND SOURCES

1. **Occurrence and Environmental Concentrations (μg/g)**   3, 4, 6, 42, 29, 47
  Relative terrestrial abundance—#12
  Chief minerals—Rhodomite (Mn silicate), braunite (Mn_2O_3), rhodochrosite
    ($MnCO_3$), Mn nodules (Mn, Fe, Ni, Co, Fe oxides)
  Earth's crust—0.3 (average)
  Rocks—50-1100 (sandstones-limestone)
  Soils—850 (average)
  Freshwater—0.012 (average)
  Seawater — 0.001-0.002

2. **Organismal Concentrations (μg/g)**   4, 42, 46, 47
  Plants—Marine: 53 (average); land: 630 (average)
  Animals—Marine: 1-60; land: 0.2 (average)
  Man—0.2 (average)
  Special concentrators—Diatoms, sponges, molluscs, some plants
  Indicators—Plants: intravenal chlorosis, in Mn deficiency

3. **Dietary Sources (Variability due to Environment)**   5, 12, 8, 26, 42, 42a,
    36, 46, 52
  High (mg/100 g) 1.0-10.0
    Meat/Organs—Snails
    Nuts/Seeds—Sunflower seeds, coconuts, peanuts, pecans, walnuts, chest-
      nuts, hazelnuts, almonds, brazils
    Fruits—Blueberries, olives, avocados
    Vegetables—Corn germ, corn, parsley
    Grains—Wheat, wheat germ and bran, rice, barley, oats, oat bran, buck-
      wheat, rye
    Miscellaneous—Kelp, cloves, tea
  Medium (mg/100 g) 0.10-1.00
    Seafood—Clams
    Meat/Organs—Liver (beef, pork)

Fruits—Peach, rhubarb, pineapples, bananas, (black-, cran-, straw-, rasp-) berries

Vegetables—Pumpkin, peas, eggplant, string beans, okra, cauliflower, cassava, cabbage, brussels sprouts, asparagus, lima benas, beets, kale, yams, potatoes, onions, carrots, lettuce, spinach, broccoli, green peppers, watercress

Miscellaneous—Yeast, bone meal, molasses, raw sugar, sugar cane

Low (mg/100 g) 0-0.10

Seafood—Shrimp, whitefish, cod, halibut, herring, haddock, halibut, oysters, mackerel

Meat/Organs—Eggs, beef, chicken, sheep, pork

Fruits—Watermelons, pears, oranges, grapefruit, tangerines, lemons, grapes, apricots, cherries, cantaloupes, apples, prunes, plums, honeydew

Vegetables—Tomatoes, cucumbers, radishes

Dairy products—Cheese (American, cottage, swiss), milk, butter

Miscellaneous—Corn oil, lard

CHEMISTRY

1. **Atomic Properties (Element)**   6, 7, 9, 30, 49

   Periodic table group no.—VIIB, period 4

   Category of element—Transition, metal

   Atomic weight—54.94

   Atomic number—25

   Atomic radius (metallic)—1.333 Å, 1.365 Å

   Electron shells—2, 8, 13, 2

   Orbital electrons—$3s^2$, $3p^6$, $3d^5$, $4s^2$

   Natural isotopes—Mn^{55} (100%)

   Long-lived radioactive isotopes—Mn^{53} (2×10^6 yr), Mn^{54} (303 days), Mn^{52} (5.7 days), Mn^{56} (2.6 hr)

2. **Ionic Properties (Biological Forms)**   6, 7, 9, 30, 49

   Oxidation states (valences)—Mn^{2+}, Mn^{3+} (Mn^{4+}, Mn^{6+}, Mn^{7+})

   Ionic radius (Å)—Mn^{2+} : 0.83; Mn^{3+} : 0.52

   Oxidation potentials—$MN^0 \rightarrow Mn^{2+}$ (1.18 v); $Mn^{2+} \rightarrow Mn^{3+}$ (−1.51 v)

   Reducing/Oxidizing forms—Mn^{2+}/(Mn^{5+}, Mn^{7+})

   Unstable in aqueous solutions—Mn^{3+}

3. **Molecular Properties (Biological Forms)**   6, 7, 9, 16, 25, 30, 43, 49
   Covalent radius (Å)—Mn^{2+} (1.6), Mn^{3+} (?)
   Coordination numbers—Mn^{2+} (4), Mn^{3+} (6)
   Stereochemistry—Mn^{2+} (square, octahedral), Mn^{3+} (octahedral)
   Electron transfer compounds—No data
   Typical molecular complexes—$[Mn(H_2O)_4]^{2+}$, $[Mn(H_2O)_6]^{2+}$, $[Mn(C_2O_4)_3]^{3-}$,
   $[Mn(SCN)_6]^{4-}$

4. **Analytical Methods**   3, 30, 31, 40, 55, 47
   Physical—Atomic absorption, neutron activation
   Chemical—Spectrophotometric (pyridylazonaphthol)
   Hair/Nail analysis—Feasible, widely used
   Comments—Lack of reference standards for comparison of methods gives un-
   certainty

5. **Chemical Properties of Compounds**   6, 7, 9, 49, 54
   See Table 11.1

MEDICINAL AND NUTRITIONAL ROLE

1. **Units of Measurement**
   Weight—μg (microgram); 1 mg (milligram) = 1000 μg = 0.001 g
   Concentration—ppm (parts per million) = $\mu g/g$; $\mu g\%$ = $\mu g/100$ ml

2. **Human Body Fluid Levels (Normal) ($\mu g/100$ ml)**   1, 2, 37, 46
   Blood—1.2-2.6 (1.9)
   Plasma/Serum—1.6-3.2 (2.4)
   Urine—0.47-6.5 (3.5)
   Serum levels may be affected by corticoids

3. **Human Tissue Levels ($\mu g/g$)**   4, 8, 24, 46, 47
   Hair—0.14-0.45
   Bone—0.30
   Muscle—0.09
   Liver—1.68
   Nerve—0.34

4. **Important Dietary Levels (mg/day)**   27, 30, 37, 39, 46
   Average dietary intake—2.5-7.0
   Deficiency limits—<0.71
   Toxic limit—>1000

Table 11.1.   Properties of Manganese Compounds

Mn = 2 + (manganic)	REACTIONS			SOLUBILITY			
	Heat °C	Air	Water	g/100 cc H$_2$O	Alc.	Eth.	Acid
Mn sulfate, MnSO$_4$ · 4H$_2$O	−4 H$_2$O 400°	efflor.	alk.	105.3⁰	I	NA	NA
Mn acetate Mn(CH$_3$COO)$_2$	NA	NA	NA	S	S	NA	NA

Mn = 2 + (manganic)	Density	MW hyd./anh.	MP °C	XL Form	Color XL/Powd.	Appearance Commercial Form	% Element h./anh.
Mn sulfate, MnSO$_4$ · 4H$_2$O	2.10	223.1/151.0	700°	rhomb. monocl.	pink/?	C	24.6/36.4
Mn acetate Mn(CH$_3$COO)$_2$	1.74	−/173.0	NA	NA	br./?	C	−/31.8

Abbreviations: br = brown; others as in earlier tables.

5. **Estimated Human Daily Balance (average American diet, 70 kg ♂, 30 yr)   27, 30, 42, 46**
   Average intake—3800 μg/day (3735 food, 64 water, 1 air)
   Average output—3800 μg/day (3731 feces, 30 urine, 39 sweat)
   Net gain/loss—Balance (normally)

6. **Indications for Supplementation of Above Diet   27, 30, 42, 46**
   Healthy normal—None
   Special conditions—None reported

7. **Factors Affecting Availability from Diet   17, 27, 37, 46**
   Decreased
        See absorption section, inhibitors
        Refining of foods, e.g., wheat
        Alkaline soils
   Increased
        See absorption section, synergizers
        Fe deficiency
        Acid soils
        Organic forms of Fe
        Water content

8. **Deficiency Symptoms   21, 37, 30, 36, 46**
   Man—Glucose intolerance
   Animals—Impaired growth, skeletal abnormalities, impaired reproduction, ataxia of newborn, defects of lipid and CHO metabolism

9. **Effects of Dietary Excess (Salts or Concentrates)   19, 33, 36, 39, 46**
   Acute—Animals: retarded growth; Ca loss in feces; severe rickets; anorexia; impotency; muscle fatigue
   Chronic—Humans: manganism (similar to Parkinson's disease); nephritis; cirrhosis (liver); anorexia; muscle fatigue, rigidity; impotency; leukopenia; anemia; monocytosis; tremors; hallucinations; insomnia; slurred speech; mental confusion

METABOLIC ROLE

1. **Intestinal Absorption   17, 30, 37, 39, 46**
   Chemical forms—Mn^{2+}, Mn^{3+} salts, chelates
        Preferred valence—Mn^{3+}
        Poorly absorbed—Mn^{2+} (converted to Mn^{3+})
        Well absorbed—Chelated forms

Sites—Small intestine
Efficiency—3-4%
Active transport—None reported
Synergizers—Ethanol
Antagonists
    Competitors—Fe, Co
    Sequestrants—PO_4, SO_4, protein

2. **Blood Carriers**   17, 30, 37, 46
    Transmanganin, transferrin, α_2 macroglobulin, corticoid complexes

3. **Half-Life of Element in Blood**   8, 17, 37, 46
    <1 hr

4. **Target (Initial) Sites**   17, 30, 37, 46
    Tissues—Liver, pancreas, kidney, intestine
    Cells—Mitochondia, nuclei

5. **Storage**   17, 30, 37, 46
    Sites—Liver, bone marrow
    Forms—Porphyrin complex (RBCs), liver mitochondrial Mn (enzymes, metal-
    ' loproteins)

6. **Homeostatic Mechanisms**   17, 30, 37, 42, 46
    Relative efficiency in element retention—80-100%
    Kidney participation—Small
    Intestinal participation—Reabsorption, some excretion via pancreas, con-
        trolled excretion in bile
    Liver (bile participation—enterohepatic circulation via bile

7. **Specific Functions (via Cofactors/Metalloenzymes/Metalloproteins/Ions)**
    17, 21, 25, 30, 37, 46
    Molecular level
        Enzyme activator or cofactor
        Component of enzymes—Structural or binding site
    Cellular level
        Mucopolysaccharide synthesis (chondroitin-SO_4)
        Mitochondrial integrity (membranes)
        Cholesterol synthesis
        RNA synthesis (DNA polymerase)
        Lipotropic agent—Choline metabolism
        Catecholamine synthesis

Organismal level
    See physiological functions
    Maintains: cartilage, gonads, pancreas, liver functions; endocrine func-
        tions; reproductive, protective functions
    Improves: growth, health, longevity   )

8. Metalloenzymes, Cofactors, Metalloproteins   8, 10, 25, 30, 37, 35, 46

System Types	Organ	Metalloenzyme/Protein	Co-factors	System Function
Metallo-enzyme	Liver (chick) (milk)	Pyruvate carboxylase (Mn^{2+})	biotin	CHO (oxaloacetate) metabolism
	Liver (chick)	Superoxide dismutase (Mn^{2+})	Cu, Fe, Zn	Destruction of superoxides
Metallo-protein	Liver (bird)	Avimanganin (Mn^{3+})	—	Storage (?)
	Liver (milk)	Farnesyl pyrophosphate synthetase—Mn^{2+}	—	Cholesterol synthesis
Mn-Specific enzyme	Mammary gland	Glycosyl transferase—Mn^{2+}	—	Glucose utilization
Nonspecific enzyme	Various	Hydrolases, kinases, trans-ferases, peptidases, arginase, phosphatases, DNA polymerase	Mn	Degradative and biosynthetic

9. Excretion   21, 30, 39, 37, 42, 46
Chemical forms—Bile compounds, fecal complexes
Organs
    Kidney (urine)—ca. 1% (increased by corticoids)
    Intestine (feces)   ⎫
    Liver (bile, intestine) ⎬ 98%
                          ⎭
    Skin (sweat)—ca. 1%

MISCELLANEOUS

1. Relationship to Other Minerals   27, 30, 37, 46
Mg—Can substitute for Mn as cofactor, certain enzymes
Cr—Improves glucose tolerance (similar to Mn)
Cu ⎫
Zn ⎬ Co-metals in superoxide dismutases
Fe ⎭

Fe, Cu, V, Mg—Metabolic antagonists
Zn—Metabolic synergist
Ca, PO_4, Fe, Co—Absorption antagonists

2. **Relationship to Vitamins**   27, 36, 37, 46
K—Synergist in blood clotting
$\left.\begin{array}{c} C \\ B_1 \end{array}\right\}$ Synergists in acetylcholine synthesis
Biotin—Cofactor for pyruvate carboxylase
Choline—Synergist in lipotropic action

3. **Relationship to Hormones**   37, 46, 51
Cortisol—Mn ligand found in tissues (mice)
Estrogens—Increase Mn serum levels (chicks)
Insulin—Mn involved in pancreatic homeostasis
T4—Mn involved in synthesis
Norepinephrine, epinephrine—Catecholamine synthesis involvement
L-Dopa—Relieves Mn toxicity, causes accumulation of Mn in liver

4. **Unusual Features**   37, 30, 36, 50, 46
Mn reported used in treatment of schizophrenia
Similarity observed between Mn poisoning and Parkinson's disease symptoms
Rheumatoid arthritis has increased Mn in RBC
RBCs have Mn in porphyrin complex
Excess Mn acts as neurotoxin
Some bacteria use Mn in respiration
Birds require more Mn than mammals
Some metalloenzymes have Mn^{3+}; others have Mn^{2+}

5. **Possible Relationship of Deficiency Symptoms to Metabolic Action**   27, 30, 36, 37, 46
$\left.\begin{array}{l} \text{Skeletal abnormalities} \\ \text{Impaired growth} \end{array}\right\}$ Poor cartilage formation
Impaired reproduction—Cholesterol synthesis, sex hormone synthesis defective
Ataxia of newborn—Myelin synthesis, mucopolysaccharide synthesis
Lipid metabolic defects—Lipotropic action, cholesterol synthesis defective
CHO metabolic defects—Maintenance of pancreas and insulin defective

Chapter 12. Iodine (I)

Iodine is found in all plants and animals, but plants do not seem to require it. Although I is essential for normal growth, development, and life span in humans, life can continue for a while without it. Its ultimate mode of molecular action is still unknown although its effects are known on an organismic scale. Iodine is required only as the thyroid hormones (T3, T4); as the iodide ion it has very little biological activity until it is transformed by the thyroid into T3 and T4. The thyroid hormone is thus in effect the vitamin form of iodine synthesized in the body. Its chief effects as T4 are the stimulation of protein, fat, and CHO metabolism and growth and development of the body, and it works very closely with the growth hormone and insulin. It is absorbed extremely efficiently as iodide or T4.

Iodine is found plentifully in foods, air, and water near the seashore, but is likely to be lacking in inland geographical areas, where it can be obtained in iodized salt and "imported" seafoods. The average American diet can provide sufficient iodine to compensate for the body losses. Iodine has some toxicity in large doses.

There is no evidence available to justify supplementation of a normal American diet with I other than in the geographical cases mentioned above and in cases of special individual needs (e.g., hypothyroidism).

GENERAL INFORMATION

1. **Dietary and Medicinal Forms**   37, 49, 53, 54
   Element—Iodine, nonmetal; sometimes used medicinally
   Inorganic salts—Iodide: sodium cuprous and potassium iodate: sodium and
      potassium
   Mineralovitamin—Thyroxin (T4), triodothyronine (T3) (also are hormones)
   Organic forms—T4, T3, T2, iodinated proteins
   Medicinal forms—Over 1000 known

2. **History of Biological Significance**   8, 21, 37, 46, 50, 53
   1811—Courtois: discovered I in seaweed
   1830—Prevost: noted association of goiter and low I in water supply
   1850—Chatin: discovered human I requirement
   1895—Baumann: discovered organic I in thyroid gland
   1918—Kimball and Marine: reduced goiter with dietary I
   1919—Kendall and Osterberg: isolated thyroxine (T4); contains I
   1928—Chesney: discovered goitrogens in food
   1948—Wolff and Chaikoff: found synthesis of T4 by thyroid stopped by high
      dietary I
   1952—Gross and Pitt-Rivers: demonstrated triiodothyronine (T3) in thyroid
   1964—Wayne et al.: established minimum safe dose for I (dietary)

3. **Physiological (Blood) Forms**   17, 21, 37, 46, 50, 53
   Iodide (I⁻), T4, T3, plasma protein complexes (PBI), (prealbumin, albumin,
      and T4-binding globulin)

4. **Synergistic Agents**   30, 35, 37, 39, 46
   Metabolic—(as T4, T3) progesterone, MSH, STH, prolactin, oxytocin, vaso-
      pressin, cortisol, histamine, serotonin, insulin, epinephrine, norepineph-
      rine
   Absorption—Amino acids

5. **Antagonistic Agents**   30, 35, 37, 39, 46
   Metabolic—*T4 action* (Mg^{2+}, ouabain, PTH); *T4 synthesis:* thiouracil, resorci-
      nol, Co^{2+}, thiocyanates, thioureas, glucosinolates
   Absorption—As *iodide* (cyanide, perchlorates, nitrates, thiocyanates, reducing
      agents); as *organic I* (Hb, liver, soybean and cottonseed meal)

6. **Physiological Functions (Maintenance of Systems/Components)**   17, 21, 30,
      37, 46, 50
   [via T4 (thyroxine) except where noted]
   Circulatory—↑ hematopoiesis, calorigenic on heart
   Excretory—Calorigenic on kidneys; salt balance maintenance

Respiratory—↑ BMR and O_2 consumption

Digestive—(I) ↑ salivary gland secretion; ↑ motility and absorption of gastro-intestinal tract

Nervous—Development and sensitization of nervous system

Special sensory—Development of visual and sound organs

Reproductive—Fertility, lactation, gametogenesis, maturation of organs maintenance

Endocrine—Synergizes STH, component of T3, T4 (hormones); excess I inhibits T4 secretion

Blood—↓ cholesterol, ↓ blood lipids

Muscular—Increased mitochondrial activity in muscle; calorigenic action

Skeletal—Bone growth (with STH)

Integument—Skin homeostasis

Immune—Inflammatory response, mast cells immunoglobulin (M) homeo-stasis

Metabolic—Calorigenesis; CHO, lipid, protein metabolism, ↑ BMR

Detoxification—Liver homeostasis; Pb + Hg removal

Growth—+

Health—+

Longevity—+

7. **Body Content**   8, 12, 21, 35, 42, 46
mg/70 kg = 12-20; μg/g = 0.17-0.30

8. **Relative Organ Concentrations (T4)**   12, 21, 42, 46
Thyroid > salivary, stomach, mammary gland, pituitary, ovary > hair > liver > lung > kidney > lymph nodes > testis, brain > muscle

9. **Deficiencies**   21, 30, 36, 37, 46
Man: cretinism, myxedema, goiter (simple and exophthalmic), Hashimoto's disease, Gull's disease, hypothyroidism

10. **Excess and Other Conditions**   21, 30, 36, 37, 39, 38, 46
Man: Grave's disease, thyrotoxicosis, thyroiditis, goiter (excess), hyper-thyroidism, hypersensitivity, idiosyncratic reactions

11. **Essentiality (as T4)**   1, 17, 37, 38, 46
Man—Vital, good health, normal life span
Other species—All vertebrates, no invertebrates

12. **Major Commercial Uses (Biological Interface)**   6, 22, 30, 54
Element—Germicides, antiseptics, catalysts, reagent, lubricants
Compounds—Feeds, table salt additive, photo emulsions, sanitizers (iodo-phors), dyes (erythrosin)

13. **Medicinal Applications**   18, 27, 30, 37, 53, 54
    Element—Topical anti-infective, counterirritant, absorptive aid, antihypo-
        thyroid
    Salts—Expectorant, iodine supplement, antihypothyroid
    Veterinary uses—Pb/Hg poisoning, bursal enlargements, actinobacillosis,
        actinomycosis

14. **Hazards and Toxicity**   19, 30, 37, 39, 41, 46
    Element
        Inhalation—Irritation of bronchial membranes, pulmonary edema
        Skin—Intense irritant
    Compounds
        Inhalation—Pulmonary edema, asthma, bronchospasm, hypotension,
            nausea, vomiting, diarrhea
        Skin—Irritation
        Oral toxicity—See nutrition section, dietary excess
    Carcinogenicity/Mutagenicity = −/− (anticarcinogenic)

DISTRIBUTION AND SOURCES

1. **Occurrence and Environmental Concentrations** (μg/g)   3, 4, 6, 29, 42, 47
    Relative terrestrial abundance—#63
    Chief minerals—saltpeter (sodium iodate and periodate)
    Geographical localization—Concentrated near seacoasts
    Earth's crust—0.3 μg/g
    Rocks—0.5-2.2 (igneous-shales)
    Soils—5.0
    Freshwater—0.002
    Seawater—0.06

2. **Organismal Concentrations** (μg/g)   4, 42, 46, 47
    Plants—Marine: 30-1500; land: 0.42
    Animals—Marine: 1-150; land: 0.43
    Man—0.20
    Special concentrators—Brown algae, diatoms, some sponges, corals, tunicates

3. **Dietary Sources (Variability due to Environment)**   8, 26, 36, 42, 46, 52
    High (mg/100 g) 30-500
        Seafood—Cod, oysters, clams, haddock, lobster, shrimp, flounder, hali-
            but, herring
        Nuts/Seeds—Sunflower seeds

Miscellaneous—Kelp, Irish moss, cod-liver oil, mushrooms
Medium (mg/100 g) 10-50
 Seafood—Eel, catfish, sea bass, sardines, tuna, mackerel, abalone, crab,
  sea trout, salmon, perch, sole, bluefish
 Meat/Organs—Eggs, beef liver
 Nuts/Seeds—Peanuts
 Fruits—Pineapple
 Vegetables—Spinach, turnip greens, chard, pickles, asparagus
 Dairy products—Cheddar cheese
 Miscellaneous—Chocolate, bone meal, iodized salt, mayonnaise
Low (mg/100 g) 1-10
 Seafood—Carp, river bass, lake trout, river perch
 Nuts/Seeds—Walnuts, almonds, cashews
 Grains—Rice, wheat, barley, oats, rye, wheat germ
 Fruits—Raisins, pears, apples, cranberries, bananas, cantaloupe, grapefruit,
  lemons, peaches
 Vegetables—Soybeans, carrots, turnips, potatoes, cabbage, peas, beans,
  tomatoes, green peppers, corn, squash, sweet potatoes, pumpkin,
  cauliflower, beets, onions, cucumber, lettuce, avocados, broccoli,
  collards, mustard greens
 Dairy products—Milk, cheese (cheddar, cottage), butter
 Miscellaneous—Honey, margarine, molasses

CHEMISTRY

1. **Atomic Properties (Element)**   6, 7, 9, 30, 49
 Periodic table group no.—VII-A, period 5
 Category of element—Nonmetal, halogen
 Atomic weight—53
 Atomic number—126.90
 Atomic radius (metallic)—Nonmetal
 Electron shells—2, 8, 18, 18, 7
 Orbital electrons—$4s^2$, $4p^6$, $4d^{10}$, $5s^2$, $5p^5$
 Natural isotopes—I^{127} (100%)
 Long-lived radioactive isotopes—I^{124} (4.2 days), I^{125} (60 days), I^{126} (13 days),
  I^{129} (1.7 × 10^7 yr), I^{131} (8.1 days)

2. **Ionic Properties (Biological Forms)**   6, 7, 9, 30, 49
   Oxidation states (valences)—+ (1, 3, 5, 7), −1
   Ionic radius (Å)—2.16-2.22
   Oxidation potentials—$I^- \rightarrow I^0$ (−0.535 v); $I^0 \rightarrow I^{5+}$ (−1.195 v)

3. **Molecular Properties (Biological Forms)**   6, 7, 9, 16, 25, 30, 43, 49
   Covalent radius (Å)—1.33-1.36
   Coordination numbers—1, 2
   Stereochemistry—1, linear; 2, planar
   Electron transfer compounds—I_2NCS^-
   Typical molecular complexes—$I_2O_9^{4-}$, IO_4^{2-}, IO_3^{--}, I_3^-, $[(C_6H_5)_2I]^+$, $[HgI_4]^{2-}$

4. **Analytical Methods**   3, 30, 31, 40, 47, 55
   Physical—Atomic absorption, X-ray fluorescence, mass spectrometry
   Chemical—Spectrophotometric: starch-iodine
   Hair/Nail analysis—High I in hair
   Comments—Problems due to volatility of sample, and I; variability due to
   lack of standards

5. **Chemical Properties of Compounds**   6, 7, 9, 49, 54
   See Table 12.1

MEDICINAL AND NUTRITIONAL ROLE

1. **Units of Measurement**
   Weight—μg (microgram); 1 mg (milligram) = 1000 μg
   Concentration—ppm (parts per million) = μg/g; μg% = μg/100 ml

2. **Human Body Fluid Levels (Normal) (μg/100 ml)**   1, 2, 12, 37, 46
   Blood—2.5-16.9 (9.7)
   Plasma/Serum—5.9-7.7 (7.0)
   Urine—0.47-32.7 (16.6)

3. **Human Tissue Levels (μg/g)**   4, 8, 24, 46, 47
   Hair—0.45-1.30
   Bone—0.27
   Liver—0.20
   Muscle—0.01
   Nerve—0.02

Table 12.1. Properties of Iodine Compounds

| | REACTIONS | | | SOLUBILITY | | | | | | | | | Appearance | |
	Heat °C	Air	Water	g/100 cc H_2O	Alc.	Eth.	Acid	Density	MW hyd./anh.	MP °C	XL Form	Color XL/Powd.	Commercial Form	% Element h./anh.
Na iodide, NaI	BP 1304°	deliq.	alk. pH 8-9	184^{25}	S	NA	NA	3.67	–/149.9	651°	cubic	col./wh.	C, G	–/84.7
K iodide, KI	BP 1330°	deliq.	alk. pH 7-9	144^{20}	S	SS	NA	3.12	–/166.0	686°	cubic hex.	col./wh.	C, G, P	–/76.5
K iodate, KIO_3	d. > 100°	NA	NA	8.5^{20}	I	NA	NA	3.89	–/214.0	560°	monocl.	col./wh.	C, P	–/18.3

4. **Important Dietary Levels (μg/day)**   5, 21, 27, 30, 37, 39
   Recommended dietary allowance—130 (δ); 100 ($\female$)
   Deficiency limits—50-75
   Toxic limit—1000

5. **Estimated Human Daily Balance (average American diet, 70 kg δ, 30 yr)**   27,
   30, 42, 46
   Average intake—205 μg/day (195 food, 5 water, 5 air)   } seashore
   Average output—205 μg/day (175 urine, 20 feces, 6 sweat, 2 hair) } proximity
   Net gain/loss—Balanced (assuming seashore proximity)

6. **Indications for Supplementation of Above Diet**   5, 27, 30, 42, 46
   Healthy normal—In inland areas, goiter belts
   Special conditions—Presence of I deficiency

7. **Factors Affecting Availability from Diet**   17, 21, 27, 37, 46, 53
   Decreased
      Inland areas (water, air, local foods)
      Cooking foods
      Goitrogens in foods
      Increased fecal output
      See absorption, antagonists
   Increased
      Proximity to seashore
      Seafood diet
      Iodized salt
      Iodophors in cleaning
      Food additives—Kelp, alginates, etc.
      See absorption, synergizers

8. **Deficiency Symptoms**   21, 30, 36, 37, 46
   Man: Tumors of pituitary, decreased BMR, accumulation of mucoprotein,
      increase in blood lipids and cholesterol, increase in liver gluconeogenesis,
      extracellular retention of NaCl and H_2O

9. **Effects of Dietary Excess of Supplements, Salts or Concentrates**   19, 33, 36,
   39, 46
   Acute—Gastrointestinal irritation, angioedema, cutaneous hemorrhage,
      hypersensitivity, serum sickness
   Chronic—(Iodism) brassy taste, burning sensation of mouth and throat,
      head-cold symptoms, pulmonary edema, inflammation of oral cavity,
      skin lesions, gastric irritation, diarrhea

METABOLIC ROLE

1. **Intestinal Absorption**   17, 30, 35, 37, 39, 46
   Chemical forms—Iodide, iodinated amino acids
      Preferred valence——1
      Poorly absorbed—Organic (except iodinated amino acids—convert to iodide)
      Well absorbed—Iodide, iodinated amino acids
   Sites—Gastrointestinal tract
   Efficiency—100%
   Active transport—Yes
   Synergizers—Amino acids
   Antagonists—Iodide: NO_3^-, SCN^-, CN^-, ClO_4^-, reducing agents; iodinated amino acids: Hb, liver, soybean and cottonseed meal

2. **Blood Carriers**   17, 30, 37, 46
   Plasma protein complexes: prealbumin, albumin, acid glycoprotein and T4-binding globulin

3. **Half-Life of Element in Blood**   8, 17, 37, 46
   6-7 hr (rat)

4. **Target (Initial) Sites**   17, 30, 37, 46
   Tissues—Thyroid, salivary and mammary gland, stomach, others
   Cells—Cytosol, mitochondria

5. **Storage**   17, 30, 37, 46
   Sites—Thyroid; small amounts (salivary, mammary, gastric)
   Forms—Thyroglobulin (colloid)

6. **Homeostatic Mechanisms**   17, 30, 37, 42, 46
   Relative efficiency in element retention—30-50% est.
   Kidney participation (chief excretory organ)—Passive reabsorption
   Intestinal participation—Recycling (active transport)
   Liver (bile) participation—Enterohepatic circulation

7. **Specific Functions (via Cofactors/Metalloenzymes/Mineraloproteins/Ions)**
      17, 21, 25, 30, 37, 46, 58
   Molecular level (as T4)
      Regulates redox potential
      Component of T4, T3
      Enzyme activator
      Hormone—Regulator of metabolism

Uncoupler of oxidative phosphorylation
Metal chelator
Cellular level (as T4, via cyclic AMP)
   Increases protein synthesis (muscle, kidney, liver, reticulocytes)
   Increases protein catabolism (brain, spleen, testis)
   Increases glucose and fat catabolism
   Increases Na pump action—Calorigenic
   Swells mitochondria—Increases oxidation rate
   Decreases mucoprotein synthesis
Organismal level (as T4)
   Stimulates—Hematopoiesis, gametogenesis, lactation, intestinal absorption
   Regulates—Growth, differentiation, electrolyte balance, heat production,
      BMR, O_2 consumption
   Sensitizes—Nervous system

8. Enzymes, Cofactors, Mineraloproteins   8, 10, 11, 15, 25, 30, 35, 37, 46

System Types	Organ	Metalloenzyme/Protein	Cofactors	System Function
Cofactor	Liver, muscle	RNA polymerase	Mg, T4	Ribosomal RNA synthesis
	Liver, fat, thyroid	Adenyl cyclase	Mg, T4	Cyclic AMP synthesis
	Salivary, thyroid, stomach	ATP-ase (K, Na)	Mg, T4, K, Na	Iodide transport
	Thyroid	Thyroid peroxidase	I⁻	Iodothyronine synthesis
	Lymph nodes, leukocytes	Catalase	I⁻	Bacteriocidal
	Lymph nodes, leukocytes	Myeloperoxidase	I⁻	Bacteriocidal
	Thyroid	Mitochondrial enzyme systems	T4	TCA cycle

67 or more tissue enzymes affected in vivo.

9. Excretion   21, 30, 37, 39, 42, 46
Chemical forms—Iodide, organic fecal complexes
Organs
   Kidney (urine)—90-97% (increased by cortisol)
   Intestine (feces)
   Liver (bile, intestine)   3-10% (enterohepatic circulation via saliva, gastric juice, bile; liver chief organ of T4 breakdown)

   Skin (sweat)—Very small

MISCELLANEOUS

1. **Relationship to Other Minerals**   27, 30, 37, 46, 53
   Mg—Cofactor for T4-activated enzymes
   Br
   NO$_3$ } Iodide transport inhibitors
   ClO$_4$
   Co^{2+}—Metabolic antagonist

2. **Relationship to Vitamins**   27, 36, 37, 46, 53
   A—T4 needed for liver synthesis of vitamin A
   C—Synergist in cold survival
   B$_{12}$—Absorption aided by T4
   Niacin—Synergist in mitochondrial metabolism
   B-complex—Deficiency develops in hyperthyroidism

3. **Relationship to Hormones**   37, 46, 53
   TSH—Stimulates production of T4
   Cortisol—Increases renal output of iodide
   FSH—Inhibited by T4
   Estradiol—Increases PBI
   Testosterone—Decreases PBI
   STH—Synergizes T4 (also progesterone, insulin, oxytocin, vasopressin, pro-
      lactin)
   Serotonin—Increases iodide in skin
   MSH, ACTH—Increase iodine uptake by thyroid
   PTH—Antagonist to T4

4. **Unusual Features**   21, 30, 36, 37, 46, 50, 53
   Iodine not essential for plants but present (some accumulate it)
   Some tumors are very sensitive to iodoacetate (toxic)
   Iodide concentrates in granuloma cells
   Mast cells rupture in high iodide concentrations
   Goitrogens (thiouracil, thioureas) inhibit T4 synthesis or thyroid absorption
      of I$^-$
   Some iodine compounds act as enzyme inhibitors (e.g., iodoacetate)
   Brain, testis, spleen are not responsive to T4
   T3 has four times potency of T4

5. **Possible Relationship of Deficiency Symptoms to Metabolic Action**   21, 30,
      27, 36, 37, 46, 53
   Decreased BMR—T4 stimulates BMR
   High lipid and cholesterol—T4 stimulates fat catabolism
   Retention of NaCl and H$_2$O—T4 regulates electrolyte balance
   Mucoprotein increase—T4 decreases mucoprotein synthesis
   Liver gluconeogenesis—T4 increases CHO catabolism and BMR

Chapter 13. Fluorine (F)

Fluorine has been shown to be essential for growth of some animals and can be considered essential for humans on the basis of its proven beneficial effects on dental health and crystal structure of bone. Its universal presence in all tissues suggests that it plays a major role in metabolism in addition to its role in fortification of bone and tooth structure. There is some evidence of its having an effect on calcium metabolism and energy metabolism indirectly by acting on the Ca or Mg cofactors of the enzyme systems involved. Fluoride serves as a Mg and Ca sequestrant and may therefore regulate the activity of calcium ion in its vital functions (e.g. calmodulin activities).

No additional dietary supplementation is indicated for normal average American adult diets for individuals not having special needs. Aging individuals may need fluoride in cases of accelerated Ca loss and osteoporosis. Children definitely require it.

GENERAL INFORMATION

1. **Dietary and Medicinal Forms**   37, 39, 53, 54
   Element—Fluorine, gas; not used medicinally
   Inorganic salts—Stannous fluoride (SnF_2), sodium fluoride (NaF), potassium fluoride (KF)
   Organic forms—Fluorapatite (bone meal) $[Ca_{10}(PO_4)_6F_2]$

2. **History of Biological Significance**   8, 21, 32, 46, 50, 53
   1901—Eager: no dental decay in children with mottled teeth
   1942—Dean: caries incidence proportional to F concentration in drinking water

1967—Marthaler: fluoride safe and effective cariostatic agent

1968—Schroeder et al.: mice with F in drinking water show increased longevity and weight

1970—Weidmann and Weatherell: growing bones incorporate more F than adult bones

1972—Schwarz and Milne: rats show increased growth with F in diet

1972—Messer et al.: F protects against anemias of pregnancy in mice

1973—Joseph and Tydd: F enhances rate of wound healing

3. **Physiological (Blood) Forms**   17, 21, 37, 46, 50, 53
Ionic—F$^-$; complexes with plasma proteins

4. **Synergistic Agents**   30, 35, 37, 39, 46
Metabolic—Fe, Mg, Mo
Absorption—Fats

5. **Antagonistic Agents**   30, 35, 37, 39, 46
Metabolic—Na, Mg, Ca, Cl
Absorption—Al, Ca, Mg, Cl, Fe

6. **Possible or Demonstrated Physiological Functions** (Maintenance of Systems/ Components)   17, 21, 30, 37, 46, 50
Circulatory—Involved in calcification of aorta
Excretory—Fecal Ca and Mg excretions promoted (sequestering agent)
Respiratory—Hematopoiesis in pregnancy (mice)
Digestive—Intestinal absorption of Fe (mice)
Nervous—Sensitizer (?)
Special sensory—Antiotosclerotic
Reproductive—Fertility (mice) maintenance
Endocrine—Activation of adenyl cyclase
Blood—Antianemic (pregnant mice), anticoagulant
Muscular—Prevention of soft tissue calcification
Skeletal—Anti-senile osteoporosis; stability and structure of bone; dental caries prevention, enamel structure
Integument—Increase of wound healing rates
Immune—Indirect via Ca or Mg regulation
Metabolic—Ca metabolism homeostasis; activiation of liver enzymes; enzyme inhibitor
Detoxification—Sequestration of metals
Growth—+ (mice, rats)
Health—+ (bone and tooth structure)

Longevity—+ (osteoporosis)

7. **Body Content**   8, 12, 21, 35, 42, 46
mg/70 kg = 2.6-6.5; μg/g = 37.0-93.0

8. **Relative Organ Concentrations**   12, 21, 42, 46
Bones > teeth [cementum > bone > dentine > enamel] > kidney > aorta >
thyroid

9. **Deficiencies**   21, 30, 36, 37, 46
Man—Osteoporosis, otosclerosis, dental caries
Animal—Calcinosis (dogs)

10. **Excess Conditions**   21, 30, 36, 37, 38, 39, 46
Man—Mottled teeth, osteosclerosis, fluorosis, genu valgam
Animals—Fluorosis (rats, dogs, guinea pigs)

11. **Essentiality**   1, 17, 37, 38, 46
Man—Vitality not clearly demonstrated; essential for growth,
longevity
Other species—Some: fungi, vertebrates

12. **Major Commercial Uses** (Biological Interface)   6, 22, 30, 54
Element—Rocket fuels
Compounds—Fluorocarbons, pesticides, preservatives, electroplating, paper
coating, glass manufacture and etching

13. **Medicinal Applications**   18, 27, 30, 37, 53, 54
Dentifrices, anticaries—SnF_2
Water fluoridation—NaF
Anthelmintic, acaricide (veterinary)—NaF
Bone imaging agent—F^{18} (radioactive)

14. **Hazards and Toxicity**   19, 30, 37, 39, 41, 46, 54
Element—Toxic
Inhalation—Industrial fumes (metal refining, coal), caustic action
Contact—Caustic action on skin, mucous membranes
Compounds—Toxic
Inhalation- Industrial fumes (metal refining, coal) caustic action
Contact—Reactive compounds caustic action
Oral toxicity—See nutrition section, dietary excess
Carcinogenicity/Mutagenicity = —/—

DISTRIBUTION AND SOURCES

1. **Occurrence and Environmental Concentrations** (μg/g)   3, 4, 6, 29, 42, 47
   Relative terrestrial abundance—#13
   Chief minerals—Fluorspar (CaF_2); cryolite (Na_3AlF_6); fluorapatite [$3Ca_3$ $(PO_4)_2 \cdot CaF_2$]
   Earth's crust—700
   Rocks—270-740 (sandstones-shales)
   Soils—30-300
   Freshwater—.09
   Seawater—1.3

2. **Organismal Concentrations** (μg/g)   4, 42, 46, 47
   Plants—Marine: 4.5; land: 0.5-40
   Animals—Marine: 2.0; land: 150-500
   Man—37.0-93.0
   Special concentrators—Sponge, mollusc, fish bones

3. **Dietary Sources** (Variability due to Environment)   8, 26, 36, 42, 46, 52
   High (μg/100 g) 1000-10,000
       Seafood—Mackerel, sardines
       Meat/Organs—Salt pork
       Miscellaneous—Tea infusion, bone meal, sea salt
   Medium (μg/100) 100-1000
       Seafood—Codfish, crab, herring, salmon, shrimp
       Meat/Organs—Beef, chicken, eggs, lamb
       Nuts/Seeds—Sunflower seeds
       Grains—Wheat germ
       Vegetables—Kale, potatoes, soybeans, spinach, watercress
       Dairy products—Butter, cheese
       Miscellaneous—Honey
   Low (μg/100 g) 1-100
       Seafood—Tuna, oysters
       Meat/Organs—Veal, pork, calf liver
       Nuts/Seeds—Filberts, almonds, hazelnuts
       Grains—Wheat, rice, oats

Fruits—Gooseberries, grapefruit, grapes, oranges, apples, apricots, bananas, cantaloupe, cherries, figs, rhubarb, strawberries, peaches, pears, pineapples, plums

Vegetables—Cabbage, carrots, celery, corn, cucumbers, eggplant, onions, parsley, turnips, radishes, tomatoes, peas, green beans, beets

Dairy products—Milk

Miscellaneous—Chocolate

CHEMISTRY

1. **Atomic Properties** (Element)   6, 7, 9, 30, 49
   Periodic table group no.—VII-A, period 2
   Category of element—Nonmetal, gas
   Atomic weight—19.00
   Atomic number—9
   Atomic radius—0.717 Å
   Electron shells—2, 7
   Orbital electrons—$1s^2$, $2s^2$, $2p^5$
   Natural isotopes—F^{19} (100%)
   Long-lived radioactive isotopes—F^{17} (66 sec), F^{18} (200 min)

2. **Ionic Properties** (Biological Forms)   6, 7, 9, 30, 49
   Oxidation states (valences)—F^-
   Ionic radius (Å)—1.36
   Oxidation potentials—$F^0 \rightarrow F^-$ (+2.85 v)

3. **Molecular Properties** (Biological Forms)   6, 7, 9, 16, 25, 30, 43, 49
   Covalent radius (Å)—0.64
   Coordination number—1
   Stereochemistry—Linear
   Electron transfer compounds—None
   Typical molecular complexes—OsF_6^{2-}, AlF_6^{2-}

4. **Analytical Methods**   3, 30, 31, 40, 47, 55
   Physical—Neutron activation, nuclear magnetic resonance, mass spectroscopy
   Chemical—Spectrophotometric (eriochrome-cyanin-R)
   Hair/Nail analysis—Not reported
   Comments—Atomic absorption not feasible; volatility of sample a problem; no reference standards

5. **Chemical Properties of Compounds**   6, 7, 9, 49, 54
   See Table 13.1

Table 13.1.   Properties of Fluorine Compounds

	REACTIONS			SOLUBILITY			
	Heat °C	Air	Water	g/100 cc H_2O	Alc.	Eth.	Acid
Na fluoride, NaF	BP 1695°	NA	alk. pH 7.4	4.22^{18}	I	NA	NA
K fluoride, KF	BP 1505°	deliq.	NA	96.4^{21}	I	NA	NA

	Density	MW hyd./anh.	MP °C	XL Form	Color XL/Powd.	Appearance Commercial Form	% Element h./anh.
Na fluoride, NaF	2.56	–/42.0	988°	cubic tetrag.	NA	C	–/45.2
K fluoride, KF	2.48	–/58.1	858°	cubic	col./wh.	P	–/32.7

Abbreviations: tetrag. = tetragonal; others as in earlier tables.

MEDICINAL AND NUTRITIONAL ROLE

1. **Units of Measurement**
   Weight—μg (microgram): 1 mg (milligram) = 1000 μg
   Concentration—ppm (parts per million) = μg/g; μg% = μg/100 ml

2. **Human Body Fluid Levels** (Normal) (μg/100 ml)　　1, 2, 12, 37, 46
   Blood—4.0-36.0 (18.0)
   Plasma/Serum—2.8
   Urine—32.7-467 (102.7)

3. **Human Tissue Levels** (μg/g)　　4, 8, 24, 46, 47
   Hair—No data
   Bone—300-600
   Liver—0.8 ⎫
   Muscle—1.0 ⎬ Mammalian
   Nerve—0.2 ⎭

4. **Important Dietary Levels**　　5, 21, 27, 30, 37, 39, 46
   Estimated dietary levels—0.31-3.1 mg/day
   Deficiency limit—1.0 mg/day
   Toxic limit—20-80 mg/day
   Recommended levels in water—1 mg/liter (1 μg/g) (1.5 mg/day)
   Lethal limit—2000 mg/day
   Recommended dietary intake—1.5-4.0 mg/day

5. **Estimated Human Daily Balance** (average American diet, 70 kg ♂, 30 yr)　　27,
   30, 42, 46
   Average intake—2400 μg/day (1000 food, 1400 water)
   Average output—2380 μg/day (1600 urine, 150 feces, 650 sweat)
   Net gain/loss—20 gain (body concentrates F in bones)

6. **Indications for Supplementation of Above Diet**　　5, 21, 27, 30, 42, 46
   Healthy normal—None
   Special conditions—Osteoporosis, dental caries, otosclerosis, pre-puberty

7. **Factors Affecting Availability from Diet**　　17, 21, 27, 37, 46, 53
   Decreased
   　　See absorption section, antagonists
   　　Drinking water low in F
   　　Cooking in low-F water
   Increased
   　　See absorption section, synergizers
   　　F deficiency

Soluble forms
Fat in diet
Excessive heating of Teflon-coated ware
High-F drinking water

8. **Deficiency Symptoms**   21, 30, 36, 37, 46
Man—Dental caries, osteoporosis, calcification of aorta
Animals—Anemia, infertility, poor growth

9. **Effects of Dietary Excess** (Salts or Concentrates)   19, 33, 36, 39, 46
Acute—Lethal amount: 2000 mg/day
    Sublethal—Weakness, gastrointestinal symptoms
    Lethal—Salivation, nausea, abdominal pain, vomiting, diarrhea, hypocal-
        cemia, hypoglycemia, irritability, convulsions, death from paralysis or
        cardiac failure
Chronic—Mottled enamel, osteosclerosis, calcification of ligaments, crippling
    fluorosis

METABOLIC ROLE

1. **Intestinal Absorption**   17, 30, 35, 37, 39, 46
Chemical forms—Fluoride ion (F^-)
    Preferred valence—F^-
    Poorly absorbed—$[Ca_{10}(PO_4)_6F_2]$ (bone meal), CaF_2, Na_3AlF_6
    Well absorbed—NaF, Na_2SiF_6
Sites—Gastrointestinal tract
Efficiency—80-90%
Active transport—No
Synergizers—Fats
Antagonists—Al, Ca, Mg, Cl

2. **Blood Carriers**   17, 30, 37, 46
Ionic fluoride and bound forms (protein)

3. **Half-Life of Element in Blood**   17, 21, 37, 46
30% excreted in 5-6 hr

4. **Target (Initial) Sites**   17, 30, 37, 46
Tissues—All, especially calcified tissues
Cells—Cytoplasm, mitochondria

5. **Storage**   17, 30, 37, 46
Sites—Bone, teeth, (aorta, kidney—small amounts)
Forms—Fluorapatite

6. Homeostatic Mechanisms   17, 30, 37, 42, 46
Relative efficiency in element retention—Est. 10-20% (skeletal structure)
Kidney participation—None, passive excretion
Intestinal participation—None
Liver (bile) participation—None
Skeletal pool of F—Actively maintains plasma F^-

7. Specific Functions (via Cofactors/Metalloenzymes/Mineralo-Proteins/Ions)
   17, 21, 25, 30, 37, 46
Molecular level
   Activates enzymes
   Replaces HCO_3^- in bone
   Substitutes for OH^- in enamel hydroxyapatite
   Removes Mg also Ca cofactors for enzymes
Cellular level
   Activates adenyl cyclase, α amylase
   Immobilizes Ca, Mg
   In excess inhibits respiratory enzymes
Organismal level
   Acts as anticoagulant
   Promotes Ca retention
   Strengthens bone
   Hardens teeth, preventing dental caries
   Prevents soft tissue calcification
   Increases wound healing

8. Metalloenzymes, Cofactors, Mineraloproteins   8, 10, 11, 15, 25, 30, 35,
   37, 46

System Types	Organ	Metalloenzyme/Protein	Cofactors	System Function
Cofactors	Tissues	Amylase	Mg, Ca, F	Carbohydrase
(F^-)	Fat cells	Adenyl cyclase	F, Mg	Cyclic AMP production
Cofactor inhibitors	Nerves	Cholinesterase	Ca, Mg, Co, Mn	Esterase
(F^-)	Testicles	Hyaluronidase	Fe, Mn	Carbohydrase
	Leukocytes	Enolase	Mg, Mn, Zn	Glycolysis
	Liver	Uricase	Mn, Cu	Purine metabolism
	Tissues	Phosphoglucomutase	Mg	Transphosphatase
	Pancreas	DNA nucleases	Mg, Mn, Ca	DNA digestion
	Pancreas	Ribonuclease	?	RNA digestion
	Tissues	Acid phosphatase	?	Phosphate removal
	Tissues	Pyrophosphatase II	Mg, Mn	Pyrophosphate splitting

9. **Excretion**   21, 30, 37, 39, 42, 46

    Chemical forms—Ionic (fluoride)

    Organs—Kidney (urine): 60-70%; intestine (feces): 6-7%; liver (bile, intestine): Negligible; skin, sweat: 25-30%

MISCELLANEOUS

1. **Relationship to Other Minerals**   27, 30, 37, 46, 53

    Mg—Metabolic and absorption antagonist; metabolic synergist

    Ca—Metabolic and absorption antagonist

    Fe—Absorption antagonist; metabolic synergist

    Al—Absorption antagonist

    Cl—Absorption and metabolic antagonist

    HCO_3^-—Replaced by F in bone

    Mo—Synergistic in tooth development

2. **Relationship to Vitamins**   27, 36, 37, 46, 53

    Vitamin D—Antagonist in Ca absorption (intestinal)

3. **Relationship to Hormones**   37, 46, 53

    Cyclic AMP—Synthesis stimulated by F

    PTH ⎫

    TCT ⎬ Bone metabolism synergists or antagonists of F

4. **Unusual Features**   21, 30, 36, 37, 46, 50, 53

    Most electronegative of all elements

    Most effective mineral in development of teeth

    Affects gastric emptying in presence of fats

    Inhibits many enzymes (control of Ca cofactors (?))

    Half-life in bone estimated at 2 yr

    Very effective sequestering agent

    Evidence of nerve tissue sensitivity to F

    High losses of F in sweat

5. **Possible Relationship of Deficiency Symptoms to Metabolic Action**   21, 27, 30, 36, 37, 46, 53

    Dental caries—Hardening of enamel by F

    Osteoporosis—Solubilization of bone by F loss

    Aortic calcification—Solubilization of bone by loss of F; also high serum Ca

Chapter 14. Selenium (Se)

Selenium in the inorganic form has limited application because of its toxicity. Its organic biologically active or vitamin form is a Se-complex of either an amino acid or fatty acid. Selenium has been shown to be required by various animals for good health and a normal life span and is implicated in Vitamin E function. Presumably this is true for humans as for other animals, but it has not yet been conclusively demonstrated by clinical studies. The presence of Se in a key enzyme in humans, glutathione peroxidase, appears to indicate a requirement for selenium in the human diet. The exact amount required is unknown, however; the trace amounts required and environmental conditions (i.e., variable regional soil and dietary concentrations) make it difficult to suggest the extent of dietary supplementation for any one region. The average American diet contains approximately 62-150 μg/day Se with losses of about 150 μg/day, leaving a variable negative balance. This 150 μg/day could be obtained in the regular diet from concentrated sources such as tuna, wheat germ, brazil nuts, liver or brewer's yeast. Selenium strongly complexes heavy metals and may be a natural detoxifier. It thus plays a role in metabolism of toxic as well as essential heavy metals. Selenium has a very narrow "window" of biological usefulness, since its toxicity range begins above 0.5 μg/g. It is reduced in living systems. (In contrast, S is oxidized). Additional major functions of Se in addition to its synergism with vitamin E are expected to be found in the near future, since unidentified selenium compounds have been found in mitochondria and muscle.

There is a possibility that Se supplementation of the human diet may be proved beneficial for special physiological states such as aging, smog exposure, and heavy metal contamination. Selenium should be obtained in food forms such as brazil nuts or brewer's yeast because selenium salts are usually toxic. Adequate vitamin E in the diet is necessary for full synergistic performance of selenium.

GENERAL INFORMATION

1. **Dietary and Medicinal Forms**   37, 49, 53, 54
   Element—Selenium, nonmetal; not used medicinally
   Inorganic salts—Sodium (selenate, selenite); Na_2SeO_9, Na_2SeO_3
   Mineralovitamin—Factor-3 (?)
   Chelated forms—Selenomethionine, selenocystine, factor-3

2. **History of Biological Significance**   8, 21, 35, 37, 50, 53, 46, 56
   1860—Madison: first described "alkali disease" (Se excess) in cattle
   1933—Robinson: toxic cattle feeds contain Se
   1934—Beath et al.: Se causes "blind staggers" (Se excess) in cattle
   1957—Schwarz and Folts: Se prevents dietary liver necrosis in rats
   1958—Nesheim and Scott: Se deficiency causes exudative diathesis in chicks
   1964—Walter et al.: gizzard myopathy in turkeys is a Se deficiency condition
   1969—Parizek et al.: selenite decreases toxicity of $HgCl_2$ in chicks
   1970—Thompson and Scott: chick's requirement of Se is independent of vitamin E
   1973—Rotruck: glutathione peroxidase is a Se enzyme (rats)
   1975—Awasthi et al.: human glutathione peroxidase contains Se

3. **Physiological (Blood) Forms**   17, 21, 37, 46, 50, 53, 56
   GPX (glutathione peroxidase RBC, plasma), selenomethionine, selenocystine

4. **Synergistic Agents**   30, 35, 37, 39, 46, 56
   Metabolic—Vitamin E, vitamin C, glutathione
   Absorption—Amino acids, peptides, proteins

5. **Antagonistic Agents**   30, 35, 37, 39, 46, 56
   Metabolic—Ag, As, Cd, Hg, Tl
   Absorption—Hg, Cu, Ag, Cd, SO_4, Tl

6. **Possible or Demonstrated Physiological Functions** (Maintenance of Systems/Components)   17, 21, 30, 37, 46, 50, 56
   Circulatory—Heart muscle and arteriole homeostasis (chicks)
   Excretory—Protection from toxic metals, complex excretion
   Respiratory—RBC-O_2 transport

Digestive—Intestinal homeostasis (chicks); pancreatic homeostasis
Nervous—Protection from Hg
Special sensory—Corneal clarity (chicks)
Reproductive—antiteratogenic (Cd), sperm motility and maturation, fertility,
  viability
Endocrine—Synergizes with sex hormones
Blood—RBC membranes, stability
Muscular—Muscle homeostasis (lamb)
Skeletal—Teeth maintenance (ewe)
Integument—Keratin, skin, hair, connective tissue maintenance
Immune—↑ immune response (mice)
Metabolic—Lipid and sulfhydryl metabolism; antinecrotic for liver (pigs)
Detoxification—Synergist in cytochrome P450 system; detoxifier: Hg, Cd,
  As, Ag, peroxides
Growth—+ ⎫
Health—+   ⎬ Chicks, lambs, pigs, rats
Longevity—+ ⎭

7. **Body Content**   8, 12, 21, 35, 42, 46, 56
   mg/70 kg = 14; μg/g = 0.2

8. **Relative Organ Concentrations**   12, 21, 42, 46, 56
   Liver > testicle > muscle > kidney, lung > brain, ovary

9. **Deficiencies**   21, 30, 36, 37, 46, 56
   Man—kwashiorkor (secondary?), neonatal jaundice (?), alcoholic hepatic
     failure (?), acanthocytosis (?), Glanzmann's thrombasthenia (?)
   Animals—Muscular dystrophy (chicks, lambs), white muscle disease (lambs),
     pancreatic fibrosis (chicks), hepatosis dietetica (pigs), liver necrosis (rats),
     exudative diathesis (chicks)

10. **Excess Conditions**   21, 30, 36, 38, 39, 37, 46, 56
    Animals: Selenosis (horses, cattle, pigs); blind staggers, alkali disease (horses,
      cattle, pigs)
    Man: Mottled teeth

11. **Essentiality**   1, 37, 17, 38, 46
    Man—Need not clearly demonstrated
    Other species—Some vertebrates (chicks, lambs, pigs, rats): need for normal
      health, life span; certain microorganisms

12. **Major Commercial Uses** (Biological Interface)   6, 22, 30, 54, 56
    Element—Electrode alloys, rectifiers, photo cells, semiconductors
    Compounds—Photography, insecticides, glass manufacture, alkaloidal reagent,
      electroplating, lubricant, catalyst, vulcanizing agent, pigment

13. **Medicinal Applications**   18, 27, 30, 37, 53, 54
    Nutritional factor (sodium selenite)
    Topical antiseborrheic (Se sulfides)
    Topical antieczema agent (Se sulfides)
    Diagnostic agent (Se[75]-methionine)—Scanning pancreas and PTH glands

14. **Hazards and Toxicity**   19, 30, 37, 39, 41, 46, 54, 56
    Element—Relatively nontoxic
       Inhalation (dust, fumes)—Garlic breath, skin rash, indigestion, psycho-
          logical symptoms
       Topical—Poorly absorbed
    Compounds—H_2Se extremely toxic [$H_2Se > SeO_3^{2-} > SeO_4^{2-} > Se$-a.a. $>$
    $(CH_3)_2Se$]
       Inhalation (liver chief organ affected)—Pallor, nervousness, depression,
          garlic breath, gastrointestinal disturbance, dermatitis, liver injury, den-
          tal caries
       Topical—Poorly absorbed
       Oral toxicity—See nutrition section, dietary excess
    Carcinogenicity/Mutagenicity = $-/\pm$ [anticarcinogenic (?)]

DISTRIBUTION AND SOURCES

1. **Occurrence and Environmental Concentrations** ($\mu g/g$)   3, 4, 6, 29, 42, 47,
    56
    Relative terrestrial abundance—#69
    Chief Minerals—Crooksite [$(Cu, Tl, Ag)_2Se$] ; clausthalite (PbSe)
    Geographic distribution—Low soil concentrations on east and west coasts of
       United States
    Earth's crust—.05-.09
    Rocks—.05-.06 (igneous, sandstones-shales)
    Soils—.01-2.0
    Freshwater—.001-.300
    Seawater—.0005-.00010

2. **Organismal Concentrations** ($\mu g/g$)   4, 34, 42, 46, 47, 56
    Plants—Marine: 0.8; land: 0.1-0.5
    Animals—Marine: 0.1-0.5; land: 1.7
    Man—0.2
    Special concentrators—*Astragalus, Conopsis*
    Indicator plants—*Astragalus, Conopsis*

3. **Dietary Sources** (Variability due to Environment)   8, 26, 28, 36, 42, 52, 46, 56

High (μg/100 g) 30-100
   Seafood—Oysters, tuna, mackerel, herring, lobsters, scallops, shrimp, pike, trout, carp, cod, flounder, salmon
   Meat/Organs—Liver (chicken, pork, turkey, beef), kidney (beef, lamb, pig)
   Nuts/Seeds—Brazil, cashew, peanut
   Grains—Wheat germ, bran and flour; brown rice; barley
   Miscellaneous—Brewer's yeast
Medium (μg/100 g) 10-30
   Meat/Organs—Beef, lamb, liver, heart, egg, beef, chicken, pork, lamb
   Nuts/Seeds—Walnuts
   Grains—White rice, oats
   Vegetables—Alfalfa, garlic, lentils (dry)
   Dairy products—Cheddar cheese
   Miscellaneous—Sugar cane, molasses, mushrooms
Low (μg/100 g) 1-10
   Meat/Organs—Egg white
   Nuts/Seeds—Hazel, chestnuts, almonds
   Fruits—Raisins, satsumas, apples, bananas, pineapple, oranges, peaches, pears
   Vegetables—Lettuce, okra, turnips, tomatoes, cabbages, kidney beans, soybeans, radishes, corn, carrots, cassavas, onions, yams, green beans, potatoes, cauliflower
   Dairy products—Milk, cheese (American, cottage, swiss), butter, cream
   Miscellaneous—White and brown sugar, torula yeast, beer, margarine

CHEMISTRY

1. **Atomic Properties** (Element)   6, 7, 9, 30, 49, 56
   Periodic table group no.—VI-A, period 4
   Category of element—Nonmetal, metalloid
   Atomic weight—78.96
   Atomic number—34
   Atomic radius—1.66, 1.73 Å
   Electron shells—2, 8, 18, 6
   Orbital electrons—$3s^2$, $3p^6$, $3d^{10}$, $4s^2$, $4p^4$
   Natural isotopes—Se^{74} (.9%), Se^{76} (9.0%), Se^{77} (7.6%), Se^{78} (23.5%), Se^{80} (49.8%), Se^{82} (9.2%)

Long-lived radioactive isotopes—Se^{72} (8.4 days), Se^{73} (7.1 hr), Se^{75} (120 days), Se^{79} (6.5 × 10^4 yr)

2. **Ionic Properties** (Biological Forms)   6, 7, 9, 30, 49, 56
   Oxidation states (valences)—Se^{2-}, Se^{4+} (SeO_3), Se^{6+} (SeO_4)
   Ionic radius (Å)—Se^{2-}, 1.91; Se^{4+}, 0.50; Se^{6+}, 0.42
   Oxidation potentials
   $Se^0 \rightarrow Se^{2-}$: −0.78 v (basic), −0.36-0.40 v (acidic)
   $Se^0 \rightarrow Se^{4+}$: +0.35 v (basic), −0.74 v (acidic)
   $Se^{4+} \rightarrow Se^{6+}$: −0.03 v (basic), −1.15 v (acidic)

3. **Molecular Properties** (Biological Forms)   6, 7, 9, 16, 25, 30, 43, 44, 56
   Covalent radius (Å)—1.17
   Coordination numbers —Se^{2-}: (2), Se^{4+}: (3), Se^{6+}: (4)
   Stereochemistry—Se^{2-} (angular), Se^{4+} (pyramidal), Se^{6+} (tetrahedral)
   Electron transfer compounds—Selenite, glutathione, selenopersulfide (?)
   Typical molecular complexes—$(SeCN)^-$; $(CH_3)_3Se^+$; G-S-Se-H (glutathione selenopersulfide)

4. **Analytical Methods**   3, 30, 31, 40, 47, 55, 56
   Physical—Flameless atomic absorption, neutron activation
   Chemical—Spectrophotometric (3,3′ diaminobenzidine)
   Hair/Nail analysis—Se relatively high in human nails; hair analysis is utilized
   Comments—Volatilization of Se compounds presents problems; divergent results from various labs; no reference standards

5. **Chemical Properties of Compounds**   6, 7, 9, 49, 54
   See Table 14.1

MEDICINAL AND NUTRITIONAL ROLE

1. **Units of Measurement**
   Weight—μg (microgram); 1 mg (milligram) = 1000 μg = .001 g
   Concentration—ppm (parts per million) = μg/g; μg% = μg/100 ml

2. **Human Body Fluid Levels** (Normal) (μg/100 ml)   1, 2, 4, 12, 35, 37, 46, 56
   Blood—10.0-34.0 (20.6)
   Plasma/Serum—1.8
   Urine—0.0-9.3 (2.3)

Table 14.1.   Properties of Selenium Compounds

	Density	MW hyd./anh.	MP °C	REACTIONS			SOLUBILITY			Appearance Commercial Form				% Element h./anh.
				Heat °C	Air	Water	g/100 cc H_2O	Color XL/Powd.	XL Form		Alc.	Eth.	Acid	
Na selenate $Na_2SeO_4 \cdot 10H_2O$ (Se = 6+ selenate)	1.60-1.62	369.1/ 188.9	NA	trans. 32°	NA	NA	43.5^{20}	col./wh.	monocl.	C	NA	NA	NA	21.4/ 41.8
Na selenite $Na_2SeO_3 \cdot 5H_2O$ (Se = 4+ selenite)	NA	263.0/ 173.0	NA	NA	efflor.	NA	S	col./wh.	tetrag. prisms	C	I	NA	NA	30.0/ 45.7

Abbreviations: as in earlier tables.

3. **Human Tissue Levels** (μg/g)   4, 8, 24, 46, 47
   Hair—0.58-0.76
   Bone—0.03
   Liver—0.30
   Muscle—0.11
   Nerve—0.09

4. **Important Dietary Levels** (μg/day) (depends on vitamin E content)   5, 21,
      30, 27, 37, 39, 46
   Safe dietary range—0.03-0.40
   Deficiency limit—<0.03
   Toxic limit—>0.4

5. **Estimated Human Daily Balance** (average American diet, 70 kg ♂, 30 yr)   27,
      30, 42, 46
   Average intake—62-150 μg/day (62-150 food; water, air negligible)
   Average output—150 μg/day (20 feces, 50 urine, 80 sweat)
   Net gain/loss—0-88 μg/day; negative balance possible
   Recommended daily intake—50-200 μg/d

6. **Indications for Supplementation of Above Diet**   5, 30, 27, 21, 42, 46
   Healthy normal—Some evidence for supplementation available; adequate vita-
      min E needed
   Special conditions—Possibly smog exposure, aging, heavy metal contamination

7. **Factors Affecting Availability from Diet**   17, 21, 27, 37, 46, 53
   Decreased
      See absorption section, antagonists
      Food processing, water cooking
      Se-deficient soils for food plants
      Hg-contaminated animal food sources
      Animal protein diet—Fish, poultry, meat
   Increased
      See absorption section, synergizers
      High protein diet (plant)
      Se-sufficient soils for food plants
      Chelated forms of Se
      Plant protein diet—Alfalfa, soybean, yeast

8. **Deficiency Symptoms**   21, 30, 36, 37, 46
   Man—Neonatal jaundice (?), alcoholic liver failure (?), acanthocytosis (?),
      thrombasthenia (?)
   Animals—(May be interrelated with vitamin E deficiency)
      General—High mortality, poor growth, infertility
      Chicks—Edema, hemorrhages, pancreas degeneration, poor feathering

Rats—Liver necrosis, cataracts, hair loss

Pigs—Edema, pigmentation, muscle degeneration

Cattle, sheep—Weight loss, diarrhea, periodontal disease, muscle degeneration, nutritional muscular dystrophy

Monkeys—Weight loss, hair loss, listlessness, liver necrosis, nephrosis, heart and skeletal muscle degeneration (preliminary data)

9. **Effects of Dietary Excess** (Selenosis) (Salts or Concentrates)   19, 33, 36, 39, 46

Animals:

Acute—"Blind staggers"; blindness; abdominal pain; salivation, grating of teeth; myelitis; respiratory failure; anorexia; weakness

Chronic—"Alkali disease"; dullness; dental caries; loss of weight, hair, vitality; sloughing hoofs; stiffness of joints; heart atrophy; liver necrosis (cirrhosis); anemia (microcytic, hypochromic); slow growth; birth defects; long-bone erosion (arthritic)

METABOLIC ROLE

1. **Intestinal Absorption**   17, 30, 35, 37, 39, 46

Chemical forms—Selenite, Se-methionine, Se-cysteine

Preferred valence—Se^{4+} $(SeO_3)^{2-}$

Poorly absorbed—Se, Na_2Se, Se-methionine

Well absorbed—Na_2SeO_3,' Na_2SeO_4, Se-cystine, factor-3

Sites—Duodenum

Efficiency—44-70%

Active transport—No data

Synergizers—Amino acids, peptides, proteins

Antagonists—Hg, Cu, Ag, Cd, SO_4, Tl, linseed oil meal

2. **Blood Carriers**   17, 30, 37, 46

β lipoprotein, α globulins, RBCs, serum albumin

3. **Half-Life of Element in Blood**   8, 17, 37, 46

ca. 24 hr (mouse)

4. **Target (Initial) Sites**   17, 30, 37, 46

Tissues—Liver, kidney, pancreas, heart, bones, RBC, WBC

Cells—Cytosol $>$ mitochondria $>$ microsomal

5. **Storage**   17, 30, 37, 46

Sites (short term)—Liver, kidney, skeletal muscle, bone, RBC, testes, brain

Forms—Tissue proteins, enzymes, peptides

6. **Homeostatic Mechanisms**   17, 30, 37, 46, 42
Relative efficiency in element retention—Est. 0-5%
Kidney participation—No regulation (↑ excretion by anabolic steroids)
Intestinal participation—No regulation
Liver (bile) participation—No regulation (↑ excretion by dietary As)

7. **Specific Functions** (via Cofactors/Metalloenzymes/Mineralo-Proteins/Ions)
   17, 21, 25, 30, 37, 46, 53, 56
Molecular level
   Sulfhydryl agent
   Water-soluble antioxidant (via GPX: Glutathione Peroxidase)
   Synergist to vitamin E
Cellular level
   Destruction of peroxides (via GPX)
   Causes swelling of mitochondria
   Protection of cell membranes
   Electron transfer agent
   Glutathione metabolism
Organismal level
   See physiological functions
   Maintenance: circulatory system, integument, digestive organs, reproductive systems
   Detoxification: heavy metals, peroxides

8. **Metalloenzymes, Cofactors, Mineraloproteins**   8, 10, 11, 15, 25, 30, 35, 37, 46, 56

System Types	Organ	Enzyme/Protein	Co-factors	System Function
Metallo-enzyme	Various organs	Glutathione peroxidase	Fe	Destruction of peroxides
	Skeletal muscle	Aryl sulfatase	?	Phenol-sulfate metabolism
	Skeletal muscle	B-glucuronidase	?	Glucuronide metabolism
	Skeletal muscle	Lactic dehydrogenase	?	Destruction of lactic acid
	Skeletal muscle	Glutamic-oxalic transaminase	?	Interconversion of amino acids

9. **Excretion**   21, 30, 37, 39, 42, 46
Chemical forms—Trimethyl selenomium, dimethyl selenide, U-2 (reductive methylation in liver)
Organs—Kidney (urine): ca. 80% (↑ by anabolic steroids and SO_4); intestine (feces): ca. 20%; liver (bile, intestine): ↑ by arsenite; skin: sweat (may be large); other: expired air route in excess

MISCELLANEOUS

1. **Relationship to Other Minerals**   14, 27, 30, 37, 46, 53
   Hg, Cu, Ag, Cd, Tl, SO_4—Antagonists to Se (absorption)
   Hg, Tl, Cd, Ag, As—Metabolic antagonists to Se
   As—Causes biliary excretion of Se
   SO_4—Increases urinary output of Se
   Hg—Potentiates toxicity of trimethyl selenomium
   Fe—Found in glutathione peroxidase (Se)

2. **Relationship to Vitamins**   27, 36, 37, 46, 53
   E—Synergist as antioxidant
   C—Synergist as antioxidant
   Niacin—Glutathione functions require it (NAD)
   CoQ—Se involved in synthesis of CoQ

3. **Relationship to Hormones**   14, 37, 46, 53
   Anabolic steroids—Control excretion of trimethyl selenomium
   Prostaglandins E and F—Conversion from G form requires glutathione PX

4. **Unusual Features**   14, 21, 30, 36, 37, 46, 50, 53
   Se found in: tRNA (Se-uridine), lamb-muscle protein
   Methionine used in detoxification of excess Se
   Not needed in plants that accumulate Se
   Dimethyl selenide more toxic in male than female
   Se more adverse to reproductive functions in female than male
   Se reduced in vivo while *S* is oxidized in vivo
   Accumulator plants (*Astragalus*) have up to 15,000 μg/g
   High losses of Se in sweat

5. **Possible Relationship of Deficiency Symptoms to Metabolic Action**   14, 21,
      30, 27, 36, 37, 46, 53
   Acanthocytosis—Deterioration of lipid metabolism in liver
   Neonatal jaundice—Breakdown of RBC membranes
   Alcoholic liver failure—Breakdown of liver cell membranes
   Thrombasthenia—Deterioration of platelet membranes
   Kwashiorkor—Growing individuals require more Se than adults

Chapter 15. Molybdenum (Mo)

Molybdenum has not been shown to have an organic vitamin-like form although it does form complexes easily. Its main importance is in certain plants, where it is essential for nitrogen fixation enzymes in root nodule bacteria. Thus it is vital for protein production by leguminous plants. A mammalian enzyme in which Mo is a vital constituent (xanthine oxidase) exists for production of uric acid and Mo has synergistic interactive effects on Fe, and SO_4 metabolism. A strong antagonism to Cu has been found. Molybdenum has not yet been found to be essential for humans, but chicks and ruminants have been found to require it in their diet for growth and normal life span. However, since it is present in all tissues, an essential role in humans may be discovered in future investigations.

No evidence is available to justify dietary supplementation of molybdenum in humans. The human requirement is so low that it is easily satisfied by ordinary dietary levels.

GENERAL INFORMATION

1. **Dietary and Medicinal Forms**   37, 49, 53, 54
   Element—Molybdenum metal; not used medicinally
   Inorganic salts—Sodium molybdate (Na_2MoO_4), ammonium molybdate ($NH_4)_6$ (Mo_7O_{24})
   Metallovitamin—No data
   Chelated forms—No data

167

2. **History of Biological Significance**   8, 21, 37, 46, 50, 53
    1932—Ter Meulen: Mo is present in plants and animals
    1953—Westerfeld et al.: xanthine oxidase requires Mo for activity
    1954—Westerfeld and Richert: tungsten is antagonistic to Mo
    1954—Mahler et al.: aldehyde oxidase requires Mo for activity
    1954—Nicholas and Nason: nitrate reductase contains Mo
    1956—Higgins et al.: chicks on tungstate require Mo
    1957—Leach and Norris: highly depleted chicks show Mo requirement
    1958—Ellis et al.: found improved cellulose digestibility in lambs using Mo
        supplement
    1959—Underwood: Mo toxicity (in cattle and sheep) is reversed by $CuSO_4$
    1967—Hart and Bray: tissue concentrations of xanthine oxidase are related
        to Mo intake

3. **Physiological (Blood) Forms**   17, 21, 37, 46, 50, 53
    Plasma protein—Cu-Mo complexes, molybdate ion $(MoO_4)^{2-}$

4. **Synergistic Agents** (Animals)   30, 35, 37, 39, 46
    Metabolic—Cu^{2+}, Fe^{2+}, F^-
    Absorption—No data

5. **Antagonistic Agents** (Animals)   30, 35, 37, 39, 46
    Metabolic—WO_4^{2-}, Cu^{2+}, Mn^{2+}, SO_4^{2-}
    Absorption—Cu^{2+}, SO_4^{2-}, methionine, protein

6. **Possible and Demonstrated Physiological Functions** (Maintenance of Sys-
        tems/Components)   17, 21, 30, 37, 46, 50
    Circulatory—No data
    Excretory—Purine catabolism (sheep, man) (xanthine oxidase)
    Respiratory—Hemoglobin synthesis (animals)
    Digestive—Cellulose digestion (ruminants)
    Nervous—No data
    Special sensory—No data
    Reproductive—Gonadal homeostasis (?) (animals)
    Endocrine—T4 levels (rabbits)
    Blood—Hemoglobin synthesis (animals)
    Muscular—No data
    Skeletal—Gout preventative (?) (man); anticariogenic (?) (man)
    Integument—Coat color and texture (cattle)
    Immune—No data
    Metabolic—Fat, aldehyde, uric acid metabolism (rat); Cu, Fe, SO_4 homeostasis
        (rat)
    Detoxification—Cu^{2+}, SO_3^{2-}, SO_2, aldehydes (rat)

Growth— + (birds)
Health— + (birds)
Longevity— + (birds)

7. **Body Content**   8, 12, 21, 35, 42, 46
mg/70 kg = 5.0-9.3; (μg/g) = .07-.13
Present in all tissues

8. **Relative Organ Concentrations**   12, 21, 42, 46
Bone > skin > liver > kidney > spleen > lung > brain, muscle

9. **Deficiencies**   21, 30, 36, 37, 46
Animals: Hypercupremia (sheep)

10. **Excess Conditions**   21, 30, 36, 37, 38, 46
Man—Gout, industrial fumes
Animals—Molybdenosis (rats, rabbits, cattle); teart, peat scours (cattle); hypocupremia (sheep)

11. **Essentiality**   1, 17, 37, 38, 46
Man—Not clearly demonstrated
Other species—All: algae, spermatophytes; some: vertebrates, bacteria, fungi

12. **Major Commercial Uses** (Biological Interface)   6, 22, 30, 54
Element—Alloys: ferromolybdenum (Fe, Mo), stainless steel (Fe, Ni, Mo, Cr, Cu)
Compounds—Lubricants, pigments, corrosion inhibitors, catalysts, reagents, photography

13. **Medicinal Applications**   27, 30, 37, 53, 54
Micronutrient
Hematinic

14. **Hazards and Toxicity**   19, 30, 37, 39, 41, 46
Element—Low order of toxicity
Inhalation—Absorbed by lungs (animals); linkage to lung diseases (?)
Skin—No data
Compounds—Moderately toxic
Inhalation (soluble compounds)—Eyes, mucous and pulmonary membranes: very irritating (rabbits)
Skin—No data
Oral toxicity—See nutrition section, dietary excess
Carcinogenicity/Mutagenicity—Weakly carcinogenic/mutagenic (?) = ±/±

DISTRIBUTION AND SOURCES

1. **Occurrence and Environmental Concentrations** (μg/g)   3, 4, 6, 29, 42, 47
   Relative terrestrial abundance—#38
   Chief minerals—Wulfenite ($PbMoO_4$); powellite [$Ca(MoW)O_4$] ; molybdenite
     (MoS_2)
   Earth's crust—1 μg/g
   Rocks—0.2-2.6 (sandstone-shales)
   Soils—2 μg/g
   Freshwater—.00035 μg/g
   Seawater—0.010-.014 μg/g

2. **Organismal Concentrations** (μg/g)   4, 42, 46, 47
   Plants—Marine: 0.45; land: 0.90
   Animals—Marine: 0.6-2.5; land: <0.2
   Man—0.1-0.2
   Special concentrators—Legumes
   Indicator plants—Wheat

3. **Dietary Sources** (Variability due to Environment)   8, 26, 36, 42, 46, 52
   High (μg/100 g) 100-400
       Meat/Organs—Pork, lamb, beef liver
       Nuts/Seeds—Sunflower
       Vegetables—Soybeans, lima beans, lentils (dry), peas
       Grains—Buckwheat, oats, barley, wheat germ, sorghum
       Miscellaneous
   Medium (μg/100 g) 10-100
       Seafood—Oysters, scallops
       Meat/Organs—Eggs, chicken heart and kidney, egg white
       Nuts/Seeds—Coconut, peanuts
       Grains—Rice, wheat, wheat bran
       Fruits—Apricots, cantaloupes, raisins
       Vegetables—Corn, green beans, yams, potatoes, spinach, zucchini
       Dairy products—Milk powder, milk
       Miscellaneous—Scotch whiskey, cocoa, flour, sugar cane, molasses
   Low (μg/100 g) 1-10
       Seafood—Fish
       Meat Organs—Beef, beef fat

Fruits—Bananas, plums, strawberries
Vegetables—Carrots, cabbage, celery, lettuce, endive, watercress
Dairy products—Butter, cheese, homogenized milk, skim milk
Miscellaneous—Tea, wine, beer, raw sugar, white sugar, lard, oils

CHEMISTRY

1. **Atomic Properties** (Element)   6, 7, 9, 30, 49
   Periodic table group no.—VI-B, period 5
   Category of element—Transition metal
   Atomic weight—95.94
   Atomic number—42
   Atomic radius (metallic)—1.362-1.390 Å
   Electron shells—2, 8, 18, 13, 1
   Orbital electrons—$4s^2$, $4p^6$, $4d^5$, $5s^1$
   Natural isotopes—Mo^{92} (15.8%), Mo^{94} (9.0%), Mo^{95} (15.7%), Mo^{96} (16.5%),
       Mo^{97} (9.5%), Mo^{98} (23.8%), Mo^{100} (9.6%)
   Long-lived radioactive isotopes—Mo^{90} (5.7 hr), Mo^{93} (7.0 hr), Mo^{93} (10^4 yr),
       Mo^{99} (66.7 hr)

2. **Ionic Properties** (Biological Forms)   6, 7, 9, 30, 49
   Oxidation states (valences)—(Mo^{4+}, Mo^{5+}), Mo^{6+}
   Ionic radius (Å)—(Mo^{4+} 0.70), Mo^{6+} 0.62
   Oxidation potentials
       $Mo^0 \rightarrow Mo^{3+}$ (+0.2 v)
       $Mo^{4+} \rightarrow Mo^{5+}$ (−0.01 v)
       $Mo^{5+} \rightarrow Mo^{6+}$ (−0.53 v)

3. **Molecular Properties** (Biological Forms) (Mo^{6+})   6, 7, 9, 16, 25, 30, 43, 49
   Covalent radius (Å)—1.30 (Mo^{6+})
   Coordination numbers—4, 5, 6
   Stereochemistry—4, tetrahedral; 5, trigonal bipyramid (?); 6, octahedral
   Electron transfer compounds—Mo-proteins, Mo-enzymes
   Typical molecular complexes—$Mo(CNS)_6^{2-}$, $Mo(CN)_8^{2-}$, $MoOCl_5^{2-}$

4. **Analytical Methods**   3, 30, 31, 40, 47, 55
   Physical—Atomic absorption (C_2H_2-N_2O), neutron activation
   Chemical—Spectrophotometric, dithiol complexes
   Hair/Nail analysis—Feasible for hair, values reported
   Comments—Lack of reference standards makes comparisons of methods
       difficult, and reliability questionable

5. **Chemical Properties of Compounds**   6, 7, 9, 49, 54
   See Table 15.1

Table 15.1.   Properties of Molybdenum Compounds

Mo = 6+ (Molybdate)	REACTIONS			SOLUBILITY			
	Heat °C	Air	Water	g/100 cc H_2O	Alc.	Eth.	Acid
Na molybdate $Na_2MoO_4 \cdot 1H_2O$	$-2\ H_2O\ 100°$	NA	alk. pH 9-10	$56.2°$	I	NA	NA
Ammonium molybdate $(NH_4)_6Mo_7O_{24} \cdot 4H_2O$	$-H_2O\ 90°$	NA	acid pH 5-6	43	I	NA	NA

Mo = 6+ (Molybdate)	Density	MW hyd./anh.	MP °C	XL Form	Color XL/Powd.	Appearance Commercial Form	% Element h./anh.
Na molybdate $Na_2MoO_4 \cdot 1H_2O$	3.28	242.0/ 205.9	NA	rhomb.	col./wh.	PL, C, P	39.6/ 46.6
Ammonium molybdate $(NH_4)_6Mo_7O_{24} \cdot 4H_2O$	2.50	1235.9/ 1163.9	d.	monocl.	gr.-yel./?	C	31.1/ 57.7

MEDICINAL AND NUTRITIONAL ROLE

1. **Units of Measurement**
   Weight—μg (microgram); 1 mg (milligram) = 1000 μg
   Concentration—ppm (parts per million) = μg% = μg/100 ml

2. **Human Body Fluid Levels** (Normal) (μg/100 ml)   1, 2, 12, 37, 46
   Blood—1.47
   Plasma/Serum—0.40
   Urine—No data

3. **Human Tissue Levels** (μg/g)   4, 8, 24, 46, 47
   Hair—0.13
   Bone—$<$2.6
   Liver—0.64
   Muscle—0.028
   Brain—0.014

4. **Important Dietary Levels**   5, 21, 27, 30, 37, 39, 46
   Estimated dietary intake—45-500 μg/day
   Deficiency limit (est.)—$<$100
   Toxic limit (est.)—$>$1000
   Recommended daily intake—150-500 μg/day

5. **Estimated Human Daily Balance** (average American diet, 70 kg δ, 30 yr)
   27, 30, 42, 96
   Average intake—300 μg/day (280 food, 16 water, air 0.1)
   Average output—300 μg/day (125 feces, 150 urine, 20 sweat)
   Net gain/loss—Balanced (approx.)

6. **Indications for Supplementation of Above Diet**   5, 27, 30, 42, 46
   Healthy normal—No data
   Special conditions—No data

7. **Factors Affecting Availability from Diet**   17, 21, 27, 37, 46, 53
   Decreased
       See absorption section, antagonists
       High-protein diet
       Acid soils for food plants
       Mo-depleted soils for food plants
       Cu or SO_4 in diet
   Increased
       See absorption section, synergizers
       Mo-enriched soils for food plants

8. **Deficiency Symptoms**   21, 30, 36, 37, 46
Man—Dental caries (?)
Animals—Depressed growth, increased mortality, excretion of xanthine (chicks); xanthine calculi (sheep)

9. **Effects of Dietary Excess** (Molybdenosis) (Salts or Concentrates)   19, 33 36, 39, 46
Acute
    Man—Severe diarrhea
    Animals—Severe gastrointestinal irritation, diarrhea; coma; death from cardiac failure
Chronic
    Man—Gout
    Animals—Cu deficiency syndromes (cattle, sheep); alopecia, dermatosis, anemia (rabbits); deficient lactation, testicular degeneration (rats); diarrhea, loss of hair color (cattle); growth retardation (general); loss of weight, anorexia, osteoporosis (general; bone joint abnormalities (general)

METABOLIC ROLE

1. **Intestinal Absorption**   17, 30, 35, 37, 39, 46
Chemical forms—MoO_4^{2-}, MoO_3, MoS_2
    Preferred valence—$Mo^{6+}(M_0O_4)^{2-}$
    Poorly absorbed—MoS_2
    Well absorbed—MoO_3, $CaMoO_4$, MoO_4^{2-}
Sites—Intestine
Efficiency—40-60%
Active transport (?)
Synergizers (?)
Antagonists—Cu^{2+}, SO_4^{2-}, methionine, protein

2. **Blood Carriers**   17, 30, 37, 46
Plasma protein—Cu-Mo complexes

3. **Half-Life of Element in Blood**   8, 17, 37, 46
95-97% decrease in 1 hr

4. **Target (Initial) Sites**   17, 30, 37, 46
Tissues—Liver, kidney, bone, all tissues
Cells—No data

5. **Storage**   17, 30, 37, 46
    Sites—Liver, kidney, bone
    Forms—No data

6. **Homeostatic Mechanisms**   17, 30, 37, 42, 46
    Relative efficiency in element retention—Relatively effective
    Kidney participation—Main route of excretion, passive
    Intestinal participation—Main reabsorptive area
    Liver (bile) participation—Enterohepatic circulation

7. **Specific Functions** (via Cofactors/Metalloenzymes/Mineralo-Proteins/Ions
        17, 21, 25, 30, 37, 46, 58
    Molecular level
        Electron transfer agent reacts with flavins
        Cofactor for five enzyme redox reactions
        Ligand binding agent
    Cellular level
        Oxidation of aldehydes
        Oxidation of purines (xanthine)
        Oxidation of sulfite
    Organismal level
        Purine metabolism
        Fat metabolism
        Sulfate metabolism (sulfite)
        Detoxication reactions (using SO_4)
        Fe + Cu metabolism

8. **Metalloenzymes, Cofactors, Metalloproteins**   8, 10, 11, 15, 25, 30, 35, 37,
        46

System Types	Organ	Metalloenzyme/ Protein	Cofactors	System Function
Cofactors	Liver, milk	Xanthine oxidase	Mo, Fe, FAD	Oxidizes purines → uric acid
	Liver	Aldehyde oxidase	Mo, Fe, FAD	Oxidation of aldehydes → acids
	Liver	Sulfite oxidase	Mo	Sulfite oxidation
	Bacteria	Nitrogenase	Mo, Fe(?), FAD(?)	Nitrogen → ammonia
	Microorganisms	Nitrogen reductase	Mo, Fe, FAD	Nitrate → nitrite

9. **Excretion**   21, 30, 37, 39, 42, 46
Chemical forms—Molybdate ion, Cu-molybdate complexes
Organs
    Kidney (urine)—40-60% ($\uparrow$ by SO_4 in diet)
    Intestine (feces)   ⎫
                      ⎬ 40%
    Liver (bile, intestine) ⎭
    Skin sweat—5-10%

MISCELLANEOUS

1. **Relationship to Other Minerals**   27, 30, 37, 46, 53
F^-—Synergist in tooth development
Fe^{2+}—Cofactor in various heme enzymes
SO_4 ⎫
WO_4 ⎬ Nutritional antagonists
Zn ⎭

2. **Relationship to Vitamins**   27, 36, 37, 46, 53
FAD (B_1)—Cofactor for xanthine and aldehyde oxidase
NAD (B_3)—Cofactor for xanthine dehydrogenase

3. **Relationship to Hormones**   37, 46, 53
Sex hormones—Sexual impotency of older male may depend on Mo (?)
T4—Levels of T4 affected by Mo

4. **Unusual Features**   21, 30, 36, 37, 46, 50, 53
Mo a powerful protein precipitator
Extremely important for N-fixing bacteria and plants
Sensitivity of Cu metabolism to Mo content of diet
Sensitivity of sheep wool pigmentation to Mo in diet
Possibly aged male sexual impotency linked to Mo deficiency
High concentrations of Mo in dental enamel
Dependence of Mo excretion on SO_4 content of diet

5. **Possible Relationship of Deficiency Symptoms to Metabolic Action**   21, 30,
    27, 36, 37, 46, 53
Dental caries—Synergism with fluoride in tooth development
Depressed growth—Purine intoxication (lack of xanthine oxidase)
Increased mortality (chicks)—Purine toxicity (lack of xanthine oxidase)
Xanthine calculi (sheep)—Lack of xanthine oxidase
Excretion of xanthine (chicks)—Lack of xanthine oxidase

REFERENCES, Part I

1. Altman, P. L., and Dittmer, D. S. (Eds.), *Biology Data Book*, Vol. III, 2nd ed., Fed. Am. Soc. Exp. Biol., Washington, D.C. (1974).
2. Altman, P. L., and Dittmer, D. S. (Eds.), *Metabolism*, Fed. Am. Soc. Exp. Biol., Washington, D.C. (1968).
3. Baker, R. A. (Ed.), *Trace Inorganics in Water*, Am. Chem. Soc., Washington, D.C. (1968).
4. Bowen, H., *Trace Elements in Biochemistry*, Academic Press, New York (1966).
5. Burton, B. T., *Human Nutrition*, 3rd ed., McGraw-Hill, New York (1976).
6. Considine, D. M. (Ed.), *Van Nostrand's Scientific Encyclopedia*, 5th ed., Van Nostrand Reinhold, New York (1976).
7. Cotton, F. A., and Wilkinson, G., *Advanced Inorganic Chemistry*, 3rd ed., Wiley-Inter-science, New York (1972).
8. Davies, I. J. T., *Clinical Significance of Essential Biological Metals*, Charles C. Thomas, Springfield, III. (1972).
9. Dean, J. A., *Lange's Handbook of Chemistry*, McGraw-Hill, New York (1972).
10. Dessy, R., Dillard, J., and Taylor, L., *Bioinorganic Chemistry*, Am. Chem. Soc., Washington, D.C. (1972).
11. Dhar, S. K. (Ed.), *Metal Ions in Biological Systems*, Plenum Press, New York (1973).
12. Diem, K. (Ed.), *Documenta Geigy Scientific Tables*, 6th ed., Geigy Pharmaceuticals, Ardsley, N. Y. (1962).
13. Dickstein, S., *Fundamentals of Cell Pharmacology*, Charles C. Thomas, Springfield, III. (1973).
14. Diplock, A. T., *Critical Reviews in Toxicology*, Vol. 4, Chemical Rubber Publishing Co., Cleveland, Ohio (1976).
15. Dixon, M., and Webb, E. C., *Enzymes*, Academic Press, New York (1964).
16. Eichorn, G. L. (Ed.), *Inorganic Biochemistry*, Vols. I and II, Elsevier, New York (1973).
17. Florkin, M. and Stotz, E. W., *Comprehensive Biochemistry*, Vol. 21, Elsevier, New York (1971).
18. Goodman, L. S., and Gilman, A. (Eds.), *The Pharmaceutical Basis of Therapeutics*, 5th ed., Macmillan, New York (1975).
19. Goyer, R. A., and Mehlman, M. A. (Eds.), *Advances in Modern Toxicology*, Vol. II, Halsted-Wiley, New York (1977).
20. Guyton, A. C., *Medical Physiology*, 5th ed., Saunders, Philadelphia (1976).
21. Hegsted, D. M. (Ed.), *Present Knowledge in Nutrition*, Nutrition Foundation, New York (1976).
22. Hempel, C. A., and Hawley, G. G., *The Encyclopedia of Chemistry*, 8th ed., Van Nostrand Reinhold, New York (1973).
23. Holvey, D. N. (Ed.), *Merck Manual*, 13th ed., Merck & Co., Rahway, N. J. (1977).
24. Hopps, H. C., Biological basis for using hair and nails for analyses, *Science of Tot. Environ.* 7:71-89 (1977).
25. Hughes, H., *Inorganic Chemistry of Biological Processes*, Wiley, New York (1973).
26. Johnson, A. H., and Peterson, M. S., *Encyclopedia of Food Technology*, Avi Publishing Co., Westport, Conn. (1974).
27. Kirschmann, J. D., *Nutrition Almanac*, McGraw-Hill, New York (1975).
28. Klayman, D. L., and Gunther, W. H. H., *Organic Selenium Compounds*, Wiley-Inter-science, New York (1973).
29. Kothny, E. L., *Trace Elements in the Environment*, Am. Chem. Soc., Washington, D.C. (1973).
30. Luckey, T. D., and Venugopal, B., *Metal Toxicity in Mammals*, Vols. I and II, Plenum Press, New York (1977).
31. Marczenko, Z., *Spectrophotometric Determination of Elements*, Halsted-Wiley, New York (1976).
32. Mahler, H. R., and Cordes, E. N., *Biological Chemistry*, 2nd ed., Harper and Row, New York (1966).
32a. Murphy, E. W., Willis, B. W., and Watt, B. K., Provisional tables on the Zinc content of foods, *J. Am. Diet. Assn.* 66:345-55 (1975).
33. Newberne, P. M. (Ed.), *Trace Substances and Health*, Part I, Marcel Dekker, New York (1976).
34. Nicholas, D. J. D., and Egan, A. R., *Trace Elements in Soil-Plant-Animal Systems*, Academic Press, New York (1975).

35. Oser, B. L. (Ed.), *Hawk's Physiological Chemistry*, 14th ed., McGraw-Hill, New York (1965).
36. Pfeiffer, C. C., *Mental and Elemental Nutrients*, Keats, New Canaan, Conn. (1975).
37. Prasad, A. S. (Ed.), *Trace Elements in Human Health and Disease*, Vols. I and II, Academic Press, New York (1976).
38. Rechcigl, M. (Ed.), *CRC Handbook in Nutrition and Food*, Sect. D, Vol. I, CRC Press, Inc., Cleveland, Ohio (1977).
39. Rechcigl, M. (Ed.), *CRC Handbook in Nutrition and Food*, Sect. E, Vol. I, CRC Press, Inc., Cleveland, Ohio (1978).
40. Sauberlich, H. E., Skala, J. H., and Dowdy, R. P., *Laboratory Tests for the Assessment of Nutritional Status*, CRC Press Inc., Cleveland, Ohio (1974).
41. Schrauzer, G. N. (Ed.), *Inorganic and Nutritional Aspects of Cancer*, Plenum Press, New York (1978).
42. Schroeder, H. A., *The Trace Elements and Man*, Devin-Adair, Old Greenwich, Conn. (1977).
42a. Schroeder, H. A., Balassa, J. J., and Tipton, I., Essential trace metals in man; Manganese, *J. Chron. Dis.* 19:545-71 (1966).
43. Sigel, H. (Ed.), *Metal Ions in Biological Systems*, Vols. I-V, Marcel Dekker, New York (1976).
44. Skoryna, S. C., and Waldron-Edward, D. (Eds.), *Intestinal Absorption of Metal Ions, Trace Elements and Radionuclides*, Pergamon, New York (1971).
45. Toepfer, E. W., Mertz, W., Roginsky, E. E., and Polansky, M. M., Chromium in foods in relation to biological activity, *J. Agr. Food Chem.* 21:1, 69-73 (1973).
46. Underwood, E J., *Trace Elements in Human and Animal Nutrition,* Academic Press, New York (1977).
47. Valkovic, M., *Trace Element Analysis*, Wiley, New York (1975).
48. Watt, B. K., and Merrill, A. L., *Composition of Foods*, Ag. Handbook #8, USDA, Washington, D.C. (1963).
49. Weast, R. C. (Ed.), *Handbook of Chemistry and Physics*, 57th ed., CRC Press, Cleveland, Ohio (1976).
50. West, E. S., Todd, W. R., Mason, H. S., and Van Bruggen, J. T., *Textbook of Biochemistry*, 4th ed., Macmillan, New York (1966).
51. Williams, R. H. (Ed.), *Textbook of Endocrinology*, 5th ed., Saunders, Philadelphia (1974).
52. Williams, R. J., *Nutrition Against Disease*, Pitman Publishing Corp., New York (1971).
53. Williams, R. J., and Lansford, E. M., *Encyclopedia of Biochemistry*, Reinhold, New York (1967).
54. Windholz, M. (Ed.), *The Merck Index*, 9th ed., Merck & Co., Rahway, N.J. (1976).
55. Winefordner, J. D., *Trace Analysis*, Wiley-Interscience, New York (1976).
56. Zingaro, R. A., and Cooper, W. C. (Eds.), *Selenium*, Van Nostrand Reinhold, New York (1974).
57. National Research Council, *Recommended Dietary Allowances*, 9th ed., Printing and Publishing Office, National Academy of Sciences, Washington, D.C. (1980).
58. World Health Organization Technical Report, *Trace Elements in Nutrition*, WHO Report #532 (1973).

Part II
Introduction to the Vitamins

The vitamins covered in the next 13 chapters represent the major vitamins now accepted and include the four fat-soluble and nine water-soluble vitamins, all essential to man. Other vitamin-like substances often mistakenly classified as vitamins include inositol, choline, vitamin F (essential fatty acids), vitamin P (bioflavonoids) and PABA. With the exception of one of the essential fatty acids (linoleic) found in vitamin F—these should be termed accessory food substances for humans, since they do not fall within the definition of vitamins for human beings as defined in the introduction. A human dietary requirement in micro-quantities for these five factors has not been definitely demonstrated although they may be demonstrated in other animals and may function as vitamins in these animals. At the time of this writing insufficient data are available to evaluate vitamin B_{17} (Laetrile) and vitamin B_{15} (pangamic acid). The fact that these two substances are extremely controversial makes it very difficult to corroborate any available data; in any case, a definite requirement of B_{17} and B_{15} for humans still needs to be demonstrated. Therefore, the above seven substances will not be covered in this edition. Linoieic acid will be covered in a later edition.

The four fat-soluble vitamins include vitamins A, D, E, and K, which are related chemically because all are synthesized via the cholesterol synthesis pathway. Vitamin A, a cyclic alcohol, has some similarity in structure to vitamins E and K, and, in addition to its cofactor function in vision, may also have other major functions in common with vitamins E and K. Vitamins E and K, being quinones, probably act at membrane sites in electron transfer, redox, or antioxidant functions. Vitamin D acts with hormone-like effects on the DNA in the nucleus, as would be expected, since chemically vitamin D is a sterol similar to the steroid hormones.

The nine water-soluble vitamins include the vitamin B complex (B_1, B_2, B_6, B_{12}, folic acid, pantothenic acid, nicotinic acid, biotin) and vitamin C (ascorbic acid), but they are dissimilar in structure although somewhat similar in action having a coenzyme action (except for vitamin C). Chemically, folic acid, pantothenic acid, and biotin are substituted amino acids, whereas B_1, B_2, B_6, B_{12}, and nicotinic acid are amines or nucleotides acting as coenzymes. Vitamin C is a hexose sugar derivative and acts as a redox and electron transfer agent.

The fat-soluble vitamins require fat or bile salts for absorption, are not excreted as rapidly as the water-soluble vitamins, and are stored to various extents. All vitamins are obtained primarily from plant sources except B_{12} which is obtained from microorganisms. Possible deficiencies in the average American diet are indicated especially for B_1, B_2, B_6, folic acid, C, and E. Therefore, supplementation with these vitamins or revision of the diet should be considered.

Major toxicity of the vitamins has been demonstrated mainly for vitamins A and D although limited toxicity has been noted for vitamins E, K, niacin, C, and B_6. The amounts of vitamins needed per day vary from microgram (B_{12}) to milligram (C) quantities. (See separate table (table 7) NRC data.) Vitamin interactions with hormones are especially noted for T4, STH, Prol, Test. with vitamins A, B_2, and C. Vitamin interactions with minerals are especially noted for PO_4^{3-} (B complex), Cu^{2+}, (B_2, B_6), and Zn^{2+}, (A, E, B_6). Relative concentrations of vitamins in blood serum range from 0.15 μg/100 ml to 1100 μg/100 ml with the remainder of the vitamins falling in between these two extremes, as shown in the accompanying table.

Vitamin Levels in Blood Serum (μg/100 ml)

Vitamin	Range	Average
A	15-65	35
D	1-3	2
E	800-1100	950
K	—	—
B_1	0.5-1.3	0.9
B_2	0.3-1.3	0.8
B_6	3.1-4.3	3.7
B_{12}	.015-.090	0.05
C	300-1000	650
Biotin	.95-1.66	1.3
Folic acid	.16-0.64	0.4
Niacin	50	50
Pantothenic acid	6-22	14

Chapter 16. Vitamin A

Vitamin A is today a mystery vitamin in many of its aspects because so little is known about its functions in the body with the notable exceptions of the eye, and mucous membranes. In the eye it functions as a key constituent of the visual pigment systems necessary for peripheral (rod) and color (cone) vision. However, recent data indicate that vitamin A may play equally important roles in other parts of the body, as, for example, in immune systems and glycoprotein systhesis (connective tissues). Major deficiency diseases are Xerophthalmia and Night Blindness.

Vitamin A is a fat-soluble vitamin, an unsaturated cyclic alcohol, which tends to accumulate in the liver (it is excreted slowly). Toxicity reports have recently indicated 50,000 I.U. daily to be toxic. This toxicity has put limits on the use of the reported selective anti-tumor activity of vitamin A at high doses. Hopefully, a chemical modification of vitamin A will be found that is non-toxic but retains its anti-tumor activity. Vitamin E and zinc act synergistically with vitamin A, whereas cortisol acts antagonistically.

Vitamin A is obtained as such from animal sources and from β-carotene in plant sources, being converted in the intestine to vitamin A. Its absorption depends on the presence of bile and fats in the intestine.

There is no indication that dietary supplementation is needed for the normal adult on an average American diet. Special conditions requiring supplementation are: pregnancy, lactation, infections, fevers, poor vision and hepatic insufficiency. High vitamin A dietary items include: liver, eggs, dairy products, carrots, spinach, kohlrabi, parsley, turnip greens, and apricots.

GENERAL INFORMATION

1. **Synonyms**   7, 16, 18, 35
   Retinol, axerophthol, biosterol, vitamin A_1, anti-xerophthalmic vitamin, anti-infective vitamin, dehydroretinol (A_2)

2. **History**   16, 18, 35
   1912—Hopkins: reported factor in milk needed for growth of rats
   1913—Osborne and Mendel: demonstrated milk factor is fat-soluble; present in other fats also
   1913-15—McCollum and Davis: identified milk factor (fat-soluble A) in butter, egg yolk
   1917—McCollum and Simmonds: found xerophthalmia in rats due to lack of fat-soluble A
   1920—Drummond: renamed fat-soluble A, vitamin A
   1930—Moore: determined carotene a precursor for vitamin A
   1930-37—Karrer et al.: isolated and synthesized vitamin A
   1935—Wald: reported visual purple in retina a complex of protein and vitamin A
   1967—Saffioti et al.: anti-tumor action of Vitamin A

3. **Physiological Forms**   16, 23, 26, 34
   Retinol (vitamin A_1) and esters
   3-Dehydroretinol (vitamin A_2) and esters
   Retinal (retinene, vitamin A aldehyde), 3-dehydroretinal (retinine-2)
   Retinoic acid
   Neovitamin A
   Neo-b-vitamin A_1 (11-*cis*-retinal (visual purple))

4. **Active Analogs and Related Compounds**   14, 16, 23, 26, 34
   α, β, γ-carotene, neo-β-carotene B, cryptoxanthine, myxoxanthine, torular-hodin, aphanicin, echinenone

5. **Inactive Analogs and Related Compounds**   14, 16, 26, 34
   Kitol, xanthophyll, lycopene

6. **Antagonists**   1, 7, 14, 16, 26, 34
   Sodium benzoate, bromobenzene, citral, oxidized derivatives of vitamin A, thyroxine (large concentrations), estrogens, vitamin E (membrane permeability), vitamin D, cortisol

7. **Synergists**   1, 7, 14, 16, 26, 34
   Vitamins B_2, B_{12}, C, E, thyroxine, testosterone, MSH, STH, Zn^{2+}, Ca^{2+}

8. **Physiological Functions**   3, 4, 14, 20, 26, 27, 34
   Growth, production of visual purple, maintenance of skin and epithelial cells, resistance to infection, gluconeogenesis, mucopolysaccharide synthesis, bone development, maintenance of myelin and membranes, maintenance of color (cone) and peripheral (rod) vision, maintenance of adrenal cortex and steroid hormone synthesis, lysosome stability

9. **Deficiency Diseases, Disorders**   3, 4, 14, 16, 26, 27a, 34
   Xerophthalmia, nyctalopia (night blindness), hemeralopia, keratomalacia, hyperkeratosis

10. **Sources for Species Requiring It (essential for man)**   1, 3, 4, 14, 26, 34
    Required by many species (all vertebrates, some fungi)
    Exogenous sources—All vertebrates and some invertebrates convert plant dietary carotenoids in gut to vitamin A, which is absorbed
    Endogenous sources—None reported

CHEMISTRY

1. **Structure**   16, 18, 19, 22, 29, 32, 34, 35

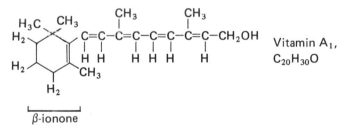

Vitamin A_1,
$C_{20}H_{30}O$

β-ionone

2. **Reactions**   3, 17, 18, 22, 29, 32, 34, 35

Heat—Labile (isomerizes)	Oxidation—Labile (isomerizes)
Acid—Labile (isomerizes)	Reduction—Stable
Alkali—Stable	Light—Labile (isomerizes) (UV
Water—Insol.	inactivates)

3. **Properties**   1, 7, 15, 17, 18, 22, 29, 32, 34

Appearance—Yellow oil	Solubility
MW—286.4	H_2O—Insol.
MP—62-64°C	Acet., Alc.—Sol.
Crystal form—Prisms	Chl., Eth.—Sol.
Salts, esters—Acetate, palmitate	Absn. max.—325-328 mμ
	Chemical nature—Unsaturated alc.
	α_D = 0 (inactive)

Important groups for activity
β-ionone ring
trans-methyl
Alcoholic hydroxyl

4. **Commercial Production**   18, 22, 29, 32, 34, 35
Chemical—Extraction of fish liver
Synthetic—From citral or β-ionone

5. **Isolation**   9, 17, 22, 29, 32, 34, 35
Sources—Fish liver oils
Method—Saponification in alcoholic KOH. Extract with ether, crystallize

6. **Determination**   14, 16, 27a, 33
Bioassay—Growth rate of rats
Physicochemical—Spectrophotometric determination of blue color on reacting with antimony trichloride or trifluoracetic acid
Radioimmunoassay of retinol-binding protein

DISTRIBUTION AND SOURCES

1. **Occurrence**   16, 19, 22, 25, 26, 29, 32, 34, 35
Plants
Fruit—Provitamin carotenoids—apricots, yellow melons, peaches, prunes
Vegetables—Provitamin carotenoids—beet greens, broccoli greens, carrots, endive, kale, lettuce, mint, mustard, parsley, pumpkins, spinach, sweet potatoes, turnip greens, cress
Nuts—Provitamin carotenoids—in small quantity in most nuts
Animals
Vitamin A in all vertebrates, and carotenoids in certain invertebrates (crustaceans) (A_2 especially in freshwater fish)
Location: Liver, heart, lungs, fat, adrenals, retina, kidney, milk, blood plasma, egg
Provitamin carotenoids found in many animals depending on diet
Hen's egg carotenoid mainly xanthophyll (inactive analog)
Microorganisms: Provitamin carotenoids in algae, fungi, bacteria. No intestinal synthesis of vitamin A

2. **Dietary Sources (Vitamin A and procarotenoids)**   3, 8, 20, 27, 30, 34, 36
High: 10,000-76,000 I.U./100 g
Liver (beef, pig, sheep, calf, chicken)

Liver oil (cod, halibut, salmon, shark, sperm whale)

Carrots, mint, kohlrabi, parsley, spinach, turnip greens, dandelion greens, palm oil

Medium: 1000-10,000 I.U./100 g

Butter, cheese (except cottage), egg yolk, margarine, dried milk, cream

White fish, eel

Kidneys (beef, pig, sheep), liver (pork)

Mangoes, apricots, yellow melons, peaches, cherries (sour), nectarines

Beet greens, broccoli, endive, kale, mustard, pumpkin, sweet potatoes, watercress, tomatoes, leek greens, chicory, chives, collards, fennel, butterhead and romaine lettuce, squash (acorn, butternut, hubbard), chard

Low: 100-1000 I.U./100 g

Milk

Herring, salmon, oyster, carp, clams, sardines

Grapes, bananas, berries (black-, goose-, rasp-, boysen-, logan-, blue-), sweet cherries, olives, oranges, avocados, prunes, kumquats, pineapples, plums, rhubarb, tangerines, red currants

Summer and zucchini squash, asparagus, beans (except kidney), brussels-sprouts, cabbages, leeks, peas, artichokes, corn, cucumbers, lentils (dry), peppers, lettuce, celery, cowpeas, rutabagas, okra

Hazelnuts, peanuts, black walnuts, cashew, pecans, pistachios

MEDICAL AND NUTRITIONAL ROLE

1. **Units**   8, 16, 17, 26, 34

   1 I.U. = 0.344 μg vitamin A acetate = 0.3 μg retinol = 0.6 μg β carotene

   1 R.E. (retinol equivalent) = 1 μg retinol

2. **Normal Blood Levels**   4, 14, 26, 33, 34

   15-65 R.E./100 ml serum

   50-215 I.U./100 ml serum

3. **Recommended Allowances**   4, 8, 21, 24, 27, 37

   Children—1300-2300 I.U./day (400-700 R.E./day)

   Adults— $\left\{ \begin{array}{l} 3300 \text{ I.U./day} \\ 1000 \text{ R.E./day} \end{array} \right\}$ (males); $\left\{ \begin{array}{l} 2640 \text{ I.U./day} \\ 800 \text{ R.E./day} \end{array} \right\}$ (females)

   Special—Pregnancy $\left\{ \begin{array}{l} 3300 \text{ I.U./day} \\ 1000 \text{ R.E./day} \end{array} \right\}$; Lactation $\left\{ \begin{array}{l} 4000 \text{ I.U./day} \\ 1200 \text{ R.E./day} \end{array} \right\}$

   Therapeutic dosage—25,000-50,000 I.U./day

4. **Administration**   8, 9, 31, 32, 35
   Injection—Parenteral
   Topical—No data
   Oral—Preferred route

5. **Factors Affecting Availability**   3, 8, 20, 27, 27a
   Decrease
       Liver damage
       Impaired intestinal conversion of carotenes
       Impaired absorption (low bile)
       Food preparation (cooking and frying—heat oxidation)
       Presence of antagonists
       Illness—increased destruction and excretion
   Increase
       Storage in body (liver)
       Intestinal conversion of carotenes—T4, insulin increase
       Absorption aids—bile, fat
       Dietary protein—mobilizes vitamin A from storage in liver

6. **Deficiency Symptoms**   3, 4, 16, 21, 24, 27, 27a, 30
   General
       Retarded growth
       Night blindness (nyctalopia)—degeneration of retina
       Hyperkeratinization of epithelial tissues
       Degenerative changes in eye epithelium (xerophthalmia, hemeralopia)
       Atrophy of odontoblasts
   Lab animals
       Poor bone and tooth development
       Resorption of fetus, atrophy of germinal epithelium
       Urolithiasis—urinary calculi

7. **Effects of Overdose, Toxicity**   3, 4, 16, 22, 26, 29, 31, 32, 34
   $> 50,000$ units/day (man)—generally toxic
   Irritability, nerve lesions, headache
   Fatigue, insomnia, painful bones and joints
   Exophthalmia, peeling of skin
   Mucous cell formation in keratinized membranes
   Hepatosplenomegaly
   Abnormal bone growth
   Loss of hair, jaundice, itchy skin, anorexia
   Decreased clotting time
   Elevated serum alkaline phosphatase

METABOLIC ROLE

1. **Biosynthesis**   3, 19, 25, 28
   Precursors
       Animals—Carotenoid conversion
           (except rat, pig, sheep, carnivores, some invertebrates and human
              infants)—cannot convert
           α, β, γ-carotenes, cryptoxanthin, myxoxanthin, torularhodin
       Plants—Cholesterol pathways—acetate, etc., aphanicin, echinenone
   Intermediates
       Plants—Mevalonic acid, squalene

2. **Production**   3, 19, 25, 28
   Species and sites
   Plants (carotenoids)
       Higher plants—Green leaves, yellow vegetables and fruits
       Some algae, fungi, bacteria—carotenoids
   Animals
       Most vertebrates (except rat, pig, sheep)
       Conversion of carotenoids to vitamin A in intestinal wall
       Some invertebrates also convert

3. **Storage Sites**   8, 9, 16, 26, 34
   Liver
   Kidney (rat, cat)

4. **Blood Carriers**   8, 14, 29, 31, 32
   α_1- and α_2-globulins, β-lipoproteins (carotenoids)
   Retinol-binding protein (retinol + esters)
   Chylomicrons in lymphatics (retinol esters)
   Serum albumin (retinoic acid)

5. **Half-life**   8, 9, 29, 31, 32, 34
   Weeks or months

6. **Target Tissues**   14, 16, 29, 31, 32, 34
   Retina, skin, bone, liver, adrenals, germinal epithelium, intestines, salivary
       glands

7. **Reactions**   5, 14, 16, 17, 28
   Coenzyme forms—Neo-b-vitamin A_1, retinoic acid

Organ	Enzyme System	Effect
Adrenal cortex	Hydroxylating—deoxycorticosterone → corticosterone	Activated
Liver	Sulfurylases—ATP + SO_4 = phospho-adenosinephosphosulfate	Activated
Intestine	Esterases—Vitamin A ester → vitamin A + fatty acid	Activated
Intestine	Synthetases—Vitamin A + Fatty acid → vitamin A ester	Activated
Liver	Dehydrogenases—neo-b-vitamin A_1 → retinene, retinal → retinoic acid	Activated
Retina	Isomerases—trans-retinene → cis-retinene (inactive)	Activated
Liver	Hydrolases—Acid phosphatase, β-glucuro-nidase, cathepsin, etc., in lysosomes on hyper- or hypo-vitaminosis A	Released

8. Mode of Action   3, 5, 6, 9, 14, 17, 22
   Cellular
      Anabolic—Synthesis of mucopolysaccharides via "active" sulfate.
         Synthesis of corticosterone
      Catabolic—No data
      Other—Precursor of retinene in retina—forms visual pigments. Maintains stability of lysosomes + cell membranes
   Organismal
      Maintenance of visual sense organs
      Maintains reproductive systems
      Maintains glucocorticoid production in adrenals
      Maintains mucous membranes
      Regulates cartilage for bone development

9. Catabolism   1, 3, 8, 9, 10, 16, 28
   Intermediates—Retinoic acid
   Excretion products
      Urine—Vitamin A (only in disease)
         fatty acid, small soluble molecules
      Breath—CO_2

MISCELLANEOUS

1. Relationship to Other Vitamins   8, 11, 13, 27, 31, 32
   Vitamin C—Plasma vitamin C levels drop on depletion of vitamin A, occurrence and action of vitamins A and C coincide often

Vitamin D—Occurs naturally with vitamin A in animal liver oils. Toxic overdose effects reduced by vitamin A

Niacin—Involved with DPN + vitamin A in activity of retinene reductase

Vitamin E—Decreases serum cholesterol in rabbit when given with vitamin A

Protects vitamin A from oxidation

Similarity of structure to vitamin A

Antagonistic to vitamin A in maintaining membrane permeability

Pantothenic acid—Promotes synthesis of vitamin A in plants

2. **Relationship to Hormones**   8, 11, 13

Thyroxine—Stimulates intestinal conversion of carotene to vitamin A

Increases vitamin A storage in liver

Antagonizes decreased basal metabolism caused by vitamin A

Increases use of vitamin A

Insulin—Stimulates intestinal conversion of carotene to vitamin A

STH—A synergist in growth

Cortisol, aldosterone, testosterone, progesterone—Decreased on vitamin A depletion (chemical adrenalectomy). Production of deoxycorticosterone and other steroids stimulated by vitamin A

Estradiol—Antagonistic to vitamin A peripherally

MSH—Decreases dark adaptation time—synergistic to vitamin A

3. **Unusual Features**   11, 13, 14, 16

Decreases serum cholesterol in large quantity administration (chicks)

Dietary protein required to mobilize liver reserves of vitamin A (Zn^{2+} synergizes)

Decreased in tumors

Coenzyme Q_{10} accumulates in A-deficient rat liver

Ubichromenol-50 accumulation in A-deficient rat liver

Retinoic acid functions as vitamin A except for visual and reproductive functions

Anti-infection properties and anti-allergic properties

Decreases basal metabolism

Detoxification of poisons in the liver aided by vitamin A

Involved in triose $\rightarrow$ glucose conversions

Anti-tumor effects limited by toxicity at high dosages

4. **Possible Relationships of Deficiency Symptoms to Metabolic Action**   11, 13, 16, 27

Growth retardation—Effects on steroid synthesis, bone growth, and membrane structure, and development of epithelial tissues

Keratinization—Effects on membranes and mucopolysaccharide biosynthesis

Bone development—Formation of chondroitin sulfate in cartilage

Reproductive failure—Effects on membranes and steroid hormones
Visual defects—Absence of retinene precursors

5. **Relationships to Minerals (See refs in specific mineral section)**
Synergists—Zn^{2+}, Ca^{2+}, I^- (as T4) small concentrations
Antagonists—I^- (as T4) large concentrations

Chapter 17. Vitamin D

Many of the major functions of vitamin D have recently been disclosed in all their complexity. Its chief function is to regulate (with PTH and TCT) the absorption and excretion in the gut and kidney of both Ca^{2+} and PO_4^{3-}. Other functions may yet be discovered. Because of the critical nature of Ca^{2+} levels in the blood, the importance of vitamin D cannot be overestimated. Owing to its sterol structure and partly endogenous synthesis, vitamin D is now regarded as a hormone by many investigators. Bone formation and metabolic regulation are involved in Ca^{2+} levels. A major deficiency disease is Rickets.

Vitamin D is a fat-soluble vitamin, a sterol similar to cholesterol, which accumulates in the liver and skin and is excreted slowly. It is converted to its active form (1,25-dihydroxycholecalciferol) in the kidney and released into the blood stream. Toxicity reports indicate doses *above* 400 I.U. (10 μg) per day (normal daily dietary intake and synthesis) can be toxic; therefore, vitamin D should be regarded as the most toxic of all the vitamins when used in excess. PTH and Ca^{2+} are its major synergists, whereas TCT is an important antagonist, functioning as part of the Ca^{2+} control system.

Vitamin D is obtained mainly from ultraviolet-irradiated skin and from dietary sources. Its absorption depends on the presence of bile and fats in the intestine.

There is no indication that dietary supplementation is needed for the normal adult on the average American diet, and exposed to sunlight for reasonable periods. Special conditions requiring supplementation are: lactation, infancy, rickets, adolescence, and lack of sunshine exposure. High dietary sources include: liver, liver oils, salt-water fish, and egg yolk.

GENERAL INFORMATION

1. **Synonyms**   7, 16, 18, 35
   Antirachitic vitamin, vitamin D_3, rachitamin, rachitasterol, cholecalciferol (D_3), activated 7-dehydrocholesterol, calciferol, ergocalciferol (D_2)

2. **History**   16, 18, 35
   1918—Mellanby: produced experimental rickets in dogs
   1919—Huldschinsky: ameliorated rachitic symptoms in children with ultraviolet irradiation
   1922—Hess: showed liver oils contain same antirachitic factor as sunlight
   1922—McCollum: increased calcium deposition in rachitic rats with cod liver oil factor
   1924—Steenbook and Hess: demonstrated irradiated foods have antirachitic properties
   1925—McCollum: named antirachitic factor vitamin D
   1931—Angus: isolated crystalline vitamin D (calciferol)
   1936—Windaus: isolated vitamin D_3 (activated 7-dehydrocholesterol)
   1971—DeLuca et al.: active form of vitamin D is 1, 25 $(OH)_2D_3$

3. **Physiological Forms**   16, 23, 26, 34
   Vitamin D_2 (calciferol, ergocalciferol), vitamin D_3 (cholecalciferol), phosphate esters of D_2, D_3, 25-hydroxycholecalciferol, 1,25-dihydroxycholecalciferol (active form), 5,25-dihydroxycholecalciferol

4. **Active Analogs and Related Compounds**   14, 16, 23, 26, 34
   Irrad. [22-dihydroergosterol (vitamin D_4), 2-dehydrostigmasterol (vitamin D_6), 7-dehydrositosterol (vitamin D_5)] ; dihydrotachysterol

5. **Inactive Analogs and Related Compounds**   14, 16, 26, 34
   Lumisterol, tachysterol, ergosterol, 7-dehydrocholesterol

6. **Antagonists**   1, 7, 14, 16, 26, 34
   Toxisterol, phytin, phlorizin, cortisone, cortisol, thyrocalcitonin, PTH, F^-, K^+, vitamin A

7. **Synergists**   1, 7, 14, 16, 26, 34
   Niacin, PTH, STH, Ca^{2+}, Mg^{2+}, Na^+, PO_4^{3-}

8. Physiological Functions   3, 4, 14, 20, 26, 27a, 34

Normal growth (via bone growth); Ca^{2+} and PO_4^{3-} absorption from intestine; antirachitic; increases tubular PO_4^{3-} reabsorption; increases citrate blood levels; maintains and activates alkaline phosphatase in bone; maintains serum calcium and phosphorus levels

9. Deficiency Diseases, Disorders   3, 4, 14, 16, 26, 27a, 34

Rickets, osteomalacia, hypoparathyroidism

10. Sources for Species Requiring It   1, 3, 4, 14, 26, 34

Required by vertebrates (essential for man) Exogenous sources—Infant vertebrates and deficient adult vertebrates

Endogenous sources—Adult vertebrates (synthesized in skin under UV irrad.—often insufficient)

CHEMISTRY

1. Structure   16, 18, 19, 22, 29, 32, 34, 35

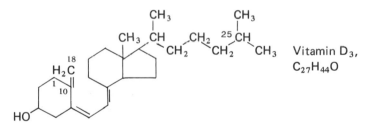

Vitamin D_3, $C_{27}H_{44}O$

2. Reactions   3, 17, 18, 22, 29, 32, 34, 35

Heat—Stable	Oxidation—Unstable
Acid—Stable	Reduction—Stable
Alkali—Stable	Light—Unstable
Water—Insol.	

3. Properties   1, 7, 15, 17, 18, 22, 29, 32, 34

Appearance—White powder

MW—384.65

MP—84-85°C

Form—Fine needles

Salts, esters

    Palmitate, 3,5-dinitrobenzoate

Important groups for activity

    C_{10}-C_{18}—Methylene (C = C)

    Alcoholic—OH

    C_1, C_{25}—OH

Solubility

    H_2O—Insol.

    Acet., alc.—Sol.

    Benz., chl., eth.—Sol.

Absn. max.—265 mμ

Chemical nature—Sterol, alc.

$\alpha_D^{20} = +102.5°$ (alc.)

4. **Commercial Production**   18, 22, 29, 32, 34, 35
Irradiation of ergosterol, 7-dehydrocholesterol
Extraction of fish liver oils

5. **Isolation**   9, 17, 22, 29, 32, 34, 35
Sources—Liver oil, irradiated yeast
Method—Saponify oil, remove vitamin A and sterols by partitioning solvents,
and adsorption chromatography, remove inactive sterols with digitonin,
crystallize as 3,5-dinitrobenzoate ester, saponify, recrystallize

6. **Determination**   14, 16, 27a, 33
Bioassay—Antirachitic test on rats
Physicochemical—Reaction with antimony trichloride; chromatography
and UV absorption

DISTRIBUTION AND SOURCES

1. **Occurrence**   16, 19, 22, 25, 26, 29, 32, 34, 35
Plants
Fruit—None
Vegetables—Grain and vegetable oils (provitamins)
Nuts—None
Animals: Tuna, halibut, codliver oils
Egg yolk, milk (irrad.), bones, intestine, blood, brain, skin, spleen, fish
liver
Shrimp, molluscs
Microorganisms: Yeast, algae, bacteria (provitamins)

2. **Dietary Sources**   3, 8, 20, 27, 30, 34, 36
High: 1000-25 $\times$ 10^6 I.U./100 g
Liver oils (bonito, tuna, lingcod, sea bass, swordfish, halibut, herring,
cod, sablefish, soupfin shark)
Medium: 100-1000 I.U./100 g
Egg yolk, margarine, lard, herring, salmon, mackerel, pilchards, sardines,
shrimp, tuna, kippers
Low: 10-100 I.U./100 g
Grain and vegetable oils
Cod roe, halibut
Butter, cream, eggs, cheeses, milk (vitamin D or irrad.)
Liver (calf, pork, lamb, beef)
Veal, horse meat, beef

MEDICAL AND NUTRITIONAL ROLE

1. **Units** 8, 16, 17, 26, 34
   1 U.S.P. = 1 I.U. = 0.025 μg vitamin D_3 (cholecalciferol); 1 μg = microgram
   1 μg D_3 = 40 I.U. D_3; 1 ng = .001 μg = nanogram

2. **Normal Blood Levels** 4, 14, 26, 33, 34
   1.0-3.0 μg/100 ml (serum); 40-120 I.U./100 ml serum
   2.6-5.8 ng/100 ml [1,25(OH)$_2$D$_3$] plasma

3. **Recommended Allowances** 4, 8, 21, 24, 27, 37
   Children—400 I.U./day
   Adults—None in equatorial zones; 200 I.U./day in temperate zones (available in normal diet)
   Special—Pregnancy, 400 I.U./day; lactation, 400 I.U./day; senility, night workers, miners, northern people
   Therapeutic dose—400-1600 I.U./day

4. **Administration** 8, 9, 31, 32, 35
   Injection—Subcutaneous, intraperitoneal, intramuscular (D_3 esters)
   Topical—Absorbed through skin
   Oral—Preferred route

5. **Factors Affecting Availability** 3, 8, 20, 27, 27a
   Decrease
   　　Liver damage
   　　Presence of antagonists
   　　Presence of phytin in gut
   　　Low bile salts in gut
   　　High pH in gut
   　　Destruction by intestinal flora
   　　Excretion in feces
   Increase
   　　Storage in liver, skin
   　　Absorption aids—Bile salts
   　　Long-acting feature (slow destruction)
   　　Decrease in pH of lower intestine
   　　Irradiation by UV

6. **Deficiency Symptoms** 3, 4, 16, 21, 24, 27, 27a, 30
   In young or experimental animals, including man
   　　Retarded growth—Rickets
   　　Malformation of long bones—Rickets

Skeletal malformation
Demineralization of bone
Decreased blood calcium and phosphorus
Increased serum alkaline phosphatase

7. **Effects of Overdose (Man), Toxicity**   3, 4, 16, 22, 26, 29, 31, 32, 34
   4000 (or more) I.U./day—Generally toxic
      Anorexia, nausea, thirst, diarrhea, renal failure
      Polyuria, muscular weakness, joint pains
      Increased serum calcium—Calcification of soft tissues (metastatic)
      Resorption of bone
      Arterial lesions and kidney injury (rats)

METABOLIC ROLE

1. **Biosynthesis**   3, 19, 25, 28
   Precursors—Animals: cholesterol (skin—UV) conversion in liver to
      $25\text{-}(OH)D_3$ in kidney to $1,25\text{-}(OH)_2 D_3$; plants: ergosterol (algae, yeast—
      UV)
   Intermediates- Plants: pre-ergocalciferol, tachysterol, 7-dehydrocholesterol
                Animals: acetate → mevalonate → squalene → cholesterol

2. **Production: Species and site**   3, 19, 25, 38
   Plants—Leaves, seeds, shoots (provitamins)
   Fungi—Various
   Bacteria—Various, but no intestinal synthesis
   Animals—Skin

3. **Storage Sites**   8, 9, 16, 26, 34
   Animals—Liver, skin

4. **Blood Carriers**   8, 14, 29, 31, 32
   Lipoproteins $(\alpha + \beta)$

5. **Half-life**   8, 9, 29, 31, 32, 34
   Long-acting (days, weeks)

6. **Target Tissues**   14, 16, 29, 31, 32, 34
   Kidney, bone, intestine, liver
   Liver—Transforms D_3 to $25 (OH) D_3$
   Kidney—Transforms $25 (OH) D_3$ to $1,25 (OH)_2 D_3$ (active form)

7. **Reactions**   5, 14, 16, 17, 28
   Reactive form—1,25-Dihydroxycholecalciferol
   Coenzyme forms—Phosphorylated vitamin D

Organ	Enzyme System	Effect
Intestine	Phytase	Activated
Serum	Alk. phosphatase—Organic phosphate (serum) → inorganic phosphate	Activated
Liver	Phosphorylase—Glycogen → glucose-1-phosphate	Activated

8. **Mode of Action**   3, 5, 6, 9, 14, 17, 22
   Cellular
       Anabolic—Increases protein synthesis in intestinal cells, esp. Ca^{2+}-binding protein
       Catabolic
       Depresses protein synthesis except in intestinal cells
       Other
           Decreases citrate oxidation
           Increases release of calcium by mitochondria
           Activates active transport of calcium by intestinal cells
           Repair of mitochondrial membrane
           Acts on DNA template to form Ca^{2+}-binding protein in intestinal cells
   Organismal
       Promotes normal bone calcification
       Increases formation of osteoclasts and capillaries in cartilage—Increases cartilage degeneration in normal bone calcification
       Regulates phosphorus and calcium metabolism—Increases calcium absorption by intestine via Ca^{2+} binding protein—Maintains normal serum calcium and phosphorus levels
       Mobilizes phosphorus from soft tissues
       Mobilizes calcium from bone in hypocalcemia (with PTH)
       Converts organic phosphates to inorganic phosphates
       Catabolic

9. **Catabolism**   1, 3, 8, 9, 10, 16, 28
   Intermediates—Similar to cholesterol conversion products: bile acids and steroid hormones
   Excretion products
       No vitamin D in urine (human)
       Animals—Excess vitamin D into feces
       Humans—70% of ingested vitamin D in feces as fecal sterols

MISCELLANEOUS

1. **Relationship to Other Vitamins**   8, 11, 13, 27, 31, 32
   Vitamin A—reduces toxic effects of vitamin D; occurs naturally with vitamin D in many fish oils
   Vitamin B_1—Increases tolerance of vitamin D

2. **Relationship to Hormones**   8, 11, 13
   Parathormone—Activity intensified by vitamin D; deficiency of vitamin D stimulates parathyroid
   Cortisone—Antagonizes effect of vitamin D on citrate metabolism
   STH—A synergist in growth

3. **Unusual Features**   11, 13, 14, 16
   Has hormonal qualities due to internal synthesis, action on DNA
   Vitamin D_2 has little activity for chickens; species differ in response
   May play role in aging calcification phenomena, especially in skin
   Absorbed through skin
   Amply available for adults from most diets and skin synthesis
   Long-acting, stored
   Furred and feathered animals obtain vitamin D in grooming and licking
   Fish thought to obtain vitamin D from marine invertebrates
   Useful in lead poisoning treatment
   Active tissue form: $1,25 \ (OH)_2 \ D_3$ is formed in kidney

4. **Possible Relationships of Deficiency Symptoms to Metabolic Action**   11, 13, 16, 27
   Decreased growth—Retarded calcification and bone growth
   Increased alkaline phosphatase—Attempt by organism to increase inorganic phosphate
   Osteomalacia—Demineralization of bone, (e.g., in pregnancy)
   Skeletal malformation—Retarded calcification

5. **Relationships to Minerals (See refs in specific mineral section)**
   Synergists—Ca^{2+}, Mg^{2+}, Na^+, PO_4^{3-}
   Antagonists—K^+, F^-
   Regulates—Absorption of PO_4^{3-} ($\uparrow$) in gut and kidney, also Ca^{2+}

Chapter 18. Vitamin E

Vitamin E is today perhaps the most mysterious of all known major vitamins, although recently some of its functions have become clearer. With the demonstration of the essentiality of Se (selenium) and its synergism with vitamin E, the antioxidant function of vitamin E seems to be the major one, although others will most likely be discovered. The cooperative action of Se and vitamin E preserves membranes from destruction by oxidation products and especially retards hemolysis of red blood cells. Vitamin E alone prevents fetal reabsorption in rats (not in humans), a reproductive function. A major deficiency disease or condition is red cell hemolysis.

Vitamin E is a fat-soluble vitamin, a complex alcohol (quinoid), which slowly accumulates in liver and fatty tissues and is excreted fairly rapidly. Toxicity reports indicate certain individuals are susceptible to high blood pressure, allergies, and Fe^{2+} metabolic derangements in the presence of excess vitamin E. Proponents of the lipid peroxidation or free-radical theory of aging claim vitamin E involvement in aging. Confirmation with controlled experiments is needed. Many claims have been made for its use in megadoses by athletes and others; these claims require confirmation because of high individual variability of response. Vitamin A and Se act synergistically with vitamin E, whereas Fe^{2+} acts antagonistically.

Vitamin E is obtained from plant sources and requires bile and fats for its efficient absorption.

There is at present some indication that dietary supplementation of vitamin E may be needed for the average American diet of a normal adult individual, especially in view of the removal or inactivation of vitamin E during food processing and its fairly rapid excretion.

Special conditions requiring supplementation are: pregnancy, newborn infancy, air pollution, diets of processed foods, and high-polyunsaturated-fat diets. High dietary vitamin E items include: wheat germ, crude vegetable and grain oils, soybeans, and yeast.

GENERAL INFORMATION

1. **Synonyms**   7, 16, 18, 35
    α-Tocopherol, antisterility vitamin, 5,7,8,-trimethyltocol, Epsilan, Ephynal, Tokopharm, factor X

2. **History**   16, 18, 35
    1922—Evans and Bishop: reported dietary factor "X" needed for normal rat reproduction
    1922—Matill: found dietary factor "X" in yeast or lettuce
    1923—Evans et al.: found factor "X" in alfalfa, wheat, oats, meat, butterfat
    1924—Sure: named factor "X" vitamin E
    1936—Evans et al.: demonstrated vitamin E belongs to tocopherol family of compounds—isolated several active tocopherols—vitamin E (α-tocopherol) most active of tocopherols
    1938—Fernholz: determined structure of vitamin E
    1938—Karrer: synthesized vitamin E
    1956—Green: discovered eighth tocopherol
    1971—Menzel et al.: vitamin E protects lungs from ozone in air pollution

3. **Physiological Forms**   16, 23, 26, 34
    d-α-tocopherol, tocopheronolactone, and their phosphate esters

4. **Active Analogs and Related Compounds**   14, 16, 23, 26, 34
    dl-α-Tocopherol, l-α-tocopherol, esters (succinate, acetate, phosphate), β, γ, ζ_1, ζ_2 tocopherols

5. **Inactive Analogs and Related Compounds**   14, 16, 26, 34
    δ, ε, η-Tocopherols

6. **Antagonists**   1, 7, 14, 16, 26, 34
    α-Tocopherol quinone, oxidants, codliver oil, thyroxine, Fe^{3+}

7. **Synergists**   1, 7, 14, 16, 26, 34
    Vitamins A, B_6, B_{12}, C, K, folic acid, estradiol, testosterone, STH, SeO_3^{2-}, Zn^{2+}

8. **Physiological Functions**   3, 4, 14, 20, 26, 27a, 34
   Biological antioxidant (esp. lipids)
   Normal growth maintenance, fertility and gestation
   Protects unsaturated fatty acids and membrane structures
   Intracellular respiration
   Maintains normal muscle metabolism
   Maintains integrity of vascular system and central nervous system
   Detoxifying agent
   Maintenance of kidney tubules, lungs, genital structures, liver and RBC
   membranes

9. **Deficiency Diseases and Disorders**   3, 4, 14, 16, 26, 27a, 34
   Laboratory animals—Degeneration of reproductive tissues, nutritional
   muscular dystrophy, encephalomalacia, liver necrosis
   Man—Skin collagenosis, red cell hemolysis, xanthomatosis, cirrhosis of
   gall bladder, steatorrhea, creatinuria, ceroid deposition in muscle

10. **Sources for Species Requiring It (Essential for man)**   1, 3, 4, 14, 26, 34
    Required by many organisms (all vertebrates, some insects and protozoa)
    Exogenous sources—Man and higher vertebrates, protozoa, some micro-
    organisms
    Endogenous sources—Plants, some microorganisms

CHEMISTRY

1. **Structure**   16, 18, 19, 22, 29, 32, 34, 35

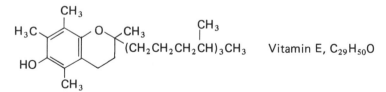

Vitamin E, $C_{29}H_{50}O$

2. **Reactions**   3, 17, 18, 22, 29, 32, 34, 35

   Heat—Labile   Oxidation—Labile
   Acid—Stable   Reduction—Stable
   Alkali—Labile   Light—Labile (esp. UV)
   Water—Insol.

3. **Properties**   1, 7, 15, 17, 18, 22, 29, 32, 34

   Appearance—Yellow oil   Solubility
   MW—430.7 H_2O—Insol.

MP—2.5-3.5°C

Crystal form—No data

Salts, esters—Succinate, acetate, phosphate

Important groups for activity

Hydroxyl (alcoholic)

Acet., Alc.—Sol.

Benz., Chl., Eth.—Sol.

Absn. max.—292 mμ (alc.)

Chemical nature: aromatic quinoid, alc.

$\alpha_D^{25} = +0.32°$ (alc.)

4. **Commercial Production**   18, 22, 29, 32, 34, 35

Molecular distillation from vegetable oils, "stripping" of vegetable oils

5. **Isolation**   9, 17, 22, 29, 32, 34, 35

Sources—Wheat germ oil, soybean oil, rice oil

Method

Saponify oil with methanolic KOH

Nonsaponifiable fraction has vitamin E, dissolve in ether

Remove sterols with digitonin precipitation

Remove xanthophylls with methanol extraction

Convert tocopherols to allophanate esters with cyanic acid

Crystallize allophanates, hydrolyze, extract vitamin E with ether

6. **Determination**   14, 16, 27a, 33

Bioassay

Rats—Prevent fetal resorption and RBC hemolysis

Chick—Liver storage

Physicochemical—Colorimetric two-dimensional paper chromatography; thin layer chromatography; fluorimetry

DISTRIBUTION AND SOURCES

1. **Occurrence**   16, 19, 22, 25, 26, 29, 32, 34, 35

Plants

Fruits—Apples, olives

Vegetables—Legumes, lettuce, spinach, corn, soybean (oil), mustard, cauliflower, green peppers, turnip greens, kale, kohlrabi, sweet potatoes

Nuts and seeds—Coconuts, peanuts, palm (oil), cottonseed

Grains—Cereals, oils (rice, wheat), oats, brown rice, wheat germ, barley, rye

Animals

Birds—Eggs

Mammals—Liver, fat, muscle, milk, pituitary, adrenals, testes

Microorganisms—Yeast

2. **Dietary Sources**   3, 8, 20, 27, 30, 34, 36
High: 50-300 mg/100 g
  Oils, crude—(cottonseed, corn soybean, safflower, wheat germ, sunflower, sesame, castor)
  Margarine, mayonnaise, sunflower seeds
Medium: 5-50 mg/100 g
  Oils, crude—(coconut, peanut, olive, codliver, palm, walnut)
  Wheat germ, apple seeds, alfalfa, barley, dry soybeans, lima beans, poppy and sesame seeds
  Chocolate, rose hips, cocoa butter, peanut butter, mint, corn, sweet potatoes
  Almonds, brazils, chestnuts, filberts, pecans, walnuts, peanuts
Low: 0.5-5 mg/100 g
  Brussels sprouts, carrots, parsnips, mustard, corn, brown rice, lettuce, cauliflower, peas, asparagus, turnip greens, kale, kohlrabi, green peppers, spinach, cabbage
  Bacon, beef, lamb, pork, veal, beef liver
  Eggs, butter, cheese
  Whole wheat flour, dried navy beans, corn meal, oatmeal, coconut, rye, oats, wheat
  Blackberries, pears, apples, olives
  Cashews, yeast

MEDICAL AND NUTRITIONAL ROLE

1. **Units**   8, 16, 17, 26, 34
1 mg d-α-tocopherol = 1.49 I.U.
1 mg dl-α-tocopherol acetate = 1 I.U.

2. **Normal Blood Levels (Man)**   4, 14, 26, 33, 34
0.8-1.1 mg/100 ml (serum); 0.22-0.24 mg/100 ml RBC

3. **Recommended Allowances**   4, 8, 21, 24, 27, 37
Children—5-7 I.U./day
Adults—8 I.U./day (females); 10 I.U./day (males)
Special—Related to unsaturated fatty acid intake: increased requirements in pregnancy and lactation, detoxification, aging, stress
Therapeutic dose—5-30 mg/day

4. **Administration**   8, 9, 31, 32, 35
Injection—Used for large dosages
Topical—No data
Oral—Preferred route

5. **Factors Affecting Availability**   3, 8, 20, 27, 27a
   Decrease
   Presence of antagonists
   Mineral oil ingestion
   Presence of vitamin E oxidation products
   Occurrence with other less active analogues
   Excretion in feces
   Impaired fat absorption
   Chemical binding in foods
   Increased destruction (stress)
   Cooking losses—Heat and O_2 labile
   Losses in frozen storage, steatorrhea, variability of natural sources
   Increase
   Storage in (adipose and muscle) tissue
   Esterification increases stability
   Use of unprocessed fresh food sources
   Absorption aids—Bile salts, oils, fats

6. **Deficiency Symptoms**   3, 4, 16, 21, 24, 27, 27a, 30
   General
   RBC hemolysis
   Creatinuria
   Xanthomatosis and cirrhosis of gall bladder
   Steatorrhea (young)
   Cystic fibrosis of pancreas (young)
   Poorly developed muscles
   Nutritional muscular dystrophy (rats, dogs, monkeys, chickens)
   Myocardial degeneration (dogs, rabbits)
   Resorption of fetus, degeneration of germ epithelium, disturbance of estrus cycle (rats)
   Hepatic necrosis (rats)
   Encephalomalacia (chickens)
   Vascular degeneration (chickens)

7. **Effects of Overdose**   3, 4, 16, 22, 26, 29, 31, 32, 34
   High blood pressure, allergies, gastrointestinal distress, nausea, derangements of Fe metabolism

METABOLIC ROLE

1. **Biosynthesis**   3, 19, 25, 28
   Precursors—Mevalonic acid—side chain (?); phenylalanine—ring (?)
   Intermediates—Tocotrienol

2. **Production: Species and sites**   3, 19, 25, 38
   Plants—Nuts, seeds, cereal germ, green leaves, legumes
   Fungi—Yeast
   Bacteria—Various

3. **Storage Sites**   8, 9, 16, 26, 34
   Muscle—Small amounts
   Adipose tissues—Small amounts
   Liver—Small amount

4. **Blood Carriers**   8, 14, 29, 31, 32
   Lipoproteins, globulins, β-lipoproteins, chylomicrons

5. **Half-life**   8, 9, 29, 31, 32, 34
   Approx. 2 weeks

6. **Target Tissues**   14, 16, 29, 31, 32, 34
   Kidneys, genital organs, muscles, liver, lungs, bone marrow, adrenals, pituitary

7. **Reactions**   5, 14, 16, 17, 28
   Data available on enzyme reactions are questionable as to extent of *direct* involvement in enzyme reactions by vitamin E. Evidently its main role in enzyme reactions is indirect by way of maintenance of reducing conditions, stabilizations of various membranes, or some other undiscovered functions.

8. **Mode of Action**   3, 5, 6, 9, 14, 17, 22
   Cellular
   　Anabolic—Maintains protein synthesis by prevention of formation of enzyme-toxic peroxides from unsaturated fatty acid
   　Catabolic—Participates in oxidation-reduction reactions via CoQ and respiratory enzyme systems
   　Other-Protects unsaturated fatty acids against oxidation; maintains structure of cellular, mitochondrial, microsomal, and lysosomal membranes
   Organismal
   　Anabolic—Increases N retention
   　Maintains kidney tubules and genital organs
   　Maintains muscle cell membranes
   　Detoxifier of toxic agents

9. **Catabolism**   1, 3, 8, 9, 10, 16, 28
   Intermediates—Tocopheryl-*p*-quinone
   Excretion products
       Breath—CO_2
       Urine—Water-soluble degradation products, tocopheronic acid glucuronate
           tocopheronolactone glucuronate, tocopheryl-*p*-quinone
       Feces—60-70% of ingested dose

MISCELLANEOUS

1. **Relationship to Other Vitamins**   8, 11, 13, 27, 31, 32
   Vitamin C—Reduces oxidized vitamin E back to vitamin E in rats; decreased synthesis of vitamin C in vitamin E-deficient animals
   Vitamin A—Conserved by vitamin E in chick; protected against oxidation by vitamin E; synergizes with vitamin E in promoting growth and disease resistance
   Vitamin B_{12} and folic acid—Act with vitamin E in treatment of macrocytic anemia; vitamin E can substitute for or potentiate vitamin B_{12}
   Vitamin K and CoQ—Very similar in structure to vitamin E
   Pantothenic acid—Promotes synthesis of vitamin E in plants

2. **Relationship to Hormones**   8, 11, 13
   FSH and LH—Production increased in vitamin E deficiency
   Testosterone—Testicular degeneration due to vitamin E deficiency in rats causes decreased production of testosterone; high content of vitamin E in testicular tissues, seminal fluid
   Cortisone—Requirements for cortisone and vitamin E increase during stress; high content of vitamin E at sites of cortisone synthesis in adrenal cortex
   STH—A synergist in growth

3. **Unusual Features**   11, 13, 14, 16
   May be involved in aging mechanisms by protecting unsaturated fatty acids and membranes against free radicals
   Only *d*-isomers occur naturally
   Vitamin E replaceable by selenium salts in therapy of rat and pig liver necrosis, and chick exudative diathesis
   Vitamin E replaceable by CoQ and antioxidants for certain symptoms of vitamin E deficiency but not for all; e.g., RBC hemolysis, resorption gestation not affected.
   Species differences in response to vitamin E treatment of similar symptoms, e.g., nutritional muscular dystrophy—rabbits positive, humans negative
   Other tocopherols only slightly active compared to vitamin E

4. Possible Relationships of Deficiency Symptoms to Metabolic Action   11, 13, 16, 27

Nutritional muscular dystrophy, creatinuria (rabbit, monkey)—Maintenance of muscle cell membranes

RBC hemolysis (man)—Maintenance of red cell membranes

Fetal resorption (rats)—Maintenance of uterine membranes and uterine nerve ganglia

Mycardial degeneration (dog, rabbit)—Maintenance of muscle cell membranes

Steatorrhea (man)—Impaired lipid absorption by intestinal cells; maintenance of intestinal cell membranes

Encephalomalacia (chick)—Maintenance of nerve and membrane structures

5. Relationships to Minerals (See refs in specific mineral section)

Synergists—Zn^{2+}, SeO_3^{2-}

Antagonists—Fe^{3+}

Chapter 19.   Vitamin K

Vitamin K is known as the blood coagulation vitamin or the antihemorrhagic vitamin. Some of its functions are not completely clear. Its chief known functions are in liver production of factors needed in clotting mechanisms; however, in lower organisms it functions as part of the energy-generating system (mitochondrial respiratory chain), and also in photosynthesis in plants. Its importance is indicated by the fatal hemorrhages that occur in its absence. A major deficiency condition would be spontaneous hemorrhage.

Vitamin K is a fat-soluble vitamin, a complex quinone, which tends to accumulate in the liver and is excreted slowly. Its toxicity when it is used in excess is well known. Its similarity to the ubiquinone structure (present in mammalian mitochondria) suggests a possible additional role of vitamin K in energy production in higher animals, similar to that already found in bacteria. Its chief synergists are Mn^{2+} and vitamin E, whereas the chief antagonist is coumarin.

Vitamin K is almost totally supplied by intestinal bacteria in man. It is also available from plant and animal sources and requires bile salts and fats for its efficient absorption.

There is no indication that average American diets for the normal adult individual are critically lacking in vitamin K. Special conditions requiring dietary supplementation are: newborn infancy, antibiotic removal of intestinal flora, and certain blood-clotting deficiencies. Items in the diet high in vitamin K are: kidney, cabbage, soybeans, spinach, and cauliflower.

GENERAL INFORMATION

1. Synonyms   7, 16, 18, 35

Antihemorrhagic vitamin, prothrombin factor, Koagulations-vitamin, phylloquinone (K_1), phytomenadione (K_1), menadione (K_3), farnoquinone (K_2), menaquinone (K_2), menaphthone (K_3)

2. History   16, 18, 35

1929—Dam: reported chicks on synthetic diet develop hemorrhagic conditions

1935—Dam: named vitamin K as the missing factor in synthetic diet

1935—Almquist and Stokstad demonstrated vitamin K present in fish meal and alfalfa

1939—Dam and Karrer: isolated vitamin K from alfalfa

1939—Doisy: isolated K_1 from alfalfa, K_2 from fish meal, and demonstrated difference

1939—MacCorquodale, Cheney, Fieser: determined structure of vitamin K_1

1939—Almquist and Klose: synthesized vitamin K_1

1941—Link et al.: discovered dicoumarol

3. Physiological Forms   16, 23, 26, 34

Plant—Vitamin K_1 (phylloquinone, phytonadione)

Animal—Vitamin $K_{2(20)}$

Bacterial—Vitamin K_2 (farnoquinone) ($K_{2(30)}K_{2(35)}$)

4. Active Analogs and Related Compounds   14, 16, 23, 26, 34

Menadiol diphosphate, menadione (vitamin K_3), menadione bisulfite Phthiocol, synkayvite, menadiol (vitamin K_4), vitamins K_5, K_6, K_7

5. Inactive Analogs and Related Compounds   14, 16, 26, 34

Reduced vitamin K

6. Antagonists   1, 7, 14, 16, 26, 34

Dicoumarol, sulfonamides, antibiotics, α-tocopherol quinone, dihydroxystearic acid glycide, salicylates, iodinin, warfarin

7. Synergists   1, 7, 14, 16, 26, 34

Vitamins E, A, C; STH, Mn^{2+}

8. Physiological Functions   3, 4, 14, 20, 26, 27a, 34

Prothrombin synthesis in liver, blood-clotting mechanisms, electron transport mechanisms, growth, photosynthetic mechanisms

9. **Deficiency Diseases, Disorders**   3, 4, 14, 16, 26, 27a, 34
   Hypoprothrombinemia, hemorrhage

10. **Sources for Species Requiring It (Essential for man)**   1, 3, 4, 14, 26, 34
    Many species require it (All vertebrates, some bacteria)
    Exogenous sources: Vertebrates, some bacteria (Intestinal bacteria provide
      it in man)
    Endogenous sources: Plants, bacteria, and all other organisms requiring it

CHEMISTRY

1. **Structure**   16, 18, 19, 22, 29, 32, 34, 35

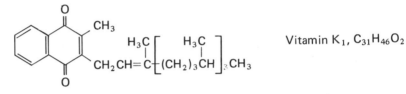

Vitamin K_1, $C_{31}H_{46}O_2$

2. **Reactions**   3, 17, 18, 22, 29, 32, 34, 35

Heat—Stable	Oxidation—Stable
Acid—(Strong) labile	Reduction—Labile
Alkali—Labile	Light—Labile
Water—Insol.	

3. **Properties**   1, 7, 15, 17, 18, 22, 29, 32, 34

Appearance—Yellow oil	Important groups for activity
MW—450.7	Menadiol nucleus
MP— −20°C	Phytyl side chain
Crystal Form—No data	*trans-Methyl* groups
Salts—Disodium phosphate	
Solubility	Absn. max.—243, 249, 260,
H_2O—Insol.	269, 325 mμ (hexane)
Acet., Alc.—Sol.	Chemical nature: Quinone
Benz., Chl., Eth.—Sol.	α_D^{20} = −0.4°C (benzene)

4. **Commercial Production**   18, 22, 29, 32, 34, 35
   Column Chromatography of fish meal extracts

5. **Isolation**   9, 17, 22, 29, 32, 34, 35
   Sources—Fish meal, alfalfa
   Method

Remove chlorophyll from petroleum ether extract by column chromatography on $ZnCO_3$

Reduce to hydroquinone using sodium hydrosulfite

Extract with petroleum ether, alkali, ether

Oxidize hydroquinone to quinone

6. **Determination** 14, 16, 27a, 33

Bioassay—Vitamin K-deficient chick assay

Physicochemical—Polarographic methods; spectrophotometry of pure solutions; prothrombin time determination; fluorimetry

DISTRIBUTION AND SOURCES

1. **Occurrence** 16, 19, 22, 25, 26, 29, 32, 34, 35

Plants:

Fruit—Orange (peel), tomato

Vegetables—Spinach, cabbage, brussels sprouts, alfalfa, cauliflower, soybean (oil)

Nuts and seeds—Hemp seed

Animals: Pork liver, eggs, milk, fish meal

Microorganisms: Intestinal bacteria, *M. phlei*

2. **Dietary Sources** 3, 8, 20, 27, 30, 34, 36

High: 100-300 μg/100 g

Cabbage, cauliflower, soybeans, spinach

Pork, beef liver, beef kidney

Medium: 10-100 μg/100 g

Potatoes, strawberries, tomatoes, alfalfa, wheat (whole, germ, bran), pine needles, egg yolk

Low: 0-10 μg/100 g

Corn, carrots, peas, parsley, mushrooms, milk

MEDICAL AND NUTRITIONAL ROLE

1. **Units** 8, 16, 17, 26, 34

0.0008 mg menadione = 20 dam units = 1 ansbacher unit = .8 μg menadione

1 μg menadione = 1.25 ansbacher units, = 25 dam units

2. **Normal Blood Levels (Man)** 4, 14, 26, 33, 34

Not reported

3. **Recommended Intakes (estimated)**   4, 8, 21, 24, 27, 37
   Children—15-60 μg/day (Supplied by intestinal bacteria normally)
   Adults—70-140 μg/day (Supplied by intestinal bacteria normally)
   Special
      Increases with external temperature
      Newborn infants with neonatal hemorrhage
      Mothers in labor
      Overdosage with anticoagulants
   Therapeutic dose—2-5 mg/day (labor); 1-2 mg/day (newborn)

4. **Administration**   8, 9, 31, 32, 35
   Injection—Intravenous, intramuscular
   Topical—No data
   Oral—Occasionally

5. **Factors Affecting Availability**   3, 8, 20, 27, 27a
   Decrease
      Biliary obstruction
      Liver damage—Cirrhosis, toxins
      Poor food preparation conditions
      Presence of antagonists
      Impaired lipid absorption in gut
      Ingestion of mineral oil
      Sterilization of gut with antibiotics and sulfa drugs
      Excretion in feces
   Increase
      Storage in liver
      Absorption aids—Bile salts

6. **Deficiency Symptoms**   3, 4, 16, 21, 24, 27, 27a, 30
   Hypoprothrombinemia—General
   Increased bleeding and hemorrhage—General
   Increased clotting time—General
   Neonatal hemorrhage—General
   Internal hemorrhage (chick)

7. **Effects of Overdose, Toxicity**   3, 4, 16, 22, 26, 29, 31, 32, 34
   Usually nontoxic, occasionally toxic
   Possible thrombosis, vomiting, porphyrinuria (man)
   Albuminuria (dog)
   Increased clotting time (rabbit)
   Cytopenia, hemoglobinemia (mouse)
   Kernicterus (menadione)

METABOLIC ROLE

1. **Biosynthesis**   3, 19, 25, 28
   Precursors—Polyacetic acid (ring); acetate (side chain)
   Intermediates—Dehydroquinic acid (ring); farnesol (side chain)

2. **Production: Species and sites**   3, 19, 25, 28
   Plants—Green leaves
   Bacteria—Intestinal (main source)

3. **Storage Sites**   8, 9, 16, 26, 34
   Liver (small)

4. **Blood Carriers**   8, 14, 29, 31, 32
   Lipoproteins

5. **Half-Life**   8, 9, 29, 31, 32, 34
   Depletion causes deficiency within 10 days in rat

6. **Target tissues**   14, 16, 29, 31, 32, 34
   Liver, vascular system

7. **Reactions**   5, 14, 16, 17, 28
   Coenzyme form—Vitamin $K_{2(20)}$, CoQ(?)

Organ	Enzyme System	Effect
	Electron transport	
Bacteria	Malate reductase	Activated
Bacteria	DPNH dehydrogenase	Activated
Liver	Vitamin K reductase	Reduction of vitamin K
Liver	Oxidative phosphorylation	Completes system
Liver	Respiratory chain	Completes system

8. **Mode of Action**   3, 5, 6, 9, 14, 17, 22
   Cellular
       Anabolic
           Prothrombin synthesis (liver)
           β-Globulin synthesis (liver)
           Photosynthesis—Hill reaction
       Catabolic—Decreases phosphate incorporation into liver RNA
       Other—Mitochondrial electron transport systems component

Organismal
  Maintenance of prothrombin and clotting factors VII, IX, X
  Control internal hemorrhage
  Anabolic—Increase nitrogen retention

9. **Catabolism**   1, 3, 8, 9, 10, 16, 28
  Intermediates—Lactones
  Excretion products—As glucuronide and sulfate conjugates in urine, bile, feces

MISCELLANEOUS

1. **Relationship to Other Vitamins**   8, 11, 13, 27, 31, 32
  Vitamin E—Synergistic to vitamin K—Maintains reduced state similar in structure to vitamin K_1 and probably interconvertible by way of CoQ and ubichromenols
  Vitamins A and C—Fragility of RBC correlated with vitamins A, C, K

2. **Relationship to Hormones**   8, 11, 13
  STH—Synergist in growth

3. **Unusual Features**   11, 13, 14, 16
  Intestinal absorption of vitamin K in chicks poor
  Side chains of vitamin K identical to those in ubiquinones (CoQ)
  Completely supplied by intestinal flora in normal adults
  Vitamin K lost on γ-irradiation of foods

4. **Possible Relationships of Deficiency Symptoms to Metabolic Action**   11, 13, 16, 27
  Hemorrhage—Decreased synthesis of prothrombin and other clotting factors by the liver

5. **Relationships to Minerals (See refs in specific mineral section)**
  Synergist—Mn^{2+}

Chapter 20. Vitamin B₁

The functions of vitamin B_1 are understood in several general categories: carbohydrate metabolism, nerve conduction, energy production and aerobic metabolism. However, the specific details in each category have yet to be completed. Its major functions are in carbohydrate metabolism where it serves as a coenzyme for decarboxylations in energy production via the Krebs cycle. It also plays a role in nerve conduction, having some function in the membranes. Its major importance is due to the fact that it directly controls aerobic metabolism by way of the Krebs cycle, at the pyruvic acid step. A major deficiency disease associated with B_1 lack is beriberi.

Vitamin B_1 is a water-soluble vitamin, a pyrimidine combined to an organic base, thiazole; it is not accumulated in the body and is excreted rapidly. Vitamin B_1 may be toxic in high concentrations. Megadoses have been administered for individual cases of depression, lumbago, sciatica, facial paralysis, and so on, but their effectiveness needs to be confirmed by controlled testing. Synergists include Mg^{2+}, Mn^{2+}, MoO_4, vitamin B_2, and vitamin B_6. Antagonists are oxythiamine and pyrithiamine.

Vitamin B_1 is obtained from plant and animal sources, but is not stored to any extent. Up to one-fourth of the human requirement may be available from intestinal bacteria. Human requirements are proportional to the amount of calories ingested. There is some indication that dietary supplementation of vitamin B_1 may be required for the normal healthy adult on an average American diet because of cooking losses and refining of cereals and grains.

Special conditions requiring supplementation are: pregnancy, lactation, heavy exercise, alcoholism, high carbohydrate intake, processed food diets, deficiency diseases (beriberi, polyneuritis, etc.), old age, gastrointestinal disturbances, and antibiotics. High dietary contents of B_1 are found in wheat germ, rice bran, soybeans, yeast (killed), and organ meats.

GENERAL INFORMATION

1. **Synonyms**   7, 16, 18, 35
   Vitamin B_1, aneurin, antineuritic factor, antiberiberi factor

2. **History**   16, 18, 35
   1897—Eijkman: ameliorated beriberi in humans by addition of rice polishings to diet
   1911—Funk: isolated dietary growth factor from rice polishings which cured beriberi; coined term "vitamine"
   1915—McCollum and Davis: proposed term "water-soluble B" for antiberiberi factor
   1920—Emmet and Luros: demonstrated two growth factors in rice polishings, including antiberiberi factor destroyed by autoclaving
   1926—Jansen and Donath: isolated crystalline antiberiberi factor from rice bran
   1927—British Medical Research Council: proposed name of B_1 for antiberiberi factor
   1936—Williams: synthesized B_1 and named it thiamine

3. **Physiological Forms**   16, 23, 26, 34
   Thiamine pyrophosphate (cocarboxylase)—Animals
   Thiamine orthophosphate—Animals
   Free thiamine—Plants

4. **Active Analogs and Related Compounds**   14, 16, 23, 26, 34
   Ethyl substituted for methyl on pyrimidine C-2
   Thiamine disulfide, acylated thiamine

5. **Inactive Analogs and Related Compounds**   14, 16, 26, 34
   Reduced thiamine

6. **Antagonists**   1, 7, 14, 16, 26, 34
   Pyrithiamine, oxythiamine, 2-*n*-butyl homologue

7. **Synergists**   1, 7, 14, 16, 26, 34
Vitamins B_{12}, B_2, B_6, niacin, pantothenic acid, STH, PO_4^{3-}, Mg^{2+}, MoO_4^{2-}

8. **Physiological Functions**   3, 4, 14, 20, 26, 27a, 34
Coenzyme in pyruvate metabolism; growth, appetite, digestion, nerve activity, gastrointestinal tonus, carbohydrate metabolism, energy production

9. **Deficiency Diseases, Disorders**   3, 4, 14, 16, 26, 27a, 34
Beriberi, opisthotonos (in birds), polyneuritis, hyperesthesia, bradycardia, edema

10. **Sources for Species Requiring It (Essential for man)**   1, 3, 4, 14, 26, 34
Some species require it for life (all vertebrates, some insects and microorganisms)
Exogenous sources—Animals, some (algae, fungi, bacteria); not much available from intestinal bacteria in man, although it is made there
Endogenous sources—Some (algae, fungi, bacteria); sheep and cattle get sufficiency from intestinal bacteria

CHEMISTRY

1. **Structure**   16, 18, 19, 22, 29, 32, 34, 35

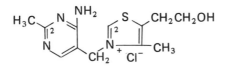

Thiamine hydrochloride, $C_2H_{17}N_4OSCl \cdot HCl$

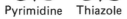

Pyrimidine   Thiazole

2. **Reactions**   3, 17, 18, 22, 29, 32, 34, 35

Heat—Labile	Oxidation—Forms thiochrome
Acid—Stable	(fluorescent)
Alkali—Unstable	Reduction—Unstable
Water—Acid (HCl)	Light—UV decomposes

3. **Properties**   1, 7, 15, 17, 18, 22, 29, 32, 34

Appearance—White crystals	Solubility
	H_2O—1 g/ml H_2O
MW—337.3 (as HCl)	Alc.—sol.
MP—244°C	Acet. Benz., Chl., Eth.—Insol.

Crystal form—Monocl. plates
Salts—Mononitrate,
   noble metals
Important groups for activity
   —OH of —CH$_2$CH$_2$OH
   C-2 of pyrimidine
   C-2 of thiazole

Absn. max.—235, 267 mμ
Chemical nature—Base, alc.,
   substituted pyrimidine
Miscellaneous—Charact. odor; pK_a =
   4.8, 9.2
α_D = 0 (inactive)

4. Commercial Production   18, 22, 29, 32, 34, 35
Synthesis
Pyrimidine + thiazole nuclei synthesized separately and then condensed
Build on pyrimidine with acetamidine

5. Isolation   9, 17, 22, 29, 32, 34, 35
Sources—Rice bran, wheat germ, yeast
Method—Aqueous extraction, adsorption on Fuller's earth; elute with
   quinine sulfate, precipitate as phosphotungstate, decompose precipi-
   tate and reprecipitate with AuCl$_3$, extract with water, precipitate from
   EtOH as hydrochloride

6. Determination   14, 16, 27a, 33
Bioassay—Yeast fermentation; polyneuritic rat—rate of cure; bacterial
   metabolism
Physicochemical—thiochrome fluorescence; polarographic; chromatographic;
   absorption at 235-267 mμ in neutral solution; at 247 in acid solution

DISTRIBUTION AND SOURCES

1. Occurrence   16, 19, 22, 25, 26, 29, 32, 34, 35
Plants
   Fruit—All, low (except gooseberries, plums, which are medium)
   Vegetables—All, low (except beans, green leafy types, cauliflower, corn,
      peas, potatoes—medium)
   Nuts—All, medium (except coconut, which is low)
   Grains—All, medium (except outer grain kernels, bran, polishings, wheat
      germ, which are high)
   Animals: All—medium (except pork, which is high, and some fish, which
      are low)
   Microorganisms: Yeast (killed)—high; intestinal bacteria not available
   Miscellaneous—Mushrooms—medium

2. **Dietary Sources**   3, 8, 20, 27, 30, 34, 36
   High: 1000-10,000 µg/100 g
   > Wheat germ, rice bran, soybean flour
   > Yeast
   > Ham
   Medium: 100-1000 µg/100 g
   > Gooseberries, plums, prunes (dry), raisins (dry), asparagus, beans (kidney, lima, snap, soy, wax), beet greens, broccoli, brussels sprouts, cauliflower, chicory, endive, corn, dandelion greens, kale, kohlrabi, leeks, lentils (dry), parsley, peas, potatoes, watercress, barley, oats, rice (brown), almonds, brazil, cashews, chestnuts, hazelnuts, peanuts, pecans, walnuts
   > Beef, calf, chicken, pork, lamb, turkey meat and organs, mushrooms
   > Eggs, milk, carp, clams, cod, lobster, mackerel, oysters, salmon
   Low: 10-100 µg/100 g
   > Apples, apricots, avocados, bananas, berries (black-, blue-, cran-, rasp-, straw-), melons (cantaloupe, water, honeydew), cherries, currants, dates (dry), figs, grapes, grapefruit, lemons, oranges, peaches, pears, pineapples, prunes, tangerines
   > Artichokes, beets, cabbage, carrots, celery, cucumbers, eggplant, lettuce, onions, parsnips, peppers, pumpkins, radishes, rhubarb, spinach, sweet potatoes, turnips, coconut, cheeses, flounder
   > Haddock, halibut, herring, pike, sardines, scallops, shrimp, trout, tuna

MEDICAL AND NUTRITIONAL ROLE

1. **Units**   8, 16, 17, 26, 34
   1 USP unit = 3 µg thiamine HCl = 1 I.U.

2. **Normal Blood Levels (Man)**   4, 14, 26, 33, 34
   0.5-1.3 µg/100 ml, serum; 3.5-11.5 g/100 ml, blood

3. **Recommended Allowances**   4, 8, 21, 24, 27, 37
   Children—0.7-1.2 mg/day
   Adults—1.0-1.1 mg/day, female; 1.2-1.5 mg/day, male
   Special—Increased requirements in pregnancy and lactation. Depends on body weight, calorie intake, intestinal synthesis and absorption, fat content of diet (increased pyruvate)
   Therapeutic dose—5-30 mg/day

4. **Administration**   8, 9, 31, 32, 35
   Injection—Intravenous, intraperitoneal

Topical—No data
Oral—Preferred route

5. **Factors Affecting Availability**   3, 8, 20, 27, 27a
   Decrease
       Cooking—Heat-labile, water-soluble
       Enzymes in food; thiaminase for vitamin breakdown
       Destruction by $CaCO_3$, K_2HPO_4, $MnSO_4$
       Nitrites, sulfites destroy
       Diuresis, gastrointestinal diseases
       Live yeast, alkali
   Increase
       Cellulose in diet increases intestinal synthesis
       Small storage capacity in heart, liver, kidney
       Bacterial synthesis in intestine (normally none)

6. **Deficiency Symptoms**   3, 4, 16, 21, 24, 27, 27a, 30
   General (man); beriberi
       Anesthesia, hyperesthesia
       Retarded growth, neuron degeneration
       Fatigue, weight loss, anorexia, gastrointestinal complaints, weakness, loss of reflexes, and vibratory sense
       Circulatory and cardiac involvement
       Mental disturbances—Depression, irritability, memory loss
       Muscular atrophy in extremities
       Increased blood pyruvate and lactate
   Lab animals
       Decreased fat stores, decreased body temperature
       Neurological disturbance—Polyneuritis, decrease in tone
       Bradycardia, cardiac enlargement, edema
       Opisthotonos (chickens, pigeons, turkey)

7. **Effects of Overdose, Toxicity**   3, 4, 16, 22, 26, 29, 31, 32, 34
   Humans—Limited toxicity, starting at approx. 125-350 mg/kg dosage; edema, nervousness, sweating, tachycardia, tremors, herpes, allergicity, fatty liver, vascular hypotension
   Rats—Sterility, B_6 deficiency

METABOLIC ROLE

1. **Biosynthesis** 3, 19, 25, 28
   Precursors—Thiazole, pyrimidine pyrophosphate
   Intermediates—Thiamine phosphate

2. **Production Sites** 3, 19, 25, 28
   Plants—Grain and cereal germ
   Bacteria—Intestinal

3. **Storage Sites** 8, 9, 16, 26, 34
   Heart, liver, kidney, brain (all small amounts)

4. **Blood Carriers** 8, 14, 29, 31, 32
   Blood cells—as cocarboxylase; serum—free B_1

5. **Half-life** 8, 9, 29, 31, 32, 34
   1 mg/day destroyed in tissues

6. **Target Tissues** 14, 16, 29, 31, 32, 34
   Heart, liver, kidney, peripheral nerves, brain

7. **Reactions** 5, 14, 16, 17, 28
   Coenzyme forms—Cocarboxylase (thiamine pyrophosphate, disphosphothia-mine); needs Mg^{2+} ion

Organ	Enzyme System	Effect
Liver, plants	Transketolase	Activated
Serum	Choline esterase	Inhibited
Liver, yeast	Thiaminokinase—thiamine → cocarboxylase	Activated
	Decarboxylases:	
Plants	Nonoxidate decarboxylation of pyruvate to OAA	Activated
Liver (mammals)	Oxidative decarboxylation of pyruvate with lipoic acid	Activated
Liver (mammals)	Phosphoroclastic cleavage of α-keto acids	Activated
Liver (mammals)	Formation of acetoin	Activated
Liver (mammals)	Oxidative decarboxylation of α-ketoglutarate to succinate	Activated

8. **Mode of Action**   3, 5, 6, 9, 14, 17, 22
   Cellular
   Anabolic—Condensations, synthesis of acetylcholine
   Catabolic—α-Keto acid decarboxylation (Krebs cycle coenzyme—ATP generation), oxidations, dismutations
   Other—Transketolation, formation of NADPH, and ribose via HMP shunt, acyl transfer agent—"active" acetaldehyde
   Organismal
   Maintenance of nerve tissues
   Maintenance of heart muscle
   Decrease blood pyruvate and lactate
   Maintain supply of ATP
   Normal growth maintenance

9. **Catabolism**   1, 3, 8, 9, 10, 16, 28
   Intermediates—pyrimidine; excretion products—pyrimidine and thiamine (.042-.420 mg/day)

MISCELLANEOUS

1. **Relationship to Other Vitamins**   8, 11, 13, 27, 31, 32
   Vitamin B_{12}—Synergistic to B_1
   Pantothenic acid, niacin, riboflavin—Energy from oxidation of carbohydrates depends on synergism with thiamine (oxidative decarboxylation)
   Vitamin C—Decreases requirement for B_1
   Vitamin B_6—Overdose of B_1 causes B_6 deficiency in rats
   Vitamin D—Tolerance increased by vitamin B_1
   Riboflavin, pyridoxine—Synergize with thiamine to produce niacin

2. **Relationship to Hormones**   8, 11, 13
   Acetylcholine—Synthesis requires vitamin B_1
   Thyroxine—Metabolic rate increase in hyperthyroidism increases B_1 requirement
   Insulin—In diabetes B_1 content of blood and liver reduced
   STH—Synergist in growth

3. **Unusual features**   11, 13, 14, 16
   Hormonal function in plants—Controls root growth
   Phosphorylation in liver, dephosphorylation in kidney
   Vitamin B enzymes easily poisoned by heavy metals, mustard gas, acetyl iodide
   Plant and animal cocarboxylases identical

Has a diuretic effect, is constipative
Can be allergenic on injection
Blood contains most cocarboxylase in leukocytes
Thiamine-sparing action by alcohol, fat, protein
Not available from intestinal bacteria

4. **Possible Relationships of Deficiency to Metabolic Action**   11, 13, 16, 27

Weight loss
Gastrointestinal complaints
Fatigue $\left.\right\}$ Flooding of system with pyruvate
Anorexia

Polyneuritis
Mental disturbances $\left.\right\}$ Decreased synthesis of acetylcholine
Circulatory and cardiac involvement

5. **Relationship to Minerals (See references in specific mineral section)**

Synergists—Mg^{2+}, Mn^{2+}, MoO_4^{2-}, PO_4^{3-}
Antagonists—$CaCO_3$, K_2HPO_4, $Mn\ SO_4$ (large concentrations will destroy B_1)

Chapter 21. Vitamin B$_2$

Vitamin B$_2$ functions principally in various coenzyme components of cellular respiration, i.e., the mitochondrial energy system. It is also concerned with fetal development, as well as maintenance of ectodermal tissues, including the eyes and skin. Its major importance stems from the fact that energy production by the mitochondria cannot proceed without those coenzymes containing vitamin B$_2$ (FAD, FMN, etc.) needed by the respiratory proteins. There is no major deficiency disease associated with B$_2$ lack as there is with B$_1$: a minor disease is cheilosis.

Vitamin B$_2$ is a slightly water-soluble vitamin, a nucleotide and substituted purine that is not stored in the body. No toxicity has been reported. There are no valid reports of any benefits derived from megadose treatment with vitamin B$_2$. It is synergistic with vitamins B$_1$, B$_6$, Fe^{2+}, Cu^{2+}, and PO$_4{}^{3-}$, and antagonized by boric acid and various flavins.

Vitamin B$_2$ is obtained from plant and animal sources, but is not stored to any extent in the body and is excreted rapidly. Although it is synthesized by the intestinal bacteria, a very small amount of this form is available. Human requirements are proportional to energy expenditure. There is some evidence that dietary supplementation of riboflavin may be required for a normal, healthy adult on the average American diet, because of its low concentration in the common foods, its low intestinal synthesis, its low solubility (poor absorption), and its destruction by ultraviolet light and alkaline conditions. Special conditions definitely requiring dietary supplementation are: pregnancy, lactation, liver malfunctions, high energy expenditure, antibiotic treatment, fevers, hyper-thyroidism, and traumatic stress. High dietary contents are found in: organ meats (esp. liver), yeast, and dairy products.

GENERAL INFORMATION

1. **Synonyms**   7, 16, 18, 35
   Vitamin B$_2$, vitamin G, lactoflavin, hepatoflavin, ovoflavin, verdoflavin, 6,7-dimethyl-9-(d-1$'$-ribityl)isoalloxazine

2. **History**   16, 18, 35
   1917—Emmet and McKim: showed dietary growth factor for rats in rice polishings
   1920—Emmett: suggested presence of several dietary growth factors in yeast concentrate, including heat-stable component and B$_1$
   1927—British Medical Research Council: proposed name of B$_2$ for heat-stable component
   1932—Warburg and Christian: isolated yellow enzyme [containing riboflavin (FMN)] from bottom yeast
   1933—Kuhn: isolated pure B$_2$ (riboflavin) from milk; recognized growth-promoting activity
   1935—Kuhn et al., Karrer et al.: achieved structure and synthesis of vitamin B$_2$; named it riboflavin
   1954—Christie et al.: determined structure and synthesized FAD

3. **Physiological Forms**   16, 23, 26, 34
   Riboflavin mononucleotide (FMN); riboflavin dinucleotide (FAD)

4. **Active Analogs and Related Compounds**   14, 16, 23, 26, 34
   Methyl-9-methyl, and 6-ethyl-7-methyl compounds, arabinoflavin

5. **Inactive Analogs and Related Compounds**   14, 16, 26, 34
   3,6,7-Trimethyl-9-(d-1$'$-ribityl)isoalloxazine

6. **Antagonists**   1, 7, 14, 16, 26, 34
   Isoriboflavin, lumiflavin, araboflavin, hydroxyethyl analogue, formyl methyl analogue, galactoflavin, flavin mono-SO$_4$, boric acid

7. **Synergists**   1, 7, 14, 16, 26, 34
   Vitamins A, B$_1$, B$_6$, B$_{12}$, niacin, pantothenic acid, folic acid, biotin, T4, insulin, STH, Fe^{2+}, Cu^{2+}, PO$_4^{3-}$, MoO$_4^{2-}$

8. **Physiological Functions**   3, 4, 14, 20, 26, 27a, 34
   Coenzyme in respiratory enzyme systems
   Constituent of flavoproteins, redox systems, respiratory enzymes
   Growth and development of fetus
   Maintenance of mucosal, epithelial, and eye tissues

9. **Deficiency Diseases, Disorders**   3, 4, 14, 16, 26, 27a, 34
   Glossitis, cheilosis, seborrheic dermatitis, corneal vascularization, anemia

10. **Sources for Species Requiring It (Essential for man)**   1, 3, 4, 14, 26, 34
    Some organisms require it (all vertebrates, some insects and microorganisms)
    Endogenous sources—Some algae, some bacteria, some fungi
    Exogenous sources—All animals, some fungi and bacteria (intestinal bacteria
      make it, but most is unavailable to man)

CHEMISTRY

1. **Structure**   16, 18, 19, 22, 29, 32, 34, 35

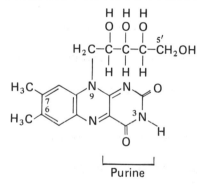

Riboflavin, $C_{17}H_{20}N_4O_6$

Purine

2. **Reactions**   3, 17, 18, 22, 29, 32, 34, 35

Heat—Blackens at 240°C	Oxidation—Decomposes
Acid—Stable	Reduction—Easily $\rightarrow$ leucoriboflavin
Alkali—Labile $\rightarrow$ lumiflavin	Light—Photolyses to lumiflavin
Water—Soluble, acidic	Intense green fluorescence 565 mμ

3. **Properties**   1, 7, 15, 17, 18, 22, 29, 32, 34

Appearance—Orange-yellow powder	Solubility
MW—376.4	H_2O—Sol. 0.01 g/100 ml
MP—282°C	Acet., Alc.—Insol.
Crystal form—Needles	Benz., Chl., Eth.—Insol.
Salts—Borate, PO_4, acetate	Absn. max.—220, 267, 336, 446 mμ

Important groups

  9-N, 5' OH

  6,7-methyl

  3-N

Miscellaneous—pI = 6

[α] $_D^{20}$ = −114° (0.1 N NaOH)

Chemical nature

  Reducing agent; nucleotide

  Substituted purine

4. **Commercial Production**   18, 22, 29, 32, 34, 35

Fermentation bacteria or yeast

Chemical synthesis from alloxan, ribose, and o-xylene

5. **Isolation**   9, 17, 22, 29, 32, 34, 35

Sources—Free—urine, whey, retina; combined—as FMN or FAD—tissues or
  egg whites

Method

  Aqueous extract of tissue treated with ether

  Fractional precipitation with picric acid

  Precipitate out proteins with ammonium sulfate

  Adsorb on Fuller's earth

  Elute with 0.1 N NaOH

  Crystallize from aqueous petroleum ether-acetone mixture

6. **Determination**   14, 16, 27a, 33

Bioassay—Rats—growth rate; microbiological—*L. caseii, L. mesenteroides*

Physiochemical—Fluorimetry, paper electrophoresis, polarography

DISTRIBUTION AND SOURCES

1. **Occurrence**   16, 19, 22, 25, 26, 29, 32, 34, 35

Plants

  Fruit—All, low

  Vegetables—All: high in tomato leaves; medium in green leafy types, corn,
    cauliflower, beans; low in others

  Nuts—All, medium except coconut (low)

  Flowers—Saffron (high)

Animals—All (liver > kidneys > heart > other tissues); high in organs,
  medium in other tissues; crustaceans—high

Microorganisms: All, esp. yeast, anerobic bacteria (high)

2. **Dietary Sources**   3, 8, 20, 27, 30, 34, 36

High: 1000-10,000 μg/100 g

  Beef (kidneys, liver), calf (kidney, liver)

  Chicken (liver)

  Pork (heart, kidneys, liver), sheep (liver, kidneys)

  Yeast (killed)

Medium: 100-1000 μg/100 g

    Avocados, currants

    Asparagus, beans (kidney, lima, snap, wax), beet greens, broccoli, brussels sprouts, cauliflower, chicory, endive, corn, dandelion greens, kale, kohlrabi, lentils (dry), parsley, parsnips, peas, soybeans (dry), spinach, turnip greens, watercress, almonds (dry), cashews, peanuts, pecans, walnuts, rice bran, wheat germ, oats, cheeses, cream, eggs, milk

    Bacon, beef, chicken, duck, goose, pork, lamb, turkey, veal, fish

Low: 10-100 μg/100 g

    Apples, apricots, bananas, blackberries, blueberries, cranberries, raspberries, strawberries, cherries, grapes, grapefruit, melons, oranges, peaches, dates (dry), figs, pears, pineapples, plums, raisins (dry), tangerines, artichokes, beets, cabbages, carrots, celery, cucumbers, eggplant, lettuce, onions, peppers, potatoes, pumpkins, radishes, sweet potatoes, tomatoes, turnips, coconuts, barley, rice

MEDICAL AND NUTRITIONAL ROLE

1. **Units**   8, 16, 17, 26, 34
   By weight, μg or mg

2. **Normal Blood Levels**   4, 14, 26, 33, 34
   0.3-1.3 μg/100 ml, serum; 4.9-10.4 μg/100 ml, blood

3. **Recommended Allowances**   4, 8, 21, 24, 27, 37
   Children—0.8-1.4 mg/day*
   Adults—1.2-1.3 mg/day female*; 1.4-1.6 mg/day male*
   Therapeutic dose—10-30 mg/day

4. **Administration**   8, 9, 31, 32, 35
   Injection—I.V.
   Topical—No data
   Oral—Preferred route

5. **Factors Affecting Availability**   3, 8, 20, 27, 27a
   Decrease
       Cooking (slightly soluble in H_2O)
       Plant foods—Lower availability, bound forms
       Decreased phosphorylation in intestines prevents absorption
       Exposure of foods to sunlight

---

*Related to caloric intake and protein levels. Increased in pregnancy, lactation. Additional sources in intestinal bacteria (small).

Enzymes for breakdown
Gastrointestinal disease
Diuresis
Increase
Storage in heart, liver, and kidneys
Very actively producing intestinal bacteria (small amount)

6. **Deficiency Symptoms**   3, 4, 16, 21, 24, 27, 27a, 30
General
Orogenital syndrome
Stomatitis
Glossitis
Cheilosis
Seborrheic dermatitis
Ocular—Photophobia, indistinct vision, corneal vascularity increased
Rats
Poor growth, ocular abnormality
Dermatitis (eczema—nostrils, eyes)
Myelin degeneration, testicular atrophy
Thymus involution
Dogs
Weight loss, fatty liver, muscle weakness
Opacity of corneal epithelium
Chicken
Egg production and hatchability decline, nerve degeneration
Monkey
Anemia, leukopenia

7. **Effects of Overdose, Toxicity**   3, 4, 16, 22, 26, 29, 32, 34
Essentially nontoxic in man
Anuria—rat
Azotemia—rat
Kidney insufficiency—rat
Paresthesia—man
Itching—man

METABOLIC ROLE

1. **Biosynthesis**   3, 19, 25, 28
Precursors—Purines, pyrimidines, ribose
Intermediates—6,7-Dimethyl-8-ribityllumazine

2. **Production Site**   3, 19, 25, 28
   Plants—Leaves, germinating seeds, root nodules
   Bacteria—Intestinal

3. **Storage Sites**   8, 9, 16, 26, 34
   Heart, liver, kidneys (small amount)

4. **Blood carriers**   8, 14, 29, 31, 32
   As nucleotides

5. **Half-life**   8, 9, 29, 31, 32, 34
   12% of intake excreted in 24 hr

6. **Target Tissues**   14, 16, 29, 31, 32, 34
   Heart, liver, kidneys, others in lesser amount

7. **Reactions**   5, 14, 16, 17, 28
   Coenzyme forms
       Redox couple: oxidized $\leftrightarrows$ reduced form
       FMN, FAD (binding to apoenzyme via cations (Fe^{2+}, Cu^{2+}, MoO_4^{2-}) to
       PO_4^{3-} of coenzyme)

Organ	Enzyme System	Effect
Liver	(1) FMN—Warburg yellow enzyme, cytochrome c reductase, l-amino acid oxidase, succinic dehydrogenase	Activated
Liver	(2) FAD—Xanthine oxidase, d-amino acid oxidase, glycine oxidase, diaphorase, fumaric dehydrogenase glucose oxidases, histaminases, aldehyde oxidase	Activated
Intestine	(3) Flavokinase—Phosphorylation of riboflavin	Activated

8. **Mode of Action**   3, 5, 6, 9, 14, 17, 22
   Cellular
       Anabolic—No data
       Catabolic—Carbohydrate metabolism
       Other—Essential complexed part of flavoproteins
           Mitochondrial electron transport system
           Oxidation-reduction enzyme systems
           Accepts 2H on isoalloxazine ring
           Part of respiratory enzyme system

Organismal
    Ectodermal maintenance—Skin and cornea
    Growth and development of fetus
    Maintenance of nervous system (myelin sheath)
    Resistance to disease

9. **Catabolism**   1, 3, 8, 9, 10, 16, 28
Intermediates—No data
Excretion products
    Urine—Free vitamin—Diurnal variations. Normally ~1/3 of dietary
        amounts excreted (0.14-1.7 mg/day)
    Feces—Uroflavin—Diurnal variations

MISCELLANEOUS

1. **Relationship to Other Vitamins**   8, 11, 13, 27, 31, 32
Vitamin A, niacin—Present with riboflavin in visual structures (retina) involved
    in visual process
Niacin—Riboflavin enzymes utilize DPN, and DPNH
Thiamine—Deficiency of B_1 leads to increased storage of riboflavin; involved
    with riboflavin in thyroxine and insulin utilization in CHO metabolism
Other B vitamins—Synergistic with riboflavin

2. **Relationship to Hormones**   8, 11, 13
ACTH—Riboflavin involved in release of ACTH from pituitary
Thyroxine, insulin—Effective only if riboflavin and thiamine are present
Thyroxine—Incorporation of iodide by sheep thyroid stimulated by FMN
Adrenal hormones—Aid in phosphorylation of riboflavin in intestines
Estradiol—Inactivation in liver decreased in riboflavin deficiency (rat)
STH—Synergist in growth

3. **Unusual Features**   11, 13, 14, 16
High levels in liver inhibit tumor formation by azo compounds in animals
Free radicals formed by light or dehydrogenation: flavine ⇋ semiquinone ⇋
    dihydroflavin
Free vitamin only in retina, urine, milk, and semen
Substitution of adenine by other purines, or pyrimidines destroys activity of
    FAD
Phosphorylation of vitamin in intestines allows absorption as FMN
Blood levels decrease during life in humans
Brain content remains constant
Available in plants as FMN and FAD
Concentrated in bull semen

4. Possible Relationships of Deficiency Symptoms to Metabolic Action   11, 13, 16, 27

Cheilosis
Glossitis
Stomatitis   } Ectodermal manifestations related to other B-vitamin
Seborrheic dermatitis { deficiencies
Corneal vascularity
Orogenital syndrome

Photophobia—Synergistic functions of vitamin A and riboflavin in visual structures

5. Relationships to Minerals   (See specific references in Minerals section)

Synergists—Fe^{3+}, Cu^{2+}, PO_4^{3-}, MoO_4^{2-}
Antagonist—Borate

Chapter 22. Vitamin B$_6$

The major functions of vitamin B$_6$ include participation in the direct line of protein, carbohydrate, and lipid metabolism, as well as its being a coenzyme constituent in amino acid metabolism and in erythrocyte formation. Its major importance stems from the fact that B$_6$ as pyridoxal phosphate coenzyme controls the various types of amino acid transformations and hence the formation of specialized proteins. There is no major deficiency disease associated with B$_6$ lack although minor diseases of the skin, microcytic hypochromic anemia, and acrodynia are well known.

Vitamin B$_6$ is a water-soluble vitamin, chemically a substituted pyridine, which appears in several chemical forms and is not stored in the body. Toxicity has been reported at higher levels (1000mg/day). It is synergistic with Zn^{2+}, Co^{2+}, Mg^{2+}, Na^+, K^+, Cu^{2+}, PO_4^{3-}, and vitamins B$_1$, B$_2$, B$_{12}$, C, E, niacin, biotin, and folic acid. It is antagonized by isoniazid, pyroxidones, penicillamine, and estrogens.

Vitamin B$_6$ is obtained from plant and animal sources, but is not stored to any extent in the body and is excreted rapidly. Although it is synthesized by the intestinal bacteria only a very small amount of it is available. Human requirements are proportional to the protein content of food. There is some evidence that dietary supplementation of vitamin B$_6$ may be required for a normal, healthy adult on the average American diet because of its low concentrations in common foods, losses on refining of foods, its low intestinal availability, its rapid excretion, its instability to light and oxidation (cooking losses), its synergism with most vitamins as well as minerals, and its central location in the metabolism of major nutrients. Special conditions requiring definite supplementation include: pregnancy, lactation, irradiation, inborn errors of metabolism, high protein diets, and stress. High dietary contents are found in: liver, herring, salmon, yeast, nuts, wheat germ, brown rice, and blackstrap molasses.

GENERAL INFORMATION

1. **Synonyms**   7, 16, 18, 35
   Pyridoxine, adermine, pyridoxol

2. **History**   16, 18, 35
   1934—György: cured a dermatitis in rats not due to B_1 or B_2 with yeast extract factor
   1938—Lepkovsky: isolated similar factor from rice bran extract
   1938—Keresztesy and Stevens: isolated and crystallized pure B_6 from rice polishings
   1938—Kohn, Wendt, and Westphal: synthesized pyridoxine, gave pyridoxine its name
   1939—Stiller, Keresztesy, and Stevens: established structure of pyridoxine
   1945—Snell: discovered pyridoxal and pyridoxamine
   1953—Snyderman et al.: first recognized and established B_6 requirement in humans

3. **Physiological Forms**   16, 23, 26, 34
   Interconvertible in vivo (pyridoxine $\rightleftharpoons$ pyridoxal $\rightleftharpoons$ pyridoxamine)
   Animals—Pyridoxal-5-phosphate (codecarboxylase); pyridoxamine phosphate
   Plants—Pyridoxol-5-phosphate, pyridoxal-5-P, pyridoxamine-P

4. **Active Analogs and Related Compounds**   14, 16, 23, 26, 34
   Pyridoxal, pyridoxamine

5. **Inactive Analogs and Related Compounds**   14, 16, 26, 34
   Nor-vitamin B_6, 4-pyridoxic acid, 5-pyridoxic acid

6. **Antagonists**   1, 7, 14, 16, 26, 34
   4-deoxypyridoxine, 4-methoxypyridoxine, toxopyrimidine, penicillamine, semicarbazide, isoniazid, estrogens, Fe^{3+}

7. **Synergists**   1, 7, 14, 16, 26, 34
   Vitamins B_1, B_2, C, E, niacin, biotin, folic acid, STH, glucagon, epinephrine, norepinephrine, Zn^{2+}, Cr^{3+}, Mg^{2+}, Na^+, K^+, Cu^{2+}, PO_4^{3-}

8. **Physiological Functions**   3, 4, 14, 20, 26, 27a, 34
   Protein, CHO, and lipid metabolism
   Coenzyme in many phases of amino acid metabolism; especially in gluconeo-
   genesis, production of neural hormones, bile acids, unsaturated fatty acids,
   and porphyrins
   Erythrocyte formation, growth

9. **Deficiency Diseases, Disorders**   3, 4, 14, 16, 26, 27a, 34
   Monkey—Arteriosclerosis
   Rats—Acrodynia
   Man—Lymphopenia, convulsions, dermatitis, irritability, nervous disorders,
   anemias, seborrheal lesions

10. **Sources for Species Requiring It (essential for man)**   1, 3, 4, 14, 26, 34
    Some organisms require B_6 (all vertebrates, some insects, protozoa, fungi,
    bacteria)
    Exogenous sources—Animals, some bacteria (intestinal bacteria make it, but
    not much is available to man)
    Endogenous sources—Plants, fungi, intestinal bacteria

CHEMISTRY

1. **Structures**   16, 18, 19, 22, 29, 32, 34, 35

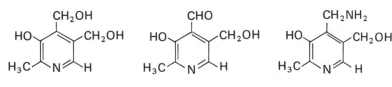

Pyridoxine, $C_8H_{11}NO_3$ Pyridoxal   Pyridoxamine

2. **Reactions**   3, 17, 18, 22, 29, 32, 34, 35

   Heat—Stable   Oxidation—Unstable
   Acid—Stable   Reduction—Unstable
   Alkali—Stable   Light—Labile (stable in acid)
   Water—Basic

3. **Properties**   1, 7, 15, 17, 18, 22, 29, 32, 34

   Appearance—White powder   Solubility
   MW—169 pyridoxine H_2O—0.2 g/ml
   MP—160° pyridoxine   Acet., Alc.—Sol.
   Crystal form—Platelets   Benz., Chl., Eth.—Insol.
   Salts—Hydrochloride, Ca^{2+} Absn. max.—256, 327 mμ pH 7.0

Important groups   Chemical nature
    —CH$_2$OH   Hydroxylated weak nitrogen base, substi-
    —N=   tuted pyridine
                                      pK_a = 5.0, 8.9
                                      α_D = 0 (inactive)

4. **Commercial Production**   18, 22, 29, 32, 34, 35
Commercially available as pyridoxine hydrochloride
Synthesized by method of Harris and Folkers; ethoxy acetylacetone con-
    densed with cyanoacetamide
Easiest route for synthesis is probably from oxazoles

5. **Isolation**   9, 17, 22, 29, 32, 34, 35
Sources—Rice polishings or bran and yeast
Methods
    Adsorb on Fuller's earth or charcoal
    Elute with Ba(OH)$_2$
    Precipitate impurities with heavy metals
    Precipitate with phosphotungstic acid

6. **Determination**   14, 16, 27a, 33
Bioassay—Animal
    Rat acrodynia test
    Rat growth and chicken growth assays
    Tryptophan loading test
    Blood cell
Bioassay—Microbial—Microbioassay
Physicochemical—Photofluorometric procedure detects 4-pyridoxic acid
    (major metabolite) in urine; chromatographic procedure to detect 4-
    pyridoxic acid

DISTRIBUTION AND SOURCES

1. **Occurrence**   16, 19, 22, 25, 26, 29, 32, 34, 35
Plants
    Fruit—All low, except bananas, avocados, grapes, pears (medium)
    Vegetables—All low or medium
    Nuts—All high
    Miscellaneous—Cereals—medium, except brown rice, wheat germ (high);
        and blackstrap molasses (high)
Animals: All medium, except herring, salmon, liver (high)
Microorganisms: All high or medium—yeast, intestinal bacteria (high); some
    other bacteria

2. **Dietary Sources**   3, 8, 20, 27, 30, 34, 36
  High: 1000-10,000 μg/100 g
    Liver (beef, calf, pork), herring, salmon
    Walnuts, peanuts, wheat germ, brown rice
    Yeast, blackstrap molasses
  Medium: 100-1000 μg/100 g
    Bananas, avocados, grapes, pears
    Barley, cabbage, carrots, corn, oats, peas, potatoes, rye, kale, tomatoes,
      turnips, yams, brussels sprouts, cauliflower, spinach, soybeans, wheat
    Beef, lamb, pork, veal (heart, brains, kidney); cod, flounder, halibut,
      mackerel, whale, sardines, tuna
    Butter, eggs
  Low: 10-100 μg/100 g
    Apples, cantaloupes, grapefruit, lemons, oranges, peaches, raisins, straw-
      berries, watermelons, cherries, currants (red)
    Asparagus, beans, beet greens, lettuce, onions
    Cheese, milk

MEDICAL AND NUTRITIONAL ROLE

1. **Units**   8, 16, 26, 34
  By weight, mg or μg

2. **Normal Blood Levels**   4, 14, 26, 33, 34
  4.6-7.2 μg/100 ml, serum; 3.1-4.3 μg/100 ml, blood

3. **Recommended Allowances**   4, 8, 21, 24, 27, 37
  Children—0.9-1.6 mg/day*
  Adults—2.0 mg/day* (females); 2.2 mg/day* (males)
  Special—Pregnancy, 2.6 mg/day; lactation, 2.5 mg/day
  Therapeutic Dose—25-100 mg/day

4. **Administration**   8, 9, 31, 32, 35
  Injection—Intravenous, subcutaneous
  Topical—No data
  Oral—Preferred route

5. **Factors Affecting Availability**   3, 8, 20, 27, 27a
  Decrease
    Administration of isoniazid

*Depends on protein content of food and inborn errors of metabolism; irradiation increases need.

30-45% loss in cooking, water-soluble
Diuresis, gastrointestinal diseases
Irradiation
Increase
Intestinal bacterial production (very small amount)
Storage in liver

6. **Deficiency Symptoms**   3, 4, 16, 21, 24, 27, 27a, 30
General
Cutaneous lesions
Anemia
Neuronal dysfunction including convulsions
Increased excretion of xanthurenic acid
Lab animals
Blood urea and urea excretion enhanced
γ-globulin and hemoglobin decreased
Urinary oxalate increased
Insulin insufficiency
Acrodynia
Demyelinization of peripheral nerves
Tonoclonic convulsion
Adrenal—Enlarged zona fasciculata
Poor reproduction

7. **Effects of Overdose, Toxicity**   3, 4, 16, 22, 26, 29, 31, 32, 34
Limited toxicity (man) (only at 3 g/kg dosage)
Convulsions at 4 g/kg (rat)

METABOLIC ROLE

1. **Biosynthesis**   3, 19, 25, 28
Precursors—Possibly glycine, serine, or glycolaldehyde
Intermediates—Unknown

2. **Production (Species and Site)**   3, 19, 25, 28
Plants—Fungi, cereal germ, seeds
Bacteria—Intestinal
Animals—None

3. **Storage Site**   8, 9, 16, 26, 34
Muscle phosphorylase (skeletal muscle) (small amount)

4. **Blood Carriers**   8, 14, 29, 31, 32
   Blood protein complexes

5. **Half-life**   8, 9, 29, 31, 32, 34
   57% of ingested dose excreted per day

6. **Target Tissues**   14, 16, 29, 31, 32, 34
   Nervous tissue, liver, lymph nodes, muscle tissue

7. **Reactions**   5, 14, 16, 17, 28
   Coenzyme forms—Codecarboxylase (pyridoxal-5-phosphate); pyridoxamine
   phosphate; Cu, Fe, Al chelates of coenzymes probably are active forms

Organ	Enzyme System	Effect
Liver	1. Transaminases (glutamic, aspartic)	Activated
Liver	2. Amino acid decarboxylases (histidine)	Activated
Liver	3. Tryptophan metabolism (kynureninase)	Activated
Liver	4. Tyrosine and phenylalanine metabolism	Activated
Muscle	5. Phosphorylases (constituent of)	Completed
Liver	6. Dehydrases (porphyrin synthesis, serine)	Activated
Liver	7. Racemases (alanine racemase)	Activated
Liver	8. Oxidases (diamine)	Activated
Liver	9. Desulfhydrases (cysteine)	Activated
Liver	10. Serine transhydroxymethylase	Activated

8. **Mode of Action**   3, 5, 6, 9, 14, 17, 22
   Cellular
       Anabolic—Unsaturated fatty acid biosynthesis
       Catabolic—Nonoxidative metabolic changes, decarboxylations, trans-
           aminations, glucogen phosphorylation
       Other—Amino acid absorption and transport, $-NH_2$ transfer (amino acids)
   Organismal
       Growth, maintenance of adrenal cortex
       Production of niacin, norepinephrine, serotonin, histamine, acetylcholine,
           γ-aminobutyric acid
       Production of bile acids (taurine synthesis)
       Erythrocyte formation, gluconeogenesis and glycogenolysis reactions

9. **Catabolism**   1, 3, 8, 9, 10, 16, 28
   Intermediates—All converted to pyridoxal
   Excretion products
       Urine—4-pyridoxic acid (0.6-11.2 mg/day); pyridoxal (.005-.40 mg/day);
           pyridoxamine (.003-.20 mg/day)
       Feces—0.5-0.8 mg/day

MISCELLANEOUS

1. **Relationship to Other Vitamins**   8, 11, 13, 27, 31, 32

   Pantothenic acid—B_6 deficiency results in lowered concentration of coenzyme A

   B_{12}—B_6 deficiency results in reduced absorption and storage of B_{12}

   Vitamin E—B_6 synergizes with E to control metabolism of unsaturated fats

   Vitamin C—Excretion of C increased in B_6 deficiency, conversion of vitamin
   C to oxalates increased, i.e., oxaluria . Helps alleviate some symptoms of
   B_6 deficiency. Synergizes with B_6 in tyrosine metabolism

   Niacin—B_6 coenzyme for niacin synthesis from tryptophan, also synergistic

   Vitamin B_1—Overdose of B_1 causes B_6 deficiency in rats, synergistic

   Vitamin B_2—Synergistic in action with B_6

   Biotin—Synergistic with B_6, B_2, and niacin in skin maintenance

2. **Relationship to Hormones**   8, 9, 11, 13, 17, 27

   Thyroxine—Decreases the activity of various pyridoxalphosphate dependent
   enzyme systems

   Insulin—Insufficiency of insulin in B_6 deficiency in animals

   Norepinephrine, acetylcholine, serotonin, epinephrine—B_6 involved in synthesis of these hormones

   ACTH—Adrenal cortex zona fasciculata enlarged (hypertrophied) on B_6
   deficiency

   B_6 possibly involved in synthesis and function of these hormones: STH,
   Estradiol-17β, Testosterone, FSH, LH, Cortisol, Aldosterone, Epinephrine, Glucagon

3. **Unusual Features**   11, 13, 14, 16, 17

   Involved in dental caries, oxaluria

   Linoleic acid relieves dermatitis symptoms of B_6 deficiency

   Presence of B_6 in phosphorylase a and b in large amounts implicates glucagon,
   epinephrine, and norepinephrine in function of B_6

   Great diversity of deficiency symptoms depending on species

   Heavy metal ion involved in binding to enzyme

   Involvement in stress, electrolyte balance, energy production, and water
   metabolism by unknown pathways

4. **Possible Relationships of Deficiency Symptoms to Metabolic Action**   11,
   13, 16, 27

   Cutaneous lesions—Synergism of B_6 with niacin and B_2 for skin maintenance

   Convulsions—Synergism of B_6 with B_1 involved in nervous tissue maintenance

   Xanthurenic acid excretion—Kynureninase requires B_6 as coenzyme

   Anemia—Synergism of B_6 with B_{12} for anti-anemic action, maintenance of
   erythrocyte production

5. **Relationships to Minerals (See refs in specific Mineral section)**
    Synergists—Zn^{2+}, Cr^{3+}, Mg^{2+}, Na^+, K^+, Cu^{2+}, PO_4^{3-}
    Antagonist—Fe^{3+}

Chapter 23. Vitamin B$_{12}$

Vitamin B$_{12}$ is unique among the vitamins in many respects: its complex corrinoid structure containing cobalt, its red color, its potency, and its method of absorption, requiring intrinsic factor. Its major functions are as coenzyme in red blood cell synthesis, protein, lipid and nucleic acid synthesis, and nerve cell maintenance. Its major importance is due to its anti-anemic action, its nervous system effects, and its methylating functions (lipotropic action). A major deficiency is pernicious anemia.

Vitamin B$_{12}$ is a water-soluble vitamin, chemically a porphyrinnucleotide, which *is* stored in the body. No toxicity has been reported at high dosage levels. It has been used in megadoses for emotionally disturbed individuals with controversial results. It is synergistic with folic acid, Intrinsic Factor, Ca^{2+}, HCl, Fe^{2+}, and Cu^{2+}, and is antagonized by vitamin C, niacin, dilantin, and estrogens.

Vitamin B$_{12}$ is obtained from animals and microorganisms, but not from plant sources. It is not excreted rapidly. Although it is synthesized in notable amounts in the intestine, none of this product is available for man.

There is no evidence that dietary supplementation of vitamin B$_{12}$ is needed for a normal, healthy adult on the average American diet, since it is available in most diets in the microquantities required (1 μg/day). Certain individuals may require more or be unable to absorb it due to lack of intrinsic factor. Special conditions requiring definite supplementation are: pregnancy, lactation, intestinal malabsorption, anorexia, old age, neuropathies, malnutrition, alcoholism, vegetarian diets, pernicious anemia, infancy, high vitamin C intake, and loss of Intrinsic Factor.

High dietary sources include: kidney, liver, brain, heart, milk, beef, egg yolk, clams, oysters, sardines, salmon, and herring.

GENERAL INFORMATION

1. **Synonyms**   7, 16, 18, 35
   Cobalamin, cyanocobalamin, antipernicious anemia vitamin

2. **History**   16, 18, 35
   1926—Minot and Murphy: controlled pernicious anemia using liver
   1944—Castle: demonstrated intrinsic factor needed to control pernicious anemia with liver
   1948—Rickes et al.: isolated and crystallized factor in liver controlling pernicious anemia
   1948—Smith and Parker: crystallized and designated liver factor as vitamin B$_{12}$
   1948—West: demonstrated clinical activity of vitamin B$_{12}$
   1955—Hodgkin et al.: determined structure of vitamin B$_{12}$

3. **Physiological Forms**   16, 23, 26, 34
   Hydroxocobalamin (vitamin B$_{12a}$), aquocobalamin (vitamin B$_{12b}$)

4. **Active Analogs and Related Compounds**   14, 16, 23, 26, 34
   Nitrocobalamin (vitamin B$_{12c}$), chlorocobalamin, thiocyanatocobalamin

5. **Inactive Analogs and Related Compounds (in Man)**   14, 16, 26, 34
   ψ-Vitamin B, factors B, C, D, E, F, G, H, I

6. **Antagonists**   1, 7, 14, 16, 26, 34
   Methylamide, ethylamide, anilide, lactone derivatives, pteridine, nicotinamide, vitamin C (excess), dilantin, estrogens

7. **Synergists**   1, 7, 14, 16, 26, 34
   Vitamins A, E, C, B$_1$, folic acid, biotin, pantothenic acid, Intrinsic Factor, Ca^{2+}, Fe^{2+}, Cu^{2+}, PO$_4^{3-}$, Co^{2+}

8. **Physiological Functions**   3, 4, 14, 20, 26, 27a, 34
   Coenzyme in nucleic acid, protein, and lipid synthesis
   Maintain growth, nucleic acid synthesis, protein synthesis, lipid synthesis, and methylations
   Maintain epithelial cells and nervous system (myelin sheath), erythropoiesis (with folic acid) and leukopoiesis

9. **Deficiency Diseases, Disorders**   3, 4, 14, 16, 26, 27a, 34
   Retarded growth, pernicious anemia, megaloblastic anemia, macrocytic and hyperchromic anemia, glossitis, spinal cord degeneration, sprue, nutritional amblyopia

10. Sources for Species Requiring It (Essential for man)   1, 3, 4, 14, 26, 34
Required by all vertebrates, some protozoa, bacteria, algae and fungi
Exogenous sources—Vertebrates, some bacteria, protozoa, algae (not available from intestinal bacteria in man)
Endogenous sources—Bacteria and actinomycetes (some)

CHEMISTRY

1. Structure   16, 18, 19, 22, 29, 32, 34, 35

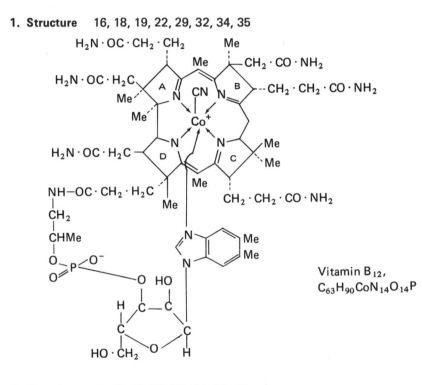

Vitamin B$_{12}$,
C$_{63}$H$_{90}$CoN$_{14}$O$_{14}$P

2. Reactions   3, 17, 18, 22, 29, 32, 34, 35

Heat—Unstable	Oxidation—Unstable
Acid—Unstable	Reduction—Unstable
Alkali—Unstable	Light—Unstable
Water—Neutral	

3. Properties   1, 7, 15, 17, 18, 22, 29, 32, 34

Appearance—Red powder
MW—1357
MP—Blackens at 190°C
Crystal form—Orthorhombic needles
Salts—Perchloric acid

Solubility
H$_2$O—1.25 g/100 ml
Alc.—Sol.
Acet., Benz., Chl., Eth.—Insol.
Absn. max.—278, 361, 550 mμ
(H$_2$O)

Important groups
   5,6-Dimethylbenzimidazole
   α-Ribothiazole

$[\alpha]_D^{23} = -59°$ (aq. soln.)
Chemical nature
   Polyacidic base
   Benzimidazole nucleotide
   Porphyrin-like corrin
   Reducing agent

4. **Commercial Production**   18, 22, 29, 32, 34, 35
Fermentation of *S. griseus* or *S. aureofaciens*
By-product of antibiotic production

5. **Isolation**   9, 17, 22, 29, 32, 34, 35
Sources—Liver, fish solubles
Method
   Extract with aqueous alcohol
   Adsorb B$_{12}$ on charcoal; elute with 65% alcohol
   Perform column chromatography on silica or alumina
   Wash with acetone; elute with alcohol
   Crystallize

6. **Determination**   14, 16, 27a, 33
Bioassay
   Microbial—*L. leichmanii, O. malhamensis, E. gracilis*
   Animal—Chick and rat, curative dose
Physicochemical—Spectrophotometry, polarography, isotope dilution

DISTRIBUTION AND SOURCES

1. **Occurrence**   16, 19, 22, 25, 26, 29, 32, 34, 35
Plants: Vegetables—very low; soybeans, green beans, beets, carrots, peas—
   very low; oats, wheat, nuts, seeds
Animals: All animals, especially in organs—Liver, kidney, heart, spleen, brain,
   stomach, intestine, eggs, milk
Microorganisms: *S. aureofaciens, B. megatherium*, protozoa, soil bacteria,
   intestinal bacteria
Miscellaneous: Seawater, sewage sludge

2. **Dietary Sources**   3, 8, 20, 27, 30, 34, 36
High: 50 μg-500 μg/100 g
   Kidney (lamb, beef)
   Liver (lamb, beef, calf, pork)
   Brain (beef)

Medium: 5-50 μg/100 g
　Kidney (rabbit)
　Liver (rabbit, chicken)
　Heart (beef, rabbit, chicken)
　Egg yolk
　Clams, sardines, salmon, crabs, oysters, herring
Low: 0.5-5 μg/100 g
　Cod, flounder, haddock, halibut, lobster, scallop, shrimp, swordfish, tuna, whale
　Beef, pork lamb, chicken
　Cheeses, milk, eggs

MEDICAL AND NUTRITIONAL ROLE

1. **Units**　8, 16, 17, 26, 34
　1 USP = 1 μg vitamin B_{12} = 11,000 LLD units (*L. lactis Dorner* units)

2. **Normal Blood Levels (Man)**　4, 14, 26, 33, 34
　.02-.09 μg/100 ml, serum; .016-.020 μg/100 ml, RBC

3. **Recommended Allowances**　4, 8, 21, 24, 27, 37
　Children—2.0-3.0 μg/day
　Adults—3.0 μg/day
　Special—Pregnancy, 4 μg/day; lactation, 4 μg/day; intestinal malabsorption or disease; anorexia; old age; neuropathies; malnutrition; alcoholism
　Therapeutic dose—1-2 μg/day (I.M.)

4. **Administration**　8, 9, 31, 32, 35
　Injection—Parenteral, intramuscular (I.M.)
　Topical—No data
　Oral—Not very effective unless intrinsic factor (enzyme) present

5. **Factors Affecting Availability**　3, 8, 20, 27, 27a
　Decrease
　　Cooking losses—Heat-labile
　　Cobalt deficiency (ruminants)
　　Intestinal malabsorption or parasites
　　Lack of Intrinsic Factor
　　Intestinal disease, aging
　　Vegetarian diet
　　Excretion in feces
　　Gastrectomy

Increase
   Administration of sorbitol
   Synthesis by intestinal bacteria (not normally available)
   Reduced temperature
   Food in stomach
   Ca^{2+} (with Intrinsic Factor)

6. **Deficiency Symptoms**   3, 4, 16, 21, 24, 27, 27a, 30
   Poor growth
   Increased hemolysis of RBCs
   Megaloblastic marrow
   Macrocytic, hyperchromic anemia
   Glossitis
   Degenerative changes in spinal cord, nervous symptoms
   Decreased blood and tissue lipids
   Disturbed carbohydrate metabolism—Excretion of methylmalonic acid
   Leukopenia
   Gastrointestinal tract changes
   Loss of hatchability $\Big\}$ Chickens
   Poor feathering
   Reproductive failure $\Big\}$ Rats
   Porphyrin whiskers
   Dermatitis $\Big\}$ Pigs
   Impaired reproduction

7. **Effects of Overdose, Toxicity**   3, 4, 16, 22, 26, 29, 31, 32, 34
   Polycythemia reported
   General lack of toxicity

METABOLIC ROLE

1. **Biosynthesis**   3, 19, 25, 28
   Precursors
      Glycine—Corrin nucleus
      δ-Aminolevulinic acid—Corrin nucleus
      Methionine—Corrin nucleus
   Intermediates
      Porphobilinogen
      α-d-Ribosides of benzimidazole
      5,6-Dimethylbenzimidazole
      α-Ribazole

2. **Production**   3, 19, 25, 28
   Species—Bacteria (some); actinomycetes (some)

3. **Storage**   8, 9, 16, 26, 34
   Liver (30-60%), lungs, kidneys, spleen

4. **Blood Carriers**   8, 14, 29, 31, 32
   α_1-Globulins (52%), α_2-globulins (21%), albumins (16%), β-globulins (7%),
   γ-globulins (6%)

5. **Half-life**   8, 9, 29, 31, 32, 34
   >1 year

6. **Target Tissues**   14, 16, 29, 31, 32, 34
   Central nervous system, kidneys, myocardium, muscle, skin, bone

7. **Reactions**   5, 14, 16, 17, 28
   Coenzyme forms
       Adenyl cobamide coenzyme (adenyl nucleoside)
       5,6-Dimethylbenzimidazolylcobamide coenzyme
       Benzimidazolylcobamide coenzyme

Organ	Enzyme System	Effect
	MUTASES	
Liver	Glutamate mutase (glutamic-aspartic)	Activated
Liver	Methylmalonyl CoA mutase (methyl malonic-succinic)	Activated
	DEHYDRASES	
Liver	Diol dehydrase (glycerol-1,3-propanediol)	Activated
Liver	Glycerol dehydrase (glycerol-β-OH-propionaldehyde)	Activated
Liver	Ethanolamine deaminase (ethanolamine-ammonia, acetaldehyde)	Activated
	TRANSMETHYLASES	
Liver	B_{12} enzyme (homocysteine-methionine) with folate	Activated
Liver	Thymidine synthesis enzymes (purine biosynthesis)	Activated
	REDUCTASES	
Liver	Methane formation enzymes	Activated
Liver	Ribonucleotide reductase (ribonucleotide-deoxyribonucleotide)	Activated
Liver	Lysine fermentation enzymes	Activated
Liver	Acetate synthesis enzymes	Activated

8. **Mode of Action**   3, 5, 6, 9, 14, 17, 22
   Cellular
     Anabolic
       DNA synthesis (nucleolar methylations, ribotide conversion)
       RNA synthesis (purine synthesis, nucleolar methylation)
       Protein synthesis (DNA synthesis, methionine synthesis)
       Synthesis of lipids
       Porphyrin synthesis
       Anabolic action—Mitosis and growth
       Choline synthesis
     Catabolic
       Carbohydrate metabolism (propionic acid)
       Lipid metabolism (glycerol, ethanolamine)
     Other
       Maintenance of membranes, esp. myelin sheath
       Maintenance of —SH groups in reduced form
       Isomerization, dehydrogenation, methylation
   Organismal
     Maintains epithelial and mucosal cells
     Maintains normal bone marrow
     Maintains normal gastrointestinal tract
     Maintains normal CNS
     Maintains erythropoiesis and leukopoiesis
     Maintains body lipids, lipotropic
     Maintains normal growth
     Improves nitrogen retention

9. **Catabolism**   1, 3, 8, 9, 10, 16, 28
   Intermediates—No body destruction
   Excretion products
     Urine—.001-.006 μg/day
     Feces—34% of ingested dose
     Bile—Some reabsorption (enterohepatic recirculation)

MISCELLANEOUS

1. **Relationship to Other Vitamins**   8, 11, 13, 31, 32
   Folic acid—Active with B$_{12}$ in nucleic acid and methionine synthesis; com-
     bined action with vitamin B$_{12}$; deficiency of folic acid increases B$_{12}$
     absorption
   Vitamin A—Uptake and utilization of carotenes increased with B$_{12}$ in diet;
     maintenance of mucosal and epithelial cells
   Vitamin B$_6$—Deficiency reduces B$_{12}$ absorption in gut

Biotin—Active with B_{12} in methylmalonyl CoA metabolism

Niacin—B_{12} deficiency causes decrease in liver NAD

Pantothenic acid—B_{12} participates in methylmalonyl CoA conversion; has sparing action on B_{12} and vice versa

Riboflavin—Possible synthesis from 5,6-dimethylbenzimidazole moiety of B_{12}

Vitamins E, C—Can substitute for vitamin B_{12} in certain conditions and synergize it; synergize vitamin B_{12} in treatment of macrocytic anemia

Vitamin B_1—Synergistic to B_{12}

Vitamin C—Antagonistic to B_{12} (vitamin C megadoses)

2. **Relationship to Hormones**   8, 9, 11, 13, 17, 27

T4—Deficiency of T4 impairs B_{12} absorption

Antithyroid antibodies in serum of B_{12}-deficient patients

Increased T4 produces loss of B_{12}

Parathormone—Pernicious anemia found coexisting with hypoparathyroidism (Ca metabolism)

STH—B_{12} needed for mitosis and growth (with folic acid)

3. **Unusual Features**   11, 13, 14, 16, 17

Cyanide group an artifact of preparation

The only vitamin synthesized in sizable amounts only by microorganisms (possibly in tumors)

Only vitamin with metal ion

Works with glutathione

Glutathione content decreased on B_{12} deficiency

Mitosis retarded in B_{12} deficiency

Requires intrinsic factor (enzyme) for activity via oral route

Increases tumor size (Rous sarcoma)

Diamagnetic properties

No acidic or basic groups revealed on titration (no pKa)

4. **Possible Relationships of Deficiency Symptoms to Metabolic Action**   11, 13, 16, 27

Degenerative changes in spinal cord—Decreased RNA synthesis

Megaloblastic marrow—Decreased DNA synthesis (with folate)

Glossitis—Decreased cell division of tongue cells

Macrocytic hyperchromic anemia—Decreased DNA synthesis of precursor cells

Decreased blood and tissue lipids—Possibly due to presence of plasma hemolytic factor in B_{12} deficiency

Disturbed CHO metabolism—Activation of methylmalonic acid mutase by B_{12}

Leukopenia—Decreased DNA synthesis in stem cells

Gastrointestinal tract changes—Decreased cell division of gastric mucosal cells

Increased hemolysis—Presence of plasma hemolytic factor in B_{12} deficiency

5. **Relationships to Minerals** (See specific refs in Minerals section)
   Synergists—Ca^{2+}, Cu^{2+}, Co^{2+}, Fe^{3+}, PO_4^{3-}, I^- (as T4)
   Co^{2+} a central atom

Chapter 24.
Ascorbic Acid (Vitamin C)

Vitamin C is probably the most controversial vitamin because of the recent claims for its ability in megadoses (a) to relieve or cure colds, cancer, heat rash, thrombophlebitis, and emotional illnesses, and (b) to detoxify environmental toxins. It functions principally as an antioxidant, in wound healing, formation of calcified tissues, growth, and capillary and adrenal gland maintenance. It is important mainly because of its antiscorbutic, antioxidant, and antistress properties, and its detoxifying actions for heavy metals and pesticides. A major dificiency disease is scurvy.

Vitamin C is a water-soluble vitamin, very unstable in water solution, chemically a modified sugar, which is stored to a small extent in the body. Its use in megadoses for the abovementioned dysfunctions has not yet found general clinical `acceptance; ongoing clinical tests may revise some negative aspects. Its toxicity in pharmacological (mega-) doses has been noted: *possible* (nephrolithiasis, oxalic aciduria, reproductive failure, vitamin C dependency, inactivation of B_{12}, loss of folic acid in urine, allergies, diarrhea, abortion, thrombosis, and uric aciduria). Its chief synergists are vitamins A and E, Zn^{2+}, Fe^{2+} and citric acid. Chief antagonists are deoxycorticosterone, estrogens, and Cu^{2+}.

Vitamin C is obtained mainly in citrus fruits, green peppers, rose hips, and other green vegetables. It is synthesized in most mammals (except humans) and is excreted rapidly although normal healthy adults on an average American diet may obtain minimum vitamin C for antiscorbutic protection. Dietary supplementation may be necessary because of its instability and because exact requirements for vitamin C have not been determined. Apparently vitamin C fulfills unique new functions at progressively higher concentration levels starting from the lowest antiscorbutic level. Because of the manifold functions of vitamin C it is likely that the present RDA (45 mg/day) is too low. Large individual variations in requirements do exist and may indicate a need for additional supplementation. Special conditions requiring definite supplementation of the diet are: scurvy, pregnancy, lactation, heavy metal intoxication, stress, trauma, allergies, old age, high protein diet, and infections. High dietary contents of vitamin C are found in: citrus fruits, rose hips, acerola berries, guavas, black currants, green peppers, parsley, kale, horseradish, collards, papayas, and strawberries.

GENERAL INFORMATION

1. **Synonyms**   7, 16, 18, 35
   Vitamin C, antiscorbutic vitamin, cevitamic acid, hexuronic acid

2. **History**   16, 18, 35
   1757—Lind: described scurvy
   1907—Holst and Frolich: produced experimental scurvy
   1928—Zilva: described antiscorbutic agents in lemon juice
   1928—Szent-Györgyi: isolated hexuronic acid from lemon juice
   1932—Waugh and King: identified hexuronic acid as antiscorbutic agent
   1933—Haworth: established configuration of hexuronic acid
   1933—Reichstein: synthesized hexuronic acid
   1933—Haworth and Szent-Györgyi: changed name of hexuronic acid to ascorbic acid

3. **Physiological Forms**   16, 23, 26, 34
   l-Ascorbic acid, dehydroascorbic acid

4. **Active Analogs and Related Compounds**   14, 16, 23, 26, 34
   l-Glucoascorbic acid, d-araboascorbic acid, l-rhamnoascorbic acid, 6-desoxy-l-ascorbic acid

5. **Inactive Analogs and Related Compounds**   14, 16, 26, 34
   d-Ascorbic acid

6. **Antagonists**   1, 7, 14, 16, 26, 34
   d-Glucoascorbic acid, deoxycorticosterone, Cu^{2+}, estrogens

7. **Synergists**   1, 7, 14, 16, 26, 34
   Vitamins A, E, B_{12}, B_6, K, pantothenic acid, testosterone, STH, folic acid, Zn^{2+}, Fe^{3+}, Ca^{2+}, Mg^{2+}, Mn^{2+}, $SeO_3{}^{2-}$

8. **Physiological Functions**   3, 4, 14, 20, 26, 27a, 34
   Absorption of iron
   Cold tolerance, maintenance of adrenal cortex
   Antioxidant
   Metabolism of tryptophan, phenylalanine, tyrosine
   Growth
   Wound healing
   Synthesis of polysaccharides and collagen
   Formation of cartilage, dentine, bone, teeth
   Maintenance of capillaries

9. **Deficiency Diseases and Disorders**   3, 4, 14, 16, 26, 27a, 34
   Scurvy, megaloblastic anemia of infancy

10. **Sources for Species Requiring It (Essential for man)**   1, 3, 4, 14, 26, 34
    Some species require it (some vertebrates, invertebrates and protozoa)
    Exogenous sources—Primates, guinea pig, flying mammals, late birds, fish,
       insects, invertebrates, protozoa
    Endogenous sources—Remainder of mammals, early birds, reptiles, amphib-
       ians, plants, algae, and bacteria

CHEMISTRY

1. **Structure**   16, 18, 19, 22, 29, 32, 34, 35

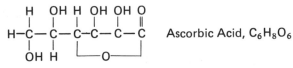

Ascorbic Acid, $C_6H_8O_6$

2. **Reactions**   3, 17, 18, 22, 29, 32, 34, 35

Heat—Labile	Oxidation—Labile
Acid—Stable	Reduction—Stable (reducing agent)
Alkali—Labile	Light—Labile
Water—Acid (pH 3) labile	

3. **Properties**   1, 7, 15, 17, 18, 22, 29, 32, 34

Appearance—White powder	Solubility
MW—176.12	H_2O—0.3 g/ml
MP—190-192°C (decomp.)	Acet., Alc.—Slightly sol.
Crystal form—Plates, needles	Benz., Chl., Eth.—Insol.
Salts—Ca, Na, metals	Absn. max.—245 mμ (acid); 265 mμ
Important groups for activity	(neutral)

Lactone ring

Enolic hydroxyls

Miscellaneous—pK_{a_1} = 4.17;

pK_{a_2} = 11.57

Redox potential—E_0^1 = +0.166 V (pH 4)

Chemical nature—Hexose acid

α_D^{25} = +20.5° (H_2O)

Miscellaneous—pK_{a_1} = 4.17; pK_{a_2} = 11.57

4. **Commercial Production**   18, 22, 29, 32, 34, 35

Microbiological—*Acetobacter suboxidans* oxidative fermentation of calcium
d-gluconate

Chemical—Oxidation of *l*-sorbose

5. **Isolation**   9, 17, 22, 29, 32, 34, 35

Sources—Adrenal cortex, citrus juices

Method—Precipitate from citrus juice as Pb-complex; crystallize from alcohol-
petroleum ether

6. **Determination**   14, 16, 27a, 33

Bioassay—Guinea pig growth or tooth structure, serum alkaline phosphatase

Physicochemical—Titration against standard oxidizing dye solution, colorimetry of excess dye; polarography

DISTRIBUTION AND SOURCES

1. **Occurrence**   16, 19, 22, 25, 26, 29, 32, 34, 35

Plants (High):

Fruit—Strawberry, citrus, pineapple, guava, black currant, West Indian
cherry

Vegetables—Cabbage, turnip greens, tomatoes, broccoli, kale, horseradish,
parsley, corn

Nuts—English walnuts (green)

Miscellaneous—Rose hips, molds

Animals: All—Retina > pituitary > corpus luteum > adrenal cortex > thymus
> liver > brain > testes > ovaries > spleen > thyroid > pancreas > salivary
glands > lungs > kidney > intestine > heart > muscle > WBC > RBC >
plasma

Microorganisms

No intestinal synthesis except in rat

Produced by certain molds

Required by bacteria, yeasts, and molds for multiplication

2. **Dietary Sources**   3, 8, 20, 27, 30, 34, 36

High: 100-300 mg/100 g

Broccoli, brussels sprouts, collards, horseradish, kale, parsley, peppers
(sweet), turnip greens

Black currant, guava, rose hips
Medium: 50-100 mg/100 g
    Beet greens, cabbages, cauliflower, chives, kohlrabi, mustard, watercress,
        spinach
    Lemons, oranges, papayas, strawberries
Low: 25-50 mg/100 g
    Asparagus, lima beans, beet greens, chard, cowpeas, mint, okra, spring
        onions, peas, potatoes, radishes, rutabagas, turnips, dandelion greens,
        fennel, soybeans, summer squash
    Gooseberries, passion fruit, grapefruit, limes, loganberries, mangoes,
        cantaloupes, honeydews, red currants, white currants, tangerines, rasp-
        berries, tomatoes, kumquats

MEDICAL AND NUTRITIONAL ROLE

1. **Units**   8, 16, 17, 26, 34
   1 I.U. = 1 U.S.P. unit = 0.05 mg *l*-ascorbic acid

2. **Normal Blood Levels**   4, 14, 26, 33, 34
   0.3-1.0 mg/100 ml, serum ⎫
   0.4-1.5 mg/100 ml, blood ⎬ vary with diet
   25 mg/100 ml, WBC ⎭

3. **Recommended Allowances**   4, 8, 21, 24, 27, 37
   Children—45 mg/day
   Adults—60 mg/day
   Special—Pregnancy (80 mg/day), lactation (100 mg/day); increased with in-
       fection, stress, trauma, allergies, old age, increased protein consumption
   Therapeutic dose—100-1000 mg/day

4. **Administration**   8, 9, 31, 32, 35
   Injection—Intramuscular, intravenous
   Topical—No data
   Oral—Preferred route

5. **Factors Affecting Availability**   3, 8, 20, 27
   Decrease
       Damage to adrenal cortex, presence of antagonists
       Food preparation (oxidation, storage, leaching, cooking)
   Increase
       Storage in body (adrenal cortex)
       Antioxidants, synergists in diet

6. **Deficiency Symptoms**   3, 4, 16, 21, 24, 27, 27a, 30
   General
   > Hyperkeratotic papules on buttocks and calves
   > Perifollicular hemorrhage, edema
   > Wound healing failure
   > Teeth and gum defects
   > Weakness, listlessness, rough skin, aching joints
   > Scorbutic bone formation

   Lab animals
   > Anemia, loss of weight
   > Abnormal collagen, no intercellular cement

7. **Effects of Overdose, Toxicity**   3, 4, 16, 22, 26, 29, 31, 32, 34
   Possible kidney stones, in gouty individuals
   Inhibitory in excess doses on cellular level (mitosis inhibited)
   Possible damage to β-cells of pancreas and decreased insulin production by dehydroascorbic acid
   Possible diarrhea, allergies, reproductive failure, vitamin C dependency, thrombosis, aciduria (oxalic, folic, uric), B_{12} inactivation

METABOLIC ROLE

1. **Biosynthesis**   3, 19, 25, 28
   Precursors—d-Mannose, d-fructose, glycerol, sucrose, d-glucose, or D-galactose
   Intermediates—UDP glucose, d-glucuronic acid, gulonic acid, l-gulonolactone, (Mn^{2+} cofactor)

2. **Production—Species and sites**   8, 9, 16, 26, 34
   All animals (except primates, guinea pig, fruit bat, late birds, insects, invertebrates, fishes)
   Organs: Kidney [reptiles, amphibians, primitive birds (chicken)], liver (mammals, song birds)
   Plants (green leaves, fruit skin)
   Cell sites—Microsomes, mitochondria, golgi

3. **Storage Sites**   8, 14, 29, 31, 32
   Adrenal cortex (small amount), liver

4. **Blood Carriers**   8, 14, 29, 31, 32
   Free in blood, especially in white blood cells

5. **Half-life**   8, 9, 29, 31, 32, 34
   16 days (man), few days (guinea pig)

6. Target Tissues   14, 16, 29, 31, 32, 34

Adrenal cortex, pituitary, ovary, connective tissue, bone, liver, teeth, gums

7. Reactions   5, 14, 16, 17, 28

Coenzyme form: Redox couple—*l*-ascorbic ⇌ dehydroascorbic acid

Organ	Enzyme Systems	Effect
	HYDROXYLATING	
Connective tissue	Proline → hydroxyproline (collagen synthesis)	Activated
Liver	Tryptophan → 5-hydroxytryptophan (tryptophan metabolism)	Activated
Adrenal cortex	Deoxycorticosterone → hydroxycorticosteroids (steroid hormone synthesis)	Activated
	OXIDATION-REDUCTION	
Liver	DPNH-cytochrome b_5 (electron transport)	Activated
Liver	Tyrosine-homogentisic acid (tyrosine metabolism)	Activated
Liver	Glutathione (reduction reaction)	Activated
Liver	Ascorbic acid oxidase (oxidation reactions)	Activated
Liver	Plasma iron-ferritin (reduction)	Activated
Liver	Amidases, proteases, glycosidases, peroxidases, esterases	Activated
Liver	Arginase, papain, liver esterase, catalase, cathepsin	Activated
Liver	Urease, b-amylase	Inhibited

8. Mode of Action   3, 5, 6, 9, 14, 17, 22

Cellular
  Anabolic
    Collagen synthesis—Proline hydroxylation
    Steroid synthesis—Accelerates acetate incorporation into cholesterol
    Serotonin, melanin synthesis
    Polysaccharide synthesis—Chondroitin sulfate incorporation
  Catabolic—Antimitotic agent
  Other
    Cellular antioxidant—Maintains membranes
    Respiration—Cellular reductions and oxidations
    Maintenance of electron transport chain in mitochondria
    Maintains low redox level for vitamin E and sulfhydryl enzymes
    Maintenance of peroxidase system (detoxification)
    Stimulates phagocytosis
Organismal
  Absorption of iron, ferritin production
  Maintenance of adrenals and ovaries (hormone biosynthesis)

Maintenance of connective tissues
Maintenance of steroid endocrine glands
Maintains stress and wound healing reactions
Maintenance of cartilage, bone, and teeth
Maintenance of capillaries, control of hemorrhage
Respiration—Maintains oxygen turnover

9. **Catabolism**   1, 3, 8, 9, 10, 16, 28
Intermediates—Diketogulonic acid, oxalic acid
Excretion products
   Urine—12-14% excreted as *l*-ascorbic acid (7-28 mg/day); 12-18% excreted
      as diketogulonic acid; 24-63% excreted as oxalic acid
   Also in feces, sweat, respiratory CO_2

MISCELLANEOUS

1. **Relationship to Other Vitamins**   8, 11, 13, 27, 31, 32
   Vitamin A—Depletion causes drop in plasma vitamin C levels; protected by
      vitamin C against oxidation
   Vitamin B_{12}—Replaced by vitamin C in lactic acid bacteria; can be replaced
      or potentiated by vitamin C; possible inactivation by megadoses of vitamin C
   Folic acid—Vitamin C decreases symptoms of folic acid deficiency, formation
      promoted by vitamin C, stimulates formation of citrovorum factor (folinic
      acid); excretion promoted by megadoses of vitamin C
   Pyridoxine—Pyridoxine-PO_4 and vitamin C related to tyrosine metabolism
   Vitamin E—Decreased synthesis and excretion of vitamin C in vitamin E-
      deficient animals, protected by vitamin C against oxidation
   Pantothenic acid—Compensated partly by vitamin C in deficiency of panto-
      thenic acid

2. **Relationship to Hormones**   8, 11, 13
   Serotonin—Produced from tryptophan under influence of vitamin C
   Thyroxine—Cold survival capacity due to vitamin C (mediated via thyroxine)
   Epinephrine, norepinephrine—Produced from tyrosine under influence of
      vitamin C; vitamin C protects against oxidation
   Deoxycorticosterone—Depresses action of vitamin C on growth of skeletal
      tissues
   Aldosterone, estradiol-17β, testosterone, cortisol—Vitamin C stimulates con-
      version of deoxycorticosterone in adrenal cortex (may be needed for
      steroid synthesis)
   Cortisone—Alleviates scorbutic symptoms in joints
   STH, ACTH, FSH, LH—High concentrations of vitamin C noted in pituitary
      tissues; STH a synergist in growth

Insulin—Dehydroascorbic acid can destroy (in megadoses) the β cells of pancreas and thereby decrease insulin production

3. **Unusual Features**   11, 13, 14, 16

Only d-form active

Antistress factor and anti-infection factor

Activates terminal oxidases in respiratory systems

Sensitivity to oxidation by heavy metals (e.g., Cu), hemochromogens, and quinones

Ease of reversible oxidation

Increased excretion due to barbiturates and drugs

Increased synthesis of vitamin C due to chloretone in vitamin C-deficient animals

Production of H_2O_2 on aerobic oxidation

Increased nitrogen assimilation by plants

Protects tissues against ionizing radiation

Prevents formation of nitrosamines from nitrites

4. **Possible Relationships of Deficiency Symptoms to Metabolic Action**   11, 13, 16, 27

Failure to produce intercellular cement—Decrease of mucopolysaccharide synthesis from glucuronic acid

Hemorrhage—Weak intercellular fibers causing capillary fragility

Poor tooth and gum structure—Decreased collagen, mucopolysaccharide synthesis; bacterial invasion

Lethargy—Decreased supply of adrenocortical and adrenal hormones

Edema—Decreased aldosterone synthesis and capillary fragility

Weight loss—Possibly decreased growth hormone level

5. **Relationships to Minerals**   (See references in specific mineral section)

Synergists—Ca^{2+}, Mg^{2+}, Zn^{2+}, Mn^{2+}, SeO_3^{2-}, I^- (as T4)

Antagonist—Cu^{2+}

Chelating agent for heavy metals

Easily oxidized by heavy metals

Chapter 25. Biotin

Biotin is one of the lesser-known vitamins, being chiefly known for its anti-avidin action in raw eggs. Its major function is as coenzyme in amino acid metabolism and maintenance of skin, hair, nerves, and sex glands. Deficiencies of this vitamin are rare in humans. Its chief importance stems from its role in growth, decarboxylations of amino acids, formation of urea, and carbohydrate metabolism.

Biotin is a slightly water-soluble vitamin, chemically a substituted amino acid. Some biotin is stored in the liver. No toxicity of large doses has been reported. Megadoses have been used experimentally in an attempt to aid hair growth but without clinical acceptance. Its chief synergists are Mn^{2+} and other B-complex vitamins, whereas its chief antagonists are avidin and desthiobiotin.

Biotin is obtained from plant, animal, and microbial sources. Its exact requirements are small, but unknown in humans. Intestinal bacteria provide most, if not all, the requirements, and it is excreted slowly. Thus there is no evidence of need for dietary supplementation for a normal, healthy adult on an average American diet. Special conditions requiring dietary supplementation are: excessive egg-white ingestion, certain cutaneous lesions, infants with seborrheic dermatitis, antibiotic and sulfa therapy, and pregnancy (possibly). Dietary items high in biotin are: yeast, liver, kidney, egg yolk, grains, and peanuts.

GENERAL INFORMATION

1. **Synonyms**   7, 16, 18, 35
   Bios IIB, protective factor X, vitamin H, egg white injury factor, CoR

2. **History** 16, 18, 35
   1924—Miller: fractionated yeast growth factor Bios into Bios, I, IIB, IIc
   1933—Allison et al.: isolated CoR (respiratory factor legume nodule bacteria)
   1934—Lease and Parsons: described egg white injury in chicks
   1936—Kögl, Tonnis: isolated growth stimulant from yeast, and egg yolk, and named it biotin
   1940—György: identified vitamin H, CoR, and biotin as equivalent
   1941—Williams et al.: found egg white injury due to antivitamin, avidin (inactivates biotin)
   1942—Du Vigneaud: characterized and determined structure of biotin
   1943—Harris: synthesized biotin

3. **Physiological Forms** 16, 23, 26, 34
   d (or +) Biotin (*cis*-form) [β-isomer, *d*(β-biotin)*cis*]
   Of eight possible stereoisomers (four *cis*, four *trans*), only one active: *d*-biotin (*cis*)
   α and β-isomers based on orientation of isomeric side chains of *cis* and *trans* forms

4. **Active Analogs and Related Compounds** 14, 16, 23, 26, 34
   Desthiobiotin in some species
   dl-Oxybiotin (microorganisms, rats, chicks)
   Biotinol (in rats)
   Biotin sulfoxide (in some)
   Biocytin (in some)

5. **Inactive Analogs and Related Compounds** 14, 16, 26, 34
   dl-Epibiotin (*cis*)
   dl-Allobiotin (*trans*)
   dl-Epiallobiotin (*trans*)
   l-Biotin (*cis*)
   α and β-isomers of these compounds

6. **Antagonists** 1, 7, 14, 16, 26, 34
   Desthiobiotin in some forms
   Ureylene phenyl
   Homobiotin
   Ureylenecyclohexyl butyric and valeric acids
   Norbiotin
   Avidin
   Lysolecithin
   Biotin sulfone

7. **Synergists** 1, 7, 14, 16, 26, 34
   Vitamins B_2, B_6, B_{12}, folic acid, pantothenic acid, STH, testosterone, Mn^{2+}

8. **Physiological Functions**   3, 4, 14, 20, 26, 27a, 34
As coenzyme for
  Carboxylation reactions
  Pyruvic oxidase
  Decarboxylation of oxaloacetic acid, succinate, aspartate, malate
  Biosynthesis of aspartate, citrulline, unsaturated fatty acids
Growth
Maintenance of skin, hair, sebaceous glands, nerves, bone marrow, sex glands

9. **Deficiency Diseases and Disorders (Man)**   3, 4, 14, 16, 26, 27a, 34
Nonspecific dermatitis
Seborrheic dermatitis in infants, furunculosis

10. **Sources for Species Requiring It (Essential for man)**   1, 3, 4, 14, 26, 34
Most organisms require it (all vertebrates, some microorganisms)
Exogenous sources—Most vertebrates, invertebrates, some bacteria and fungi
  (intestinal bacteria supply needs of man)
Endogenous sources—Higher plants, most fungi and bacteria

CHEMISTRY

1. **Structure**   16, 18, 19, 22, 29, 32, 34, 35

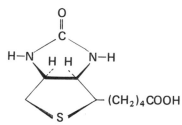

$d(\beta\text{-Biotin})(cis)$, $C_{10}H_{16}N_2O_3S$

2. **Reactions**   3, 17, 18, 22, 29, 32, 34, 35

Heat—Stable	Oxidation—Unstable
Acid—Unstable	Reduction—Forms desthiobiotin
Alkali—Unstable	Light—Stable
Water—Acidic	

3. **Properties**   1, 7, 15, 17, 18, 22, 29, 32, 34

Appearance—White powder	Solubility
MW—244.3	H_2O—0.03 g/100 ml
MP—230-32°C	Alc.—Sol.
Crystal form	Acet., Benz. Chl. Eth.—Insol.
Orthorhombic (α)	Absn. max.—234 mμ

Colorless needles (β)
Salts—Na
Important groups: HN

Chemical nature
    Diamino-, monocarboxylic acid
    Substituted amino acid
Miscellaneous-pI = 3.5
α_D^{21} = +91°C (0.1 N NaOH)

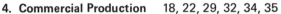

4. **Commercial Production**   18, 22, 29, 32, 34, 35
Use meso-diamino succinic acid derivative of fumaric acid for starting synthesis

5. **Isolation**   9, 17, 22, 29, 32, 34, 35
Sources—Egg yolk, liver, milk
Method—Extract with acetone, precipitate with alcohol and phosphotungstate, adsorb and elute from charcoal, precipitate with $HgCl_2$, dissolve, purify, crystallize

6. **Determination**   14, 16, 27a, 33
Bioassay
    Microbiological—*L. arabinosus*
    Rat and chick method—Growth response after biotin deficiency
Physicochemical—Polarography

DISTRIBUTION AND SOURCES

1. **Occurrence**   16, 19, 22, 25, 26, 29, 32, 34, 35
Plants
    Fruit—All low
    Vegetables—All low, except beans, peas, cauliflower
    Nuts—All medium, also cereals
Animals—All low except in organs (except liver and kidneys are high)
Microorganisms—Afford best source of biotin, especially yeast, lower fungi and bacteria

2. **Dietary Sources**   3, 8, 20, 27, 30, 34, 36
High: 100-400 μg/100 g
    Royal jelly, yeast, lamb liver, pork liver
Medium: 10-100 μg/100 g
    Wheat, rice, corn, oats, barley

Eggs, beef liver, chicken, mushrooms
Cowpeas, chick-peas, lentils, soybeans, cauliflower, chocolate
Mackerel, salmon, sardines
Almonds, peanuts, pecans, walnuts, filberts, hazelnuts
Low: 0-1 μg/100 g
    Cheese, milk
    Apples, bananas, strawberries, cantaloupes, grapefruit, grapes, oranges, peaches, watermelon, avocados
    Lima beans, beets, carrots, cabbages, corn, lettuce, onions, peas, sweet potatoes, tomatoes, spinach, beet greens
    Beef, lamb, veal, pork, tuna, halibut, oyster

MEDICAL AND NUTRITIONAL ROLE

1. **Units**   8, 16, 17, 26, 34
    By weight, μg

2. **Normal Blood Levels**   4, 14, 26, 33, 34
    0.95-1.66 μg/100 ml serum; 0.75-1.73 μg/100 ml, blood

3. **Recommended Intakes (Estimated)**   4, 8, 21, 24, 27, 37
    Children—65-120 μg/day
    Adults—100-200 μg/day estimated; may be available from intestinal bacteria and diet

4. **Administration**   8, 9, 31, 32, 35
    Injection—Parenteral, intramuscular
    Topical—No data
    Oral—Mainly used

5. **Factors Affecting Availability**   3, 8, 20, 27, 27a
    Decrease
        Presence of avidin in food
        Cooking losses
        Antibiotics
        Sulfa drugs
        Binding in foods (yeast, animals)
    Increase—Synthesis by intestinal bacteria

6. **Deficiency Symptoms**   3, 4, 16, 21, 24, 27, 27a, 30
    General
        Desquamation of the skin
        Lassitude, somnolence, muscle pain

Hyperesthesia
Seborrheic dermatitis
Alopecia, spastic gait, and kangaroo-like posture (rats and mice)
Dermatitis and perosis (chicks and turkeys)
Progressive paralysis, K^+ deficiency (dogs)
Alopecia, spasticity of hind legs (pigs)
Thinning and depigmentation of hair (monkeys)

7. **Effects of Overdose, Toxicity**   3, 4, 16, 22, 26, 29, 31, 32, 34
None noted—1 g/kg not toxic
Essentially nontoxic in man

METABOLIC ROLE

1. **Biosynthesis**   3, 19, 25, 28
Precursors—Pimelic acid, cysteine, carbamyl phosphate
Intermediates—Desthiobiotin

2. **Production: Species and sites**   3, 19, 25, 28
Plants—Seedlings, leaves
Fungi—Some
Bacteria—Intestinal, some others

3. **Storage Sites**   8, 9, 16, 26, 34
Liver

4. **Blood Carriers**   8, 14, 29, 31, 32
Unknown

5. **Half-life**   8, 9, 29, 31, 32, 34
Requires 3-4 weeks to produce human deficiency with avidin

6. **Target Tissues**   14, 16, 29, 31, 32, 34
Skin, nervous tissue, male genitalia, bone marrow, liver, kidney

7. **Reactions**   5, 14, 16, 17, 28
Coenzyme forms: CO_2-biotin-enz; d-biotin-lys-enz

Organ	Enzyme System	Effect
Liver	CARBOXYLASES Propionyl-CoA carboxylase β-methylcrotonyl-CoA-carboxylase Acetyl-CoA carboxylase Phosphoenolpyruvate carboxykinase ATP-dependent pyruvic carboxylase	Activated
Liver	TRANSCARBOXYLASES Oxalosuccinate-acetyl-CoA transcarboxylase Methylmalonyl-oxalacetic transcarboxylase	Activated
Liver	Malic enzyme	Activated
Liver	Ornithine transcarbamylase	Activated

8. **Mode of Action**   3, 5, 6, 9, 14, 17, 22
   Cellular
      Anabolic—Purine, protein, and carbohydrate synthesis; synthesis of
         aspartic acid, oleic acid, fatty acids
      Catabolic—Deamination of serine in animals; tryptophan metabolism
      Other—CO_2 fixation; ureido carbon of enzyme-bound biotin is the "active
         carbon"; implicated in carbamylation reactions
   Organismal—Growth; maintenance of sebaceous glands, nervous tissue, skin,
      blood cells, hair, male genitalia

9. **Catabolism**   1, 3, 8, 9, 10, 16, 28
   Intermediates—Little known
   Excretion products
      Urine—14-70 μg/day biotin, biocytin sulfoxide (?)
      Feces—2.5 x amount in food intake (bacterial synthesis)

MISCELLANEOUS

1. **Relationship to Other Vitamins**   8, 11, 13, 27, 31, 32
   Pantothenic acid—Indicated by depigmentation of hair in deficiency of bio-
      tin + pantothenic acid
   Vitamin C—Ascorbic acid biosynthesis requires biotin
   Vitamins B_2, B_6, niacin, A, D—Synergistic with biotin in maintenance of skin
   Niacin—Not synthesized from tryptophan in biotin deficiency
   Folic acid (with pantothenic acid and biotin)—Increased stress response in
      adrenalectomized rats

2. **Relationship to Hormones**   8, 11, 13
   Testosterone—Rat male genital system retarded in biotin deficiency (symp-
      toms develop earlier than in female)

Cortisol—Adrenocortical insufficiency noted in biotin-deficient rats
STH—Synergist in growth

3. **Unusual Features   11, 13, 14, 16**
   Binding and inactivation by avidin protein found in egg white
   Fetal tissues and cancer tissues are higher in biotin than adult tissues
   Biotin deficiency increases severity and duration of some diseases, notably
      some protozoan infections
   Oleic acid and related compounds act to replace biotin as unspecific stimu-
      latory compounds in bacteria
   Combines to lysine residues of proteins
   Only (+) isomer active
   Inactivated by rancid fats, choline

4. **Possible Relationships of Deficiency Symptoms to Metabolic Action   11,**
   13, 16, 27
   Desquamation of skin—Decreased fatty acid synthesis, synergism with A, D,
      other B vitamins
   Hyperesthesia—Increased lactic acid levels
   Lassitude, somnolence—Decreased oxidation of pyruvate
   Muscle pain—Increased lactic acid levels, decreased fatty acid synthesis
   Seborrheic dermatitis—Decreased synergism with vitamins A, D, other B
      vitamins

5. **Relationship to Minerals   (See references in specific minerals section)**
   Synergist—Mn^{2+}

Chapter 26.   Folic Acid

Folic acid is a very important vitamin. Its major functions are as coenzyme in nucleic acid synthesis and metabolism, growth, methylations, and porphyrin synthesis. Deficiencies of this vitamin are widespread. Its chief importance lies in its relationship to cell division and hence to growth and cancer, as well as to blood diseases (anemias, leukopenia) and intestinal maintenance. Anti-folic acid compounds are widely used as anti-tumor agents. Major deficiency diseases are several types of anemias.

Folic acid is a very slightly water-soluble vitamin—chemically a complex of amino acid, paraminobenzoic acid, and a pteridine. Small amounts are stored in the liver. Folic acid is nontoxic in man in quantities up to 5 mg/day. Megadoses have been used experimentally in an attempt to control epilepsy but without general clinical acceptance. Its chief synergists are vitamin C, vitamin B_{12}, niacin, pantothenic acid, Fe^{2+}, and Cu^{2+}, whereas its chief antagonists are aminopterin, methotrexate, alcohol, and estrogens.

Folic acid is obtained from plant and animal sources. Its requirements are established at 0.4 mg/day, and it is rapidly excreted. Some of it is available from intestinal bacteria, but most folic acid must be obtained from the diet. There is evidence that dietary supplementation is required for a normal, healthy individual on an average American diet, since only about half the RDA is available in the average American diet. Cooking losses and poor absorption further exacerbate the deficiency. Special conditions requiring definite dietary supplementation are: pregnancy, illness, anemias [pernicious (with B_{12}), megaloblastic, macrocytic], old age, alcoholism, mental illness and retardation, gastric disturbances, malabsorption, diarrhea, antibiotic and some anticonvulsant therapy, leukemia, cheilosis, infections, and Hodgkins' disease.

Dietary items high in folic acid are: liver, kidney, yeast, green vegetables, legumes, peanuts, mushrooms, beef, veal, and egg yolk.

GENERAL INFORMATION

1. **Synonyms**   7, 16, 18, 35
   Folacin, pteroylmonoglutamic acid, antianemia factor, *L. casei* factor, vitamin B_c, vitamin M, PGA

2. **History**   16, 18, 35
   1931—Wills: demonstrated a factor from yeast active in treating anemia
   1938—Day et al.: found yeast or liver extracts active in treating anemia in monkeys
   1939—Hogan and Parrott: prevented anemia in chicks with liver extract
   1940—Snell and Peterson: isolated *L. casei* growth factor from liver and yeast
   1941—Hutchings et al.: found *L. casei* factor also essential for chicks
   1941—Mitchell, Snell, Williams: isolated bacterial (*S. lactis R*) growth factor similar to *L. casei* factor from yeast; named it folic acid
   1943—Stokstad: reported *L. casei* factor from liver more active than that from yeast; evidence for multiple factors
   1946—Angier et al.: isolated pteroylmonoglutamic acid, proved structure, and synthesized it

3. **Physiological Forms**   16, 23, 26, 34
   Tetrahydrofolic acid, pteroyltriglutamic acid, pteroylheptaglutamic acid, *l*-folinic acid (citrovorum factor), dihydrofolic acid (5-formyl-5,6,7,8-tetrahydro-PGA) (leucovorin)

4. **Active Analogs and Related Compounds**   14, 16, 23, 26, 34
   Pteroic acid (bacteria), 10-formyl-FAH_4, 5,10-methenyl-FAH_4, diopterin, 5,10-methylene-FAH_4, 5-formimino-FAH_4, rhizopterin (bacteria), xanthopterin (bacteria), biopterin (urine), ichthyopterin (fish), leucopterin (invertebrates)

5. **Inactive Analogs and Related Compounds**   14, 16, 26, 34
   d-folinic acid

6. **Antagonists**   1, 7, 14, 16, 26, 34
   Aminopterin (4-amino-PGA), methotrexate (amethopterin), pyrimethamine, 4-amino-pteroylaspartic acid, alcohol, estrogens

7. **Synergists**   1, 7, 14, 16, 26, 34
   Biotin, pantothenic acid, niacin, vitamins B_6, B_2, C, B_1, E, B_{12}, STH, estradiol, testosterone, Fe^{2+}, Cu^{2+}

8. **Physiological Functions**   3, 4, 14, 20, 26, 27a, 34
    Synthesis of nucleic acid, coenzyme in purine-pyrimidine metabolism, serine-glycine conversion, intermediate in metabolism of purines and pyrimidines, differentiation of embryonic nervous system, one-carbon transfer mechanisms, metabolism of tyrosine and histidine, formation of active formate, and methionine, synthesis of choline

9. **Deficiency Diseases and Disorders**   3, 4, 14, 20, 26, 27a, 34
    Anemias (macrocytic, megaloblastic, pernicious), glossitis, diarrhea, gastro-intestinal lesions, intestinal malabsorption, sprue, pancytopenia

10. **Sources for Species Requiring It (Essential in man)**   1, 3, 4, 14, 26, 34
    Most animals require it (all vertebrates, some insects, protozoa, bacteria)
    Exogenous sources—Vertebrates, invertebrates, some bacteria (intestinal bacteria provide it in man, rats, dogs, pigs, rabbits, but not in monkey, guinea pig, mice, fox, chicken, geese, turkeys)
    Endogenous sources—Intestinal bacteria, fungi, yeast

CHEMISTRY

1. **Structure**   16, 18, 19, 22, 29, 32, 34, 35

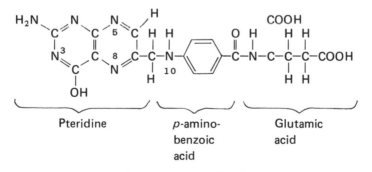

Folic acid, $C_{19}H_{19}N_7O_6$

2. **Reactions**   3, 17, 18, 22, 29, 32, 34, 35

Heat—Labile (in soln.)	Oxidation—Labile
Acid—Labile	Reduction—Stable
Alkali—Stable	Light—Labile (in soln.) to UV
Water—Stable (acid, pH 4.4)	

3. **Properties**   1, 7, 15, 17, 18, 22, 29, 32, 34

Appearance—Yellow crystals

MW—441.2

MP—Chars at 250°C

Crystal form—Lenticular

Salts—Ba, Na, Pb

Important groups for activity

Glutamic acid

N^{10}, N^5, N^3, N^8

Solubility

H_2O—0.01 mg/ml

Acet., Alc.—Insol.

Benz., Chl., Eth.—Insol.

Absn. max.—282, 350 mμ (pH 7.0)

Miscellaneous—pK_a = 8.2

α_D^{25} = ±23° (0.1 N NaOH)

Chemical nature—Purine, amino acid, benzoic acid

4. **Commercial Production**   18, 22, 29, 32, 34, 35

Extraction from yeast or liver; synthetic

5. **Isolation**   9, 17, 22, 29, 32, 34, 35

Sources—Spinach, liver, yeast, alfalfa, wheat bran

Method

Extract (aq.) liver at pH 3.0

Adsorb on norite; elute with NH_4OH-ethanol

Adsorb on superfiltrol, pH 1.3; elute with NH_4OH-ethanol

Precipitate with Ba^{2+}, pH 7.0, in alcohol

Esterify with methanol; extract with n-butanol

Adsorb on superfiltrol, pH 7; elute ester with 75% acetone

Crystallize from hot methanol; hydrolyze ester

Recrystallize from hot H_2O

6. **Determination**   14, 16, 27a, 33

Bioassay

Animal—Chick feathering, rat oviduct development

Microbial—Growth of *L. casei, S. fecalis*

Physicochemical

Enzymatic—DPNH reductase activity

Fluorometric—Fluorescence at 470 mμ

Colorimetric—Estimation of aromatic amine on cleavage

Polarographic—Paper chromatography

DISTRIBUTION AND SOURCES

1. **Occurrence**   16, 19, 22, 25, 26, 29, 32, 34, 35

Plants

Fruit—Low

Vegetables—Green leafy vegetables, dried beans

Nuts—Almonds, filberts, peanuts, walnuts
Miscellaneous—Green leaves, grass, barley, oats, rye, wheat
Animals
Liver, kidney
Butterflies (wing pigment, xanthopterin)
Fish scales (ichthyopterin)
Microorganisms: Intestinal bacteria, yeast, fungi, algae
Miscellaneous: Mushrooms

2. **Dietary Sources**   3, 8, 20, 27, 30, 34, 36
High: 90-300 μg/g
Liver (beef, lamb, pork, chicken)
Asparagus, spinach
Wheat, bran
Dry beans (lentils, limas, navy)
Yeast
Medium: 30-90 μg/100 g
Kidney (beef)
Lima beans, snap beans, broccoli, corn, beet greens, chicory, endive, kale, parsley, chard, turnip greens, watercress
Almonds, filberts, peanuts, walnuts
Barley, oats, rye, wheat
Low: 0-30 μg/100 g
Beef (muscle, heart), lamb, pork, chicken, turkey (muscle)
All fruit tested
Cheese, milk
Brazil nuts, coconuts, pecans
Wax beans, beets, brussels sprouts, cabbages, carrots, brown rice, cauliflower, celery, cucumbers, eggplant, escarole, mustard, kohlrabi, lettuce, mushrooms, okra, onions, parsnips, peas, peppers, potatoes, pumpkins, radishes, rutabagas, squash, sweet potatoes, tomatoes, turnips

MEDICAL AND NUTRITIONAL ROLE

1. **Units**   8, 16, 17, 26, 34
By weight, μg

2. **Normal Blood Levels**   4, 14, 26, 33, 34
0.4-0.6 μg/100 ml, serum; 16-64 μg/100 ml, RBC

3. **Recommended Allowances**   4, 8, 21, 24, 27, 37
Children—0.1-0.3 mg/day
Adults—0.4 mg/day
Provided by intestinal synthesis in dogs, cats, rabbits

Required by monkey, guinea pig, mice, fox, chicken, geese, turkeys, man
Special—Pregnancy, illness

4. **Administration**   8, 9, 31, 32, 35
Injection—Subcutaneous
Topical—No data
Oral—Preferred route

5. **Factors Affecting Availability**   3, 8, 20, 27, 27a
Decrease
   High urinary excretion (75% ingested)
   Destruction by certain intestinal bacteria
   Increased urinary excretion caused by vitamin C
   Sulfonamides, block intestinal synthesis
   Poor absorption
Increase—Intestinal bacterial synthesis and release: man, rats, dogs, pigs,
   rabbits

6. **Deficiency Symptoms**   3, 4, 16, 21, 24, 27, 27a, 30
Intestinal disturbances
Leukopenia
Glossitis
Thrombocytopenia
Macrocytic anemia
Pernicious anemia
Sprue
Megaloblastic erythropoiesis
Gingivitis, agranulosis (monkey)
Hydrocephalus, splenic enlargement (rats)
Endocrine disturbances, poor feathering (chick)
Lethargy, convulsions (guinea pig)

7. **Effects of Overdose, Toxicity**   3, 4, 16, 22, 26, 29, 31, 32, 34
Man—No toxicity reported
Mice—Renal damage, convulsions: LD_{50} = 600 mg/kg
Chick—Arrest cells in metaphase with high doses

METABOLIC ROLE

1. **Biosynthesis**   3, 19, 25, 28
Precursors: Para-aminobenzoic acid, glutamic acid, unknown pteridine
Intermediates: Para-aminobenzoylglutamic acid

2. **Production: Species and sites** 3, 19, 25, 28
   Plants—Leaves, seeds, cereal germ, algae
   Bacteria—Intestinal supply sufficient for man, rats, pigs, dogs, rabbits; other
      species require exogenous sources
   Fungi—Yeast

3. **Storage** 8, 9, 16, 26, 34
   Liver (small amount), spinal fluid

4. **Blood Carriers** 8, 14, 29, 31, 32
   Prefolic acid A

5. **Half-life** 8, 9, 29, 31, 32, 34
   75% of ingested folic acid excreted in urine in 24 hr

6. **Target Tissues** 14, 16, 29, 31, 32, 34
   Liver, bone marrow, lymph nodes, kidneys

7. **Reactions** 5, 14, 16, 17, 28
   Coenzyme forms: Folinic acid (citrovorum factor), 10-formyl-FH_4, 5,10-methylene-FH_4, 5-formimino-FH_4, 10-formimino-FH_4, 5-methyl-FH_4, 5-hydroxymethyl-FH_4

Organ	Enzyme System	Effect
	REDUCTASES	
Liver	Dihydrofolate reductase: $FH_2 \rightarrow FH_4$	Activated
	N^5N^{10}-Methylene-FH_4 reductase: N^5N^{10}-methylene-$FH_4 \rightarrow N^5$-methyl-FH_4	
	TRANSFERASES	
Liver	Formiminoglutamate formimino transferase: Formation of formimino glutamate	Activated
	Serine transhydroxymethylase: Glycine-serine interconversion	
	Formylglutamate formyl transferase: Formation of glutamate	
	ISOMERASES	
Liver	N^5-formyl-tetrahydrofolate isomerase: N^5-formyl-$FH_4 \rightarrow N^{10}$-formyl-FH_4	Activated
	SYNTHETASES	
Liver	Formyl tetrahydrofolate synthetase: $FH_4 \rightarrow N^{10}$-formyl-FH_4	Activated
	CONJUGASES	
Liver	Folic acid conjugase: Converts pteroyltriglutamate $\rightarrow$ PGA	Activated

8. **Mode of Action**   3, 5, 6, 9, 14, 17, 22
   Cellular
     Anabolic
       Purine and pyrimidine synthesis
       Choline synthesis
       Methionine synthesis
       Formation of lignin, nicotine, betaine
     Catabolic—Histidine metabolism, tryptophan metabolism
     Other
       Mitotic step: Metaphase → anaphase requires folic acid
       Serine-glycine interconversion
       Formiminoglutamate formation
   Organismal
     Erythropoiesis, growth
     Maintenance of sex organs
     Maintenance of intestinal tract
     Leukopoiesis
     Differentiation of nervous system

9. **Catabolism**   1, 3, 8, 9, 10, 16, 28
   Intermediates: Xanthopterin, leucopterin
   Excretion products: Urine—Biopterin, leucovorin, pteroylglutamic acid—
     2.1-21 μg/day; feces—enterohepatic circulation of folate

MISCELLANEOUS

1. **Relationship to Other Vitamins**   8, 11, 13, 27, 31, 32
   Vitamin C
     Facilitates conversion of folic to folinic acid (CF-citrovorum factor)
     Protects folinic acid from oxidation, increases urinary excretion of CF
     Fundamental role with folic acid in erythropoiesis
   Vitamin B_{12}
     Blood and marrow changes in pernicious anemia respond to folic acid or
       B_{12}
     Neurological changes in pernicious anemia involve B_{12} and folic acid
     Involved with folic acid in formation of methionine from homocysteine
   Biotin—Aids in storage and utilization of pantothenic acid in liver (with folic
     acid)
   Pantothenic acid—Utilization in CoA synthesis (with biotin and folic acid)
   Niacin
     Need folic acid for niacin metabolism
     DPNH required for production of N^5-methyl-FH_4
     DPN involved in methionine formation (with folic acid)

Vitamin B_6—Required with folic acid for serine-glycine transformations and for methionine formation

Riboflavin—Required with DPN, folic acid, vitamin B_{12}, vitamin B_6, for methionine formation

2. **Relationship to Hormones   8, 11, 13**

Estradiol—Folic acid deficiency eliminates normal response of female reproductive organs to estrogens; pregnancies not normal

Testosterone—Folic acid increases action of testosterone on development of accessory sex organs

STH—Synergist in growth

3. **Unusual Features   11, 13, 14, 16**

Folic acid antagonists used in cancer therapy with temporary remissions

Occurs in chromosomes

Distributed throughout cell

Needed for mitotic step metaphase $\rightarrow$ anaphase

Antibody formation decreased in folic acid deficiency

Choline-sparing effects

Analgesic in man—Pain threshold increased

Low intravenous toxicity in man

Antisulfonamide effects

Enterohepatic circulation of folate

Synthesized by psittacosis virus

Concentrated in spinal fluid

4. **Possible Relationships of Deficiency Symptoms to Metabolic Action   11, 13, 16, 27**

Cytopenia—Decreased nucleic acid synthesis and porphyrin synthesis

Intestinal disturbances—Indirect relationship with other vitamin deficiencies

Thrombocytopenia—Decreased nucleic acid synthesis

Leukopenia—Decreased nucleic acid synthesis

Glossitis—Indirect effect of other vitamin B deficiencies (loss of synergism)

Macrocytic anemia and pernicious anemia—Vitamin B_{12} lack and decreased porphyrin synthesis

Sprue—Indirect effect of lack of other vitamins (synergistic loss)

5. **Relationship to Minerals   (See references in specific minerals section)**

Synergists—Fe^{2+}, Cu^{2+}

Chapter 27. Niacin

Niacin is a very well-known vitamin, being associated with pellagra, a once widespread deficiency disease. Its major functions are as a coenzyme (esp. Coenz. I + II) in tissue respiration and carbohydrate and lipid metabolism. Deficiencies of this vitamin are less prevalent than they once were. Its chief importance is its relationship to energy output, disorders of the skin and digestive organs, mental disturbances, and alleviation of the major deficiency disease, pellagra.

Niacin is water-soluble, with two chemical forms, nicotinic acid and nicotinamide, both chemical derivatives of pyridine. Some niacin is stored in the liver, muscle, and the heart. Niacin has limited toxicity in megadoses with symptoms of skin flushing (nicotinic acid only), vasodilation, depression, and circulatory and central nervous system disturbances. Megadoses have been used in attempted treatments of schizophrenia by certain medical groups but without general clinical acceptance. Major synergists of niacin are: B_{12}, folic acid, Cr^{2+}, and Zn^{2+}. Antagonists include 3-acetyl pyridine and leucine.

Niacin is obtained from plant and (mainly) animal sources, and is excreted fairly rapidly. It is not available from intestinal synthesis, but a small amount is available from dietary protein-tryptophan conversion. Human requirements are based on caloric intake. There is no evidence that dietary supplementation is required for a normal, healthy adult on an average American diet. However, many special conditions exist requiring additional supplementation: pregnancy, lactation, high-caloric diets, pellagra, malnutrition, dermatosis, high serum cholesterol (?), high corn intakes, sprue, and glossitis.

Dietary items high in niacin include: peanuts, yeast, organ meats, tuna, halibut, swordfish, chicken, and turkey.

GENERAL INFORMATION

1. **Synonyms**   7, 16, 18, 35
   Nicotinic acid, nicotinamide, P-P factor, antipellagra factor, anti-blacktongue factor, B_3

2. **History**   16, 18, 35
   1867—Huber: first synthesized nicotinic acid
   1914—Funk: isolated nicotinic acid from rice polishings
   1915—Goldberger: demonstrated that pellagra is a nutritional deficiency
   1917—Chittenden and Underhill: demonstrated that canine blacktongue is similar to pellagra
   1935—Warburg and Christian: determined niacinamide essential in hydrogen transport as DPN
   1936—Euler et al.: isolated DPN and determined its structure
   1937—Elvhehjem et al.: cured blacktongue with niacinamide from liver
   1937—Fouts et al.: cured pellagra with niacinamide
   1947—Handley and Bond: established conversion of tryptophan to niacin by animal tissues

3. **Physiological Forms**   16, 23, 26, 34
   Niacinamide, NAD (DPN, Co I), NADP (TPN, Co II), N^1-methylnicotinamide

4. **Active Analogs and Related Compounds**   14, 16, 23, 26, 34
   Niacin esters, coramine, β-picoline, 3-hydroxymethylpyridine

5. **Inactive Analogs and Related Compounds**   14, 16, 26, 34
   Trigonelline

6. **Antagonists**   1, 2, 14, 16, 26, 34
   Pyridine-3-sulfonic acid (bacteria), 3-acetylpyridine, 6-aminonicotinamide, 5-thiazole carboxamide, leucine

7. **Synergists**   1, 7, 14, 16, 26, 34
   Vitamins B_1, B_2, B_6, B_{12}, D, pantothenic and folic acids, STH, Cr^{3+}, Zn^{2+}, MoO_4^{2-}, PO_4^{3-}

8. **Physiological Functions**   4, 14, 20, 26, 27a, 34
   Maintenance of NAD, NADP; hydrogen and electron transfer agents in CHO metabolism; furnish coenzymes for dehydrogenase systems; coenzyme in lipid catabolism, oxidative deamination, photosynthesis

9. **Deficiency Diseases, Disorders**   4, 14, 16, 26, 27a, 34
   Pellagra (man), blacktongue (dogs), malnutrition, dermatosis (man), glossitis, gastrointestinal and central nervous system dysfunction

10. **Sources for Species Requiring It (Essential for man)**   1, 3, 4, 14, 26, 34
    Required by some species: Some vertebrates, insects, protozoa, fungi, bacteria
    Exogenous sources: Animals, some bacteria and fungi (not available from in-
    testinal bacteria in man, but some conversion from tryptophan occurs in
    tissues)
    Endogenous sources: Plants: algae; some bacteria and fungi; animals: man
    and some species partly via tryptophan; other species completely via
    tryptophan

CHEMISTRY

1. **Structure**   16, 18, 19, 22, 29, 32, 34, 35

   Niacin, $C_6H_5O_2N$

2. **Reactions**   3, 17, 18, 22, 29, 32, 34, 35

Heat—Stable	Oxidation—Stable
Acid—Stable	Reduction—Unstable
Alkali—Stable	Light—Stable
Water—Acidic	

3. **Properties**   1, 7, 15, 17, 18, 22, 29, 32, 34

   Appearance—White crystalline
     powder
   MW—123.1
   MP—234-237°C (sublimes)
   Crystal form—Needles
   Solubility
     H_2O—1 g/100 ml
     Alc.—Sol.
     Benz., Chl., Eth., Acet.—Insol.
   Absn. max.—261.5 mμ

   Salts—HCl, metallic, Na
   Important groups
     —N on ring
     —COOH
   Chemical nature—Carboxylic acid;
     amine; substituted pyridine
   Miscellaneous—pK_a = 4.8, 12.0
   α_D = 0 (inactive)

4. **Commercial Production**   18, 22, 29, 32, 34, 35
   Hydrolysis of 3-cyanopyridine
   Oxidation of nicotine, quinoline, or collidine

5. **Isolation**   9, 17, 22, 29, 32, 34, 35
   Sources—Liver, yeast
   Method—Remove lipids with solvents; hydrolyze with acid or alkali; extract
     niacin from acidified hydrolyzate; isolate as an acid, ester, or Cu salt;
     purify by recrystallization or sublimation

6. Determination   14, 16, 27a, 33
Bioassay
Animal—Dogs, blacktongue (curative)
Microbial—*L. arabinosus*, growth
Physicochemical
Colorimetric—Cyanogen Br + reducing agent → color
Spectrophotometric—UV max. of DPN, TPN

DISTRIBUTION AND SOURCES

1. Occurrence   16, 19, 22, 25, 26, 29, 32, 34, 35
Plants:
Fruit—All low (exc. avocados and dried figs, dates, and prunes—medium)
Vegetables—All low (exc. beans, peas, potatoes, broccoli, asparagus, corn,
parsley, kale—medium)
Nuts—All medium (exc. coconuts, pecans—low)
Animals: All medium [exc. livers, kidneys, beef heart, rabbit, turkey and
chicken (white meat), tuna, halibut, swordfish—high]
Microorganisms—All high—Intestinal bacteria, some other bacteria

2. Dietary Sources   3, 8, 20, 27, 30, 34, 36
High: 10,000-100,000 μg/100 g (10-100 mg/100 g)
Peanuts (roasted), rice bran
Liver (beef, calf, chicken, pork, sheep)
Heart (calf), kidney (pork, beef)
Rabbit, turkey and chicken (white meat)
Meat extract
Tuna, halibut, swordfish
Yeast
Medium: 1000-10,000 μg/100 g (1-10 mg/100 g)
Avocados, dates (dry), figs (dry), prunes (dry)
Asparagus, beans (kidney, lima, snap, wax), broccoli, corn, kale, lentils
(dry), parsley, peas, potatoes, soybeans (dry)
Almonds (dry), cashew nuts, chestnuts, walnuts
Barley, oats, wheat, rye, brown rice, wheat germ, molasses, cheeses
(Camembert, swiss, roquefort)
Beef, veal, chicken (dark meat), duck, lamb, fish (exc. tuna, halibut,
swordfish), clams, shrimp, oysters
Mushrooms
Low: 100-1000 μg/100 g (0.1-1.0 mg/100 g)
Apples, apricots, bananas, berries (black-, blue-, cran-, rasp-, straw-),
cherries, currants, figs, grapes, grapefruit, lemons, melons, oranges,
peaches, pears, pineapples, plums, raisins (dry), tangerines

Beets, beet greens, brussels sprouts, cabbage, carrots, cauliflower, celery, chicory, endive, cucumbers, dandelion greens, eggplant, kohlrabi, lettuce, onions, parsnips, peppers, pumpkins, radishes, rhubarb, spinach, sweet potatoes, tomatoes, turnips, watercress

Coconuts, pecans

Eggs, milk

MEDICAL AND NUTRITIONAL ROLE

1. **Units**   8, 16, 17, 26, 34
By weight, mg equivalents

2. **Normal Blood Levels**   4, 14, 26, 33, 34
.05 mg/100 ml, serum; 3.0 mg/100 ml, blood

3. **Recommended Allowances**   4, 8, 21, 24, 27, 37
Children—9-16 mg equivalents/day*
Adults—16-19 mg equivalents/day—male; 13-15 mg equivalents/day—female*
Special—Pregnancy, 15 mg equivalents/day; lactation, 20 mg equivalents/day
Therapeutic dose—100-1000 mg/day (niacinamide)

4. **Administration**   8, 9, 31, 32, 35
Injection—I.V.
Topical—No data
Oral—Preferred route

5. **Factors Affecting Availability**   3, 8, 20, 27, 27a
Decrease
    Cooking losses
    Bound form in corn, greens, seeds, partially unavailable
    Oral antibiotics
    Decreased absorption—Disease
    Decreased tryptophan converted in B_6 deficiency
Increase
    Alkali treatment of cereals
    Storage in liver, possibly muscle, kidney
    Increased intestinal synthesis

6. **Deficiency Symptoms**   3, 4, 16, 21, 24, 27, 27a, 30
General (man)—Pellagra
    Retarded growth, achlorhydria

*Depends on tryptophan content of diet; allow 10 mg equivalents for each 600 mg dietary tryptophan, assume 60 g/day protein in diet has 600 mg tryptophan.

Weakness, anorexia, indigestion, lassitude, dermatitis, pigmentation, diar-
rhea, tongue erythema, irritability, headaches, insomnia, memory loss
Histological changes in central nervous system (dog, cat—blacktongue)
Drooling (dog, cat—blacktongue)
Perosis (chickens)
Poor feathering (chickens)

7. **Effects of Overdose, Toxicity**   3, 4, 16, 22, 26, 29, 31, 32, 34
Man—Limited toxicity, starting approx. 1-4 g/kg dosage with individual variations in sensitivity—Burning, itching skin; peripheral vasodilation; decreased serum cholesterol, fatty liver; stimulated central nervous system;
increased: pulse rate, respiratory rate, cerebral blood flow; decreased blood
pressure
Rat—Respiratory paralysis, ketosis
Dogs—Death
Chick—Inhibition of growth, fatty liver

METABOLIC ROLE

1. **Biosynthesis**   3, 19, 25, 28
Precursors—Tryptophan (animals, bacteria). Glycerol and succinic acid
(plants)
Intermediates—Kynurenine, hydroxyanthranilic acid, quinolinic acid

2. **Production: Species and sites**   3, 19, 25, 28
Fungi—*Neurospora*
Plants—Leaves, germinating seeds, shoots
Bacteria—Intestinal
Animals—Tissues (not intestinal)

3. **Storage**   8, 9, 16, 26, 34
Liver, heart, muscle

4. **Blood Carriers**   8, 14, 29, 31, 32
Mostly as DPN in blood corpuscles

5. **Half-life**   8, 9, 29, 31, 32, 34
1/3 of intake excreted in 24 hr

6. **Target Tissues**   14, 16, 29, 31, 32, 34
Liver (storage), heart, muscle, kidney, skin, gastrointestinal tract, spinal cord

7. Reactions   5, 14, 16, 17, 28

Coenzyme forms—(DPN, NAD) and (TPN, NADP). Act as redox couples: oxidized ⇌ reduced

Organ	Enzyme System	Effect
	More than 50 metabolic reactions known	
Liver	DEHYDROGENASES: Alcohol, lactate, malate, isocitrate, glucose-6-P-succinic, β-hydroxybutyrate, 3β-hydroxy-steroids, betaine aldehyde, glutamate, α-glycerophosphate, uridine DPG, reduced glutathione, glyceraldehyde-3-P	Activated
Liver	OXIDASES: α-Keto glutaric oxidase microsomal mixed-function oxidases (DPN + TPN), oxidation of steroids, fatty acids, drugs, and carcinogens	Activated or completed

8. Mode of Action   3, 5, 6, 9, 14, 17, 22

Cellular

Anabolic—Maintains microsomal reductive biosynthesis; photosynthesis

Catabolic

Furnishes coenzymes for lipid catabolism

Oxidative deamination

CHO metabolism—Dehydrogenation, oxidation

Key reactions in glycolysis, TCA cycle, and HMP

Other

Hydrogen and electron transfer agent

A mobile hydrogen transfer agent

Maintains respiratory chain in mitochondria

Organismal

Maintains growth

Maintains energy supply to organism from degradation of carbohydrates, proteins, and lipids

Maintains terminal section of respiratory cycle

Maintains manufacture of hormones (steroids), proteins, lipids

Stimulates gastric secretion and bile secretion

9. Catabolism   1, 3, 8, 9, 10, 16, 28

Intermediates—N^1-Methylnicotinamide (liver)

Excretion Products

Feces: Nicotinic acid

Urine: N^1-methyl-6-pyridone-3-carboxamide; nicotinamide, 0.7-3.5 mg/day; N-Methylnicotinamide, 2.8-42.0 mg/day

MISCELLANEOUS

1. **Relationship to Other Vitamins**   8, 11, 13, 31, 32
   Vitamin B_2—Flavo-proteins reoxidize NAD, NADP
   Vitamin B_6—Decreased tryptophan conversion to niacin in B_6 deficiency
   Vitamins B_1, B_2, B_6, pantothenic acid, folic acid, vitamin B_{12}—General synergism with niacin in alleviating deficiencies and in CHO metabolism
   Vitamins B_1, B_2, B_6—Needed for conversion of tryptophan to niacin

2. **Relationship to Hormones**   8, 9, 11, 13, 17, 27
   Serotonin—Reduces tryptophan conversion to niacin (in cancer cases)
   Thyroxine, insulin—Affect mitochondrial metabolism (as do DPN and TPN), and energy production from CHO metabolism
   Cortisol, testosterone, estradiol, progesterone, aldosterone—DPN and TPN involved in steroid oxidations in liver, in steroid hormone synthesis, and in cholesterol metabolism
   STH—Synergist in growth

3. **Unusual Features**   11, 13, 14, 16, 17
   Has hormonal quality, being partially internally synthesized
   Vasodilator, causes flushing (not as niacinamide)
   High-corn diets cause deficiency due to tryptophan deficiency in corn protein and unavailability of niacin in corn
   Prepared from nicotine using strong oxidizing agent
   Stereo-specific action of dehydrogenases on DPN
   Serum cholesterol lowering with large doses
   Antagonist (6-aminonicotinamide) active against some rat tumors
   Other pyridine derivatives functional in DPN and TPN
   Conversion of tryptophan not in intestines
   Toxicity of overdose preventable by feeding methionine (rats)

4. **Possible Relationships of Deficiency Symptoms to Metabolic Action**   11, 13, 16, 27
   Retarded growth—General synergism of all B vitamins
   Dermatitis, itching, pigmentation, tongue lesions; other B vitamins, esp. B_2, involved
   Irritability, mental disturbances, nervous lesions related to thiamine synergism with niacin
   Gastrointestinal lesions and disturbances related to thiamine deficiency and synergism
   Mottled liver, fatty liver are disturbances of cholesterol metabolism

5. **Relationship to Minerals**   (See specific mineral section references)
   Synergists—Zn^{2+}, Cr^{3+}, MoO_4^{2-}, PO_4^{3-}, I (as T4), SeO_3^{2-}

Chapter 28.
Pantothenic Acid

Pantothenic acid occupies a key position in metabolism. Its major function is to serve as part of coenzyme A, which is at the center of energy metabolism and fat, acetylcholine, and antibody synthesis. Deficiencies of this vitamin are difficult to find. Its chief importance stems from its relationship to energy production, stress resistance, and synergism with other B vitamins to prevent other B vitamin deficiency diseases.

Pantothenic acid is somewhat soluble in water, being chemically a complex of pantoic acid and an amino acid. Some storage occurs in the liver, heart, and kidney. Toxicity from megadoses has not been reported except for increases in blood histamine and increased sensitivity of skeletal and tooth joints. Synergists of pantothenic acid are folic acid, biotin, niacin, B_{12}, and Cr^{3+}. Antagonists are Cu^{2+}, and omega-methylpantothenic acid.

Pantothenic acid is obtained mainly from animal sources and a few plants and bacteria. It is fairly rapidly excreted, and is not available from intestinal bacteria. Exact human requirements have not been published, but according to knowledgeable estimates there is no evidence that dietary supplementation is required for a normal, healthy adult on an average American diet. Special conditions requiring dietary supplementation are: stress, aging, arthritis, illness, malabsorption, weakness, depression, streptomycin toxicity, and burning foot syndrome. Dietary items high in pantothenic acid are: yeast, liver, kidney, eggs, peanuts, wheat germ, herring, and royal jelly.

GENERAL INFORMATION

1. **Synonyms**   7, 16, 18, 35
   Chick antidermatitis factor, B_5, Bios IIa, antigray-hair factor

2. **History**   16, 18, 35
   1901—Wildiers: described Bios, essential for yeast growth
   1933—Williams: isolated crystalline Bios from yeast; named it pantothenic acid
   1938—Williams: isolated pantothenic acid from liver
   1939—Jukes determined liver antidermatitis factor (chick) identical to yeast factor
   1939—Woolley et al.: demonstrated β-alanine a vital part
   1940—Harris, Folkers, et al.: reported structure determination and synthesis of pantothenic acid; crystallization also
   1950—Lipmann et al.: discovered CoA
   1951—Lynen: characterized coenzyme A structure

3. **Physiological Forms**   16, 23, 26, 34
   Coenzyme A, pantotheine, d(+)pantothenic acid

4. **Active Analogs and Related Compounds**   14, 16, 23, 26, 34
   Pantothenyl alcohol, β-alanine (bacteria), pantotheine (LBF), pantothine, pantothenylcystine, ethylmonoacetylpantothenate, ethyl pantothenate

5. **Inactive Analogs and Related Compounds**   14, 16, 26, 34
   l-pantothenate, α-alanine analogs

6. **Antagonists**   1, 7, 14, 16, 26, 34
   Pantoyltaurine, ω-methylpantothenic acid, bis(β-pantoylaminoethyl)disulfide, 6-mercaptopurine, pantoylaminoethanethiol, Cu^{2+}

7. **Synergists**   1, 7, 14, 16, 26, 34
   Biotin, folic acid, vitamins C, B_{12}, B_1, B_2, niacin, STH, Cr^{3+}, Zn^{2+}, PO_4^{3-}

8. **Physiological Functions**   3, 4, 14, 20, 26, 27a, 34
   Part of coenzyme A in carbohydrate metabolism (2 carbon transfer-acetate, or pyruvate), lipid metabolism (biosynthesis and catabolism of fatty acids, sterols, + phospholipids), protein metabolism (acetylations of amines and amino acids), porphyrin metabolism, acetylcholine production, isoprene production

9. Deficiency Diseases, Disorders   3, 4, 14, 16, 26, 27a, 34
Dermatitis (chick), achromotrichia (rat), adrenal necrosis (rats), bloody whiskers (rat), alopecia (mice)

10. Sources for Species Requiring It (Essential for man)   1, 3, 4, 14, 26, 34
Some organisms require it (all vertebrates, some insects and microorganisms)
Endogenous sources—Higher plants
Exogenous sources—All other organisms (not available from intestinal synthesis in man)

CHEMISTRY

1. Structure   16, 18, 19, 22, 29, 32, 34, 35

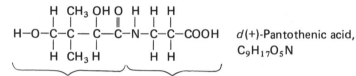

Pantoic acid   β-Alanine

d(+)-Pantothenic acid,
$C_9H_{17}O_5N$

2. Reactions   3, 17, 18, 22, 29, 32, 34, 35

Heat—Labile	Oxidation—Stable
Acid—Labile (warm)	Reduction—Stable
Alkali—Labile (warm)	Light—No data
Water—Sol. (acid)	

3. Properties   1, 7, 15, 17, 18, 22, 29, 32, 34

Appearance—Yellow viscous oil	MP—Unstable
MW—219.24	Crystal form—No data
Salts—Calcium, sodium	Absn. max.—358 mμ
Important groups for activity	Chem. nature—Conjugated amino acid,
β-amino group	polyhydroxy acid
Solubility	Optical rotation—$\alpha_D{}^{25}$ = (+37.5°)
H$_2$O—7 g/100 ml	(H$_2$O)
Acet., Alc.—Sol.	pK_a = 4.4
Benz., Chl., Eth.—Insol.	

4. Commercial Production: Synthetic   18, 22, 29, 32, 34, 35
Condensation of d-pantolactone with salt of β-alanine

5. Isolation   9, 17, 22, 29, 32, 34, 35
Sources—Rice, bran, liver, yeast
Method
   Extract liver with 90% ethyl alcohol
   Adsorb out organic bases on Fuller's earth
   Adsorb vitamin on charcoal, pH 3.6; elute with ammonia
   Form brucine salts; extract selectively with $CHCl_3$
   Convert brucine salt to calcium salt
   Purify by fractional precipitation from organic solvents

6. Determination   14, 16, 27a, 33
Bioassay
   Animal—Growth rate of chicks
   Microbiol—Growth of *L. casei*
Physicochemical—Estimate of β-alanine after hydrolysis; estimate CoA by
   citrate cleavage enzyme

DISTRIBUTION AND SOURCES

1. Occurrence   16, 19, 22, 25, 26, 29, 32, 34, 35
Plants
   Fruit—All (low)
   Vegetables—All (medium and low)
   Nuts—All (high and low)
Animals
   All (medium and high)
   Organs (brain, heart, kidney, liver)
Microorganisms
   Yeast (high); rumen bacteria in sheep and cattle
   Molds

2. Dietary Sources   3, 8, 20, 27, 30, 34, 36
High: 2.0-10.0 mg/100 g
   Beef (brain, heart, liver, kidney), pork (liver, kidney), sheep liver, chicken
      liver, lamb kidney
   Eggs
   Herring, cod ovary
   Wheat germ, bran, dried peas, peanuts
   Yeast, royal jelly
Medium: 0.5-2.0 mg/100 g
   Salmon, clams, mackerel
   Walnuts

Broccoli, soybeans, oats, lima beans, cauliflower, peas, avocado, carrots, kale, dried lentils, spinach, rice

Beef, pork (ham, bacon), chicken, lamb

Mushrooms, wheat, cheese

Low: 0.1-0.5 mg/100 g

Bananas, oranges, peaches, pears, pineapples, tomatoes, apples, grapes, grapefruit, lemons, plums

Onions, kidney beans, cabbage, lettuce, peppers, white and sweet potatoes, turnips, watercress

Almonds

Oysters, lobster, shrimp

Veal

Milk, honey, molasses

MEDICAL AND NUTRITIONAL ROLE

1. **Units**   8, 16, 17, 26, 34
   By weight, mg, μg

2. **Normal Blood Levels**   4, 14, 26, 33, 34
   6 μg/100 ml, serum; 183 μg/100 ml, blood

3. **Recommended Intakes (est.)**   4, 8, 21, 24, 27, 37
   Children—3-5 mg/day
   Adults—4-7 mg/day
   Special—Increased needs in stress situations

4. **Administration**   8, 9, 31, 32, 35
   Injection—Parenteral
   Topical—No data
   Oral—Preferred route

5. **Factors Affecting Availability**   3, 8, 20, 27, 27a
   Decrease
   Cooking—Up to 44% loss
   Heat instability
   Difficult release of bound forms
   Increase: Intestinal bacteria synthesis (very little in man)

6. **Deficiency Symptoms**   3, 4, 16, 21, 24, 27, 27a, 30
   General
   Neuromotor disturbances
   Cardiovascular disorders

Digestive disorders
Infection susceptibility
Physical weakness, depression
Stress susceptibility—rats
Skin disorders (cornea)—rats, chicks
Liver disorder—rat, chick
Reproductive failure—chick
Decreased antibody production—rat

7. **Effects of Overdose, Toxicity**   3, 4, 16, 22, 26, 29, 31, 32, 34
10 g/kg in mice, respiratory failure
Essentially nontoxic in man except for increases in blood histamine and sensitivity of joints

METABOLIC ROLE

1. **Biosynthesis**   3, 19, 25, 28
Precursors
    α-Ketoisovaleric acid (pantoic acid)
    Uracil (β-alanine)
    Aspartic acid (β-alanine)
Intermediates
    Ketopantoic acid
    Pantoic acid
    β-alanine

2. **Production:** Species and sites   3, 19, 25, 28
Plants—Green plants, fungi
Bacteria—Intestinal

3. **Storage**   8, 9, 16, 26, 34
Possibly liver, heart, kidney (all small amounts)

4. **Blood Carriers**   8, 14, 29, 31, 32
Blood proteins

5. **Half-life**   8, 9, 29, 31, 32, 34
Est. average loss: 25% of daily requirements

6. **Target tissues**   14, 16, 29, 31, 32, 34
All, esp. brain, heart, kidney, liver

7. **Reactions**   5, 14, 16, 17, 28
   Coenzyme form: CoA (adenine-3'-P-ribose-P-P-pantothenic acid-β-mercapto ethylamine)

Organ	Enzyme System	Effect
Liver	TRANSFERASE: Citrate condensing enzyme β-Ketothiolase, CoA transferase	Activated
Brain	TRANSACYLASES: Choline acetylase, lipoic transacetylase, phosphotransacetylase	Activated
Liver	ISOMERASES: Methylmalonyl isomerase, β-hydroxyacyl racemase, enoyl isomerase	Activated
Liver	ESTERASES: Acetyl CoA deacylase, succinyl CoA deacylase	Activated
Liver	HYDRASES: Enoylhydrase	Activated
Liver	SYNTHETASES: Acetic thiokinase, fatty acid thiokinases, succinic thiokinase, acetyl carboxylase, propionyl carboxylase, methyl crotonylcarboxylase	Activated
Muscle and liver	DEHYDROGENASES: Hydroxyacyldehydrogenase, pyruvate dehydrogenase, α-ketoglutarate dehydrogenase acyl dehydrogenases	Activated

8. **Mode of Action**   3, 5, 6, 9, 14, 17, 22
   Cellular
      Anabolic
         Lipid synthesis increased
         Active in synthesis of porphyrins, acetylcholine, and isoprenoid groups
         Sterol and hormone synthesis increased
      Catabolic—Regulates CHO mechanism
      Other—As coenzyme A in CHO, lipid, and protein metabolism; acyl transfer agent
   Organismal
      Fat synthesis and breakdown
      Respiratory pigment synthesis
      Water metabolism regulator
      Energy metabolism regulator

9. **Catabolism**   1, 3, 8, 9, 10, 16, 28
   Intermediates—Not destroyed in body
   Excretion Products
      Urine—Pantothenic acid (1-7 mg/day)
      Feces—Variable

MISCELLANEOUS

1. **Relationship to Other Vitamins**   8, 11, 13, 27, 31, 32
   Folic acid—Required for utilization of pantothenic acid
   Biotin—Required for utilization of pantothenic acid; acts with pantothenic acid in fatty acid biosynthesis; reduces severity of pantothenic acid deficiency in rats
   Vitamin C—Compensates partly for deficiency of pantothenic acid
   CoQ—Decreased in pantothenic acid deficiency
   Vitamin A and vitamin E—Synthesis promoted by pantothenic acid (isoprene production)
   Pantothenic acid and biotin involved in synthesis of niacin

2. **Relationship to Hormones**   8, 11, 13
   Aldosterone, deoxycorticosterone, cortisol, testosterone, progesterone— Cholesterol precursors for sterol hormones in adrenal cortex require pantothenic acid for synthesis; pantothenic acid deficiency produces cortical necrosis
   Cortisone—Relieves certain pantothenic acid deficiency symptoms in humans
   STH—Produces pantothenic acid deficiency in rats; synergist in growth

3. **Unusual Features**   11, 13, 14, 16
   Promotes amino acid uptake
   Potentiated by Zn^{2+} in preventing graying of hair in rats
   Provides resistance to stress of cold immersion
   Forms polyglutamic acid derivatives of PGA in vivo
   Deficiency of pantothenic acid in tumors
   Chick hatchability depends on pantothenic acid
   Useful in treating vertigo, postoperative shock, poisoning with isoniazid and curare
   Useful in acceleration of wound healing
   Useful in treating Addison's disease, liver cirrhosis, and diabetes

4. **Possible Relationships of Deficiency Symptoms to Metabolic Action**   11, 13, 16, 27
   Neuromotor disturbances
      Decreased phospholipid and acetylcholine synthesis
      Effect of pantothenic acid on membranes, degeneration of nerves
   Cardiovascular disorders—Disturbances of fat and CHO metabolism due to degeneration of liver
   Digestive disorders—Decreased bile acid production due to decreased sterol production; atrophy of intestinal mucosa

Infection susceptibility—Decreased antibody production due to decreased ATP synthesis

Physical weakness and depression—Decreased ATP synthesis

5. **Relationship to Minerals** **(See references in specific mineral section)**
Synergists—Cr^{3+}, Zn^{2+}, PO_4^{3-}
Antagonist—Cu^{2+}

PRINCIPAL REFERENCES, Part II

GENERAL—VITAMINS, HORMONES, etc.

1. Altman, P. L., and Dittmer, D. S. (Eds.), *Biology Data Book*, Vols. II and III, 2nd ed., Fed. Am. Soc. Exp. Biol., Washington, D.C. (1974).
2. Altman, P. L., and Dittmer, D. S. (Eds.), *Human Health and Disease*, Fed. Am. Soc. Exp. Biol., Washington, D.C. (1977).
3. Altman, P. L., and Dittmer, D. S. (Eds.), *Metabolism*, Fed. Am. Soc. Exp. Biol., Washington, D.C. (1968).
4. Berkow, R. (Ed.), *The Merck Manual*, 13th ed., Merck & Co., Rahway, N.J. (1977).
5. Boyer, P. D., and Snell, E. E. (Eds.), *Annual Reviews of Biochemistry*, Vols. 36-47, Annual Reviews, Inc., Palo Alto, Calif. (1967-78).
6. Conn, E. E., and Stumpf, P. K., *Outlines of Biochemistry*, 3rd ed., Wiley, New York (1976).
7. Dawson, R. M. C., Elliott, D. C., Elliot, W. H., and Jones, K. M. (Eds.), *Data for Biochemical Research*, 2nd ed., Oxford University Press, New York and Oxford (1969).
8. Diem, K. (Ed.), *Documenta Geigy Scientific Tables*, 6th ed., Geigy Pharmaceuticals, Ardsley, N.Y. (1962).
9. Goodman, L. S., and Gilman, A. (Eds.), *The Pharmaceutical Basis of Therapeutics*, 5th ed., Macmillan, New York (1975).
10. Greenberg, D. M. (Ed.), *Metabolic Pathways*, Vol. VII, 3rd ed., Academic Press, New York and London (1975).
11. Harris, R. S., and Thimann, K. (Eds.), *Vitamins and Hormones*, Vols. 25-34, Academic Press, New York and London (1967-76).
12. Long, C. (Ed.), *Biochemists' Handbook*, Van Nostrand Reinhold, New York (1961).
13. Needham, A. E., *The Growth Process in Animals*, Van Nostrand Reinhold, New York (1964).
14. Oser, B. L. (Ed.), *Hawk's Physiological Chemistry*, 14th ed., McGraw-Hill (Blakiston Div.), New York (1965).
15. Weast, R. C. (Ed.), *Handbook of Chemistry and Physics*, 57th ed., The Chemical Rubber Co., Cleveland, Ohio (1976).
16. West, E. S., Todd, W. R., Mason, H. S., and Van Bruggen, J. T., *Textbook of Biochemistry*, 4th ed., Macmillan, New York (1966).
17. Wilson, C. O., Gisvold, O., Doerge, R. F. (Eds.), *Textbook of Organic, Medicinal and Pharmaceutical Chemistry*, 6th ed., Lippincott, Philadelphia (1971).
18. Windholz, M. (Ed.), *The Merck Index*, 9th ed., Merck & Co., Inc., Rahway, N.J. (1976).

SPECIFIC—VITAMINS

19. Bonner, J., and Varner, J. E. (Eds.), *Plant Biochemistry*, Academic Press, New York and London (1976).
20. Burton, B. T., *The Heinz Handbook of Nutrition*, 3rd ed., H. J. Heinz Co. (McGraw-Hill), New York (1976).
21. Davidson, S., and Passmore, R., *Human Nutrition and Dietetics*, 6th ed., Williams & Wilkins, Baltimore, Md. (1975).
22. DeLuca, H. F., and Suttie, J. W. (Eds.), *The Fat-Soluble Vitamins*, University of Wisconsin Press, Madison, Wis. (1970).
23. Furia, T. E. (Ed.), *Handbook of Food Additives*, The Chemical Rubber Co., Cleveland, Ohio (1973).
24. Goodhart, R. S., and Shils, M. E., *Modern Nutrition in Health and Disease*, Lea & Febiger, Philadelphia (1973).
25. Goodwin, T. W., *The Biosynthesis of Vitamins and Related Compounds*, Academic Press, London and New York (1963).
26. Hegsted, D. M. (Ed.), *Present Knowledge in Nutrition*, 4th ed., Nutrition Foundation, New York (1976).
27. Kirschmann, J. D., *Nutrition Almanac*, McGraw-Hill, New York (1975).
27a. Marks, J., *A Guide to the Vitamins*, University Park Press, Baltimore, Md. (1975).
28. McCormick, D. B., and Wright, L. D. (Eds.), *Methods in Enzymology*, Vol. XVIII, *Vitamins and Coenzymes*, Parts A-C, Academic Press, New York and London (1970).
29. Morton, R. A. (Ed.), *Fat-Soluble Vitamins*, Pergamon Press, New York (1970).
30. Pfeiffer, C. (Ed.), *Mental and Elemental Nutrients*, Keats, New Canaan, Conn. (1975).
31. Rechcigl, M. (Ed.), *CRC Handbook in Nutrition and Food*, Sect. E, Vol. I, CRC Press, West Palm Beach, Fla. (1978).
32. Robinson, F. A., *The Vitamin Co-factors of Enzyme Systems*, Pergamon Press, New York (1966).
33. Sauberlich, H. E., *Laboratory Tests for Assessment of Nutritional Status*, CRC Press, Cleveland, Ohio (1974).
34. Sebrell, W. H., Jr., and Harris, R. S. (Eds. Vols. I-V), Gyorgy, P., and Pearson, W. N. (Eds. Vols. VI-VII), *The Vitamins*, 2nd Ed., Vols. I-VII, Academic Press, New York and London (1967).
35. Wagner, A. F., and Folkers, K., *Vitamins and Coenzymes*, Wiley (Interscience Div.), New York (1964).
36. Watt, B. L., and Merrill, A. L., *Composition of Foods*, Ag. Handbook #8 U.S. Government Printing Office (1975).
37. National Research Council, *Recommended Dietary Allowances*, 9th rev. ed., Printing and Publishing Office, National Academy of Sciences, Washington, D.C. (1980).

Part III
Introduction to the Hormones

The hormones covered in the next 23 chapters represent the 22 major hormones plus one chapter covering the eight brain (hypothalamic) releasing factors (hormones) for some of the 22 major hormones. The 22 major hormones include the five steroid adrenal/sex gland hormones, nine peptide pituitary hormones, six peptide thyroid-pancreas-ovary hormones, and two amine adrenal hormones. Only three (MSH, prolactin and oxytocin) of these 22 are not in continuous use by man; thus 19 are vitally essential over various time scales. An excess of any hormone is usually toxic to a certain degree; in addition, STH, estradiol and possibly all other steroids in large doses are carcinogenic. Besides the 22 major hormones and the 8 releasing factors, various minor and tentative natural hormones exist, such as: (1) alternate steroids with estrogenic, androgenic, glucocorticoid, and progestin activities (e.g., DOCA); (2) additional new pituitary hormones (e.g., β-lipotropin); (3) pineal hormones (e.g., melatonin); and (4) a new class of local tissue agents called "local regulators." This last group has been identified as including vascular regulators (kinins, serotonin, and prostaglandins), neurotransmitters (acetylcholine), mitogenic agents, such as NPF (nucleoprotein factor), FGF (fibroblast growth factor), NGF (nerve growth factor), and EGF (epidermal growth factor), and gastrointestinal "hormones," such as gastrin, secretin, pancreozymin, and cholecystokinin. These substances will not be covered in this edition.

The nine peptide pituitary hormones (water-soluble) include ACTH, FSH,

LH, STH, TSH, MSH, prolactin, oxytocin, and ADH.* All but prolactin and STH act by stimulating formation of an intracellular regulatory agent called cyclic AMP by adenyl cyclase in the cell membranes of the target organ, with either (1) subsequent release of steroid hormones (ACTH, FSH, LH), or T4 (TSH), or insulin (STH), or (2) tissue actions by MSH, prolactin, oxytocin, and ADH, on skin, mammary gland, ovary and kidney respectively. MSH, prolactin, and oxytocin are not utilized continuously by man and are thus unessential for everyday existence. Mode of action of STH and prolactin are presently unknown.

The five steroid fat-soluble hormones from the adrenal cortex and sex glands include cortisol, aldosterone, progesterone, testosterone, and estradiol. These hormones function by acting on the DNA of the cell nucleus of the target organ, resulting in new messenger RNA, new enzymes, and other proteins, with resulting actions by these products.

The six water-soluble peptide body-endocrine-organ hormones include insulin, glucagon, PTH, T4, TCT, and relaxin. These hormones function by stimulating formation of: (1) cyclic AMP in cell membranes (glucagon, TCT, PTH) and cyclic GMP (insulin) with subsequent reactions in the target tissues (liver, bone, cartilage, general tissues, respectively), or (2) cytoplasmic messenger RNA [T4, relaxin (?) with subsequent reactions in the thyroid and uterus-pelvis.

The two water-soluble amine hormones from the adrenal medulla (epinephrine, norepinephrine) function by stimulating formation of cyclic AMP in the cell membranes of the target organ with subsequent action in the nervous and circulatory systems. Norepinephrine also acts as a neurotransmitter in the nervous system.

The eight peptide water-soluble hypothalamic releasing factors (CRH, LRH, TRH, PIH, GRH, MIH, MRH, somatostatin) function by controlling the output of the pituitary hormones from the pituitary gland. These are very small peptides, ranging in length from 3 to 16 amino acids. Some (CRH, LRH, TRH, GRH) act by way of stimulating cyclic AMP production in pituitary cell membranes by adenyl cyclase. These are the most important controlling agents, since they are positioned at the head of the hierarchy of pituitary hormones.

Chemically, cyclic AMP is a nucleotide, similar to ATP less two PO_4^{3-} groups. It plays a very significant role in hormone action (12 of 22 major hormones) in its function as an intracellular secondary messenger. In addition to the above hormones, four of the eight hypothalamic factors plus the prostaglandins also work by way of cyclic AMP. C-AMP (cyclic AMP) functions as follows: a hormone molecule in the blood or extracellular fluid combines with a receptor site on the cell surface of the target tissues, with resultant activation of an enzyme, adenyl cyclase, to produce C-AMP, which is then released intracellularly. C-AMP acts by stimulating or inhibiting enzyme actions in the cell interior, to result in the final hormone tissue action characteristic of the target organ, e.g., synthesis of growth hormone in the pituitary. Cyclic GMP (C-GMP) is another nucleotide, which is similar to C-AMP but opposes C-AMP. The only hormone known to function via C-GMP is insulin.

*See text for abbreviations.

The prostaglandins are local extracellular regulators, cyclic unsaturated fatty acids, formed from essential fatty acids and released into the blood stream which can function to control blood pressure, vasodilation, and vasoconstriction by way of action through the C-AMP mechanism. Prostaglandins also have other pharmacological effects on kidney function, muscle contraction, hypersensitivity, asthma, edema, and so on, actions that are now the subjects of intensive research.

Hormone-mineral interactions have been specially noted with Ca^{2+}, Cu^{2+}, and Mn^{2+} (see minerals, introduction), while many hormone-vitamin interactions have been observed with vitamins A, B_2, and C (see vitamins, introduction). Relative concentrations of hormones in blood plasma range from .002 $\mu g/100$ ml (oxytocin) to 15 $\mu g/100$ ml (cortisol), with the rest of the hormones falling in between the two extremes. (See accompanying table.)

Most hormones need to be administered by injection, since oral intake results in digestive destruction of peptides and complexing of steroids except for T4, progesterone, some forms of estradiol and testosterone, and vitamin D, which acts as a hormone. Administration via the skin (topical) is sometimes used for steroid hormones.

Hormone Levels in Human Blood Plasma/Serum ($\mu g/100$ ml)

Hormone	Range	Average
STH	0.0-0.3	0.15
TSH	0.54-4.1	2.3
FSH	0.2-0.5	0.35
LH	0.1-0.2	0.15
PROL	0.5-1.0	0.75
ACTH	0.1-1.0	0.55
MSH	0.1	0.1
OXY	.00003-.0003	0.0002
ADH	.00005-.0007	0.0004
T4	3-12	7.5
PTH	0-.025	0.013
TCT	.002-.040	0.021
INS	.02-.60	0.31
GLUC	.01-.025	0.017
ALD	.0001-.001	0.0006
CORT	5-25	15
EST ♀	.005-.070	0.037
♂	.008-.020	0.014
TEST ♀	.025-.040	0.03
♂	.45-.75	0.60
PROG ♀	.10-1.0	0.60
♂	.01-.03	0.02
RELAXIN	—	—
EPIN	.002-.008	0.005
NOREP	.012-.028	0.020

Chapter 29.
Hypothalamic
Releasing Factors (Hormones)

There are five hypothalamic-derived releasing hormones acting on the anterior pituitary that are now accepted generally: GRH, TRH, LRH, CRH, and MRH, which release STH, TSH, LH (and FSH), ACTH, and MSH, respectively.* There are at present three release-inhibitory hormones, namely, somatostatin (inhibits STH), PIH (inhibits prolactin), and MIH (MSH-inhibiting). This list is being revised continuously (since intensive research and new data are being generated continuously). These are super master hormones which act as a regulatory higher level of control for the pituitary master hormones. Most feedback control mechanisms function via these releasing hormones. One of the release inhibitors, somatostatin, has many interesting properties.

All eight of these hormones are very small peptides (3-16 amino acids) with very short half-lives (4-10 min). Some have been synthesized (e.g., TRH, LRH). No toxicity data are available. Synergists include Ca^{2+} in some cases. No data are available on antagonists.

These regulatory hormones are produced mostly in the hypothalamus and stored there (with few exceptions). Releasing factors and release-inhibiting factors for these super master hormones vary with the individual hormones, noted in the text. These hormones act by stimulating or inhibiting pituitary cells to secrete the hormones, mainly by the cyclic AMP mechanism, although other pathways are also possible.

*See text for abbreviations.

CORTICOTROP(H)IN-RELEASING HORMONE (CRH)

1. Synonyms   1, 9, 18
CRF, cortical-releasing factor (hormone), (adreno) corticotrop(h)in-releasing factor

2. History   9, 18, 22, 39
1955—Saffran et al.: first demonstrated release of ACTH by crude hypothalamic extract
1962—Schally et al.: proposed structure for CRH
1963—Critchlow et al.: reported CRH preparation maintains ACTH synthesis in pituitary transplants

3. Forms   22, 37, 39
α_1, α_2, and β

4. Analogs   22, 37, 39
Vasopressin, oxytocin

5. Functions   1, 9, 22, 25, 27, 30, 37, 39
Chemical stimulant; messenger from hypothalamus to ACTH-producing cells in anterior pituitary; stimulates production of ACTH & release of ACTH

6. Structure   1, 9, 18, 22, 25, 27, 37, 39
Peptide with disulfide ring system
α_1—16 amino acids, similar to α-MSH
α_2—13 amino acids, almost identical to α-MSH
β—11 amino acids, similar to arginine vasopressin

7. MW   1, 9, 18, 22, 37, 39
Approx. 1100 (β), 1500 (α)

8. Extraction; Purification   22, 25, 27
Acid acetone, pH 1.5, extraction, precipitation with $(NH_4)_2SO_4$, chromatography, countercurrent distribution

9. Determination   1, 22, 25, 27, 37, 38
Bioassay—Release of corticosteroids in rat plasma on injection of CRH

10. Factors Affecting Release of CRH   1, 19, 22, 25, 27, 37, 39
Stimulators—Stress, low level of cortisol, sympathomimetic amines (e.g. epinephrine)
Inhibitors—Cerebral cortex factors

11. **Production Sites and Storage Location**   9, 22, 32, 37, 39
    Hypothalamus—Ventral area, neurohypophysis, median eminence

12. **Target Tissues**   1, 22, 29, 37, 39
    Anterior pituitary (ACTH-producing cells)

13. **Reactive Intermediate**   25, 27, 30, 31, 32, 37, 39
    Cyclic AMP

14. **Unusual Features**   22, 25, 27
    Very unstable, destroyed by trypsin but not by pepsin or chymotrypsin

LUTEINIZING HORMONE-RELEASING HORMONE (LRH)

1. **Synonyms**   1, 9, 18
   LRF, LH-releasing factor (hormone), (LH-RH/FSH-RH), Gonadotropin releasing hormone (Gon-RH), (GnRH)

2. **History**   9, 18, 22, 39
   1941—Guillemin: first postulated existence of LH-releasing factor
   1964—McCann and Ramirez: caused depletion of ovarian ascorbic acid with
       extracts of hypothalamus
   1964—Campbell et al.: infused hypothalamic extract into anterior pituitary
       and produced ovulation
   1971—Schally et al.: isolated LRH
   1972—Burgus et al.: determined structure of LRH
   1972—Monahan and Rivier: synthesized LRH

3. **Functions**   1, 9, 22, 25, 27, 30, 37, 39
   Chemical stimulant: messenger from hypothalamus to LH-producing cells in
       anterior pituitary, releases LH and FSH

4. **Structure**   1, 9, 18, 22, 25, 27, 37, 39
   Decapeptide—ovine—pyro Glu-His-Trp-Ser-Tyr-Gly-Leu-Arg-Pro-Gly; NH_2:
       synthesized, active in man

5. **MW**   1, 9, 18, 22, 37, 39
   1182.3

6. **Extraction; Purification**   22, 25, 27
   Acetic acid extraction, gel filtration on sephadex G-25, chromatography

7. **Determination**   1, 22, 25, 27, 37, 38
   Bioassay: depletion of ovarian vitamin C; radioimmunoassay

8. **Factors Affecting Release of LRH**   1, 19, 22, 25, 27, 37, 39
   Stimulators—Low levels of estradiol, progesterone; dopamine, clomiphene, epinephrine
   Inhibitors—High levels of testosterone, progesterone, estrogen

9. **Production Sites and Storage Location**   9, 22, 32, 37, 39
   Hypothalamus

10. **Target Tissues**   1, 22, 27, 37, 39
    Anterior pituitary (LH-producing cells)

11. **Reactive Intermediate:**   25, 27, 30, 31, 32, 37, 39
    Cyclic AMP

12. **Unusual features**   22, 25, 27
    Chymotrypsin, papain, subtilisin, themolysin destroy activity of LRH

THYROTROP(H)IN-RELEASING HORMONE (TRH)

1. **Synonyms**   1, 9, 18
   TRF, TSH-releasing factor (hormone)

2. **History**   9, 18, 22, 39
   1958—Harris and Woods: produced thyroidal I_{131} release on stimulation of hypothalamus
   1958—Nikitovich et al.: produced TSH after reimplanting pituitary graft near median eminence, but not in temporal lobe area
   1969—Folkers et al.: determined structure of porcine TRH
   1970—Flouret—synthesized TRH

3. **Antagonists**   22, 37, 39
   T3, T4 (large doses)

4. **Functions**   1, 9, 22, 25, 27, 30, 37, 39
   Chemical stimulant: messenger from hypothalamus to TSH-producing cells in anterior pituitary, prolactin release, TRH release

5. **Structure**   1, 9, 18, 22, 25, 27, 37, 39
   Procine TRH (tripeptide): L-pyroglutamyl-L-histidyl-L-proline amide

6. **MW**   1, 9, 18, 22, 37, 39
   362

7. **Extraction; Purification**   22, 25, 27
   Gel filtration, high-voltage electrophoresis

8. **Factors Affecting Release of TRH**   1, 19, 22, 25, 27, 37, 39
   Stimulators—Low level of T4, cold, stress, light, Ca^{2+} ion
   Inhibitors—No data

9. **Production Sites and Storage Location**   9, 22, 32, 37, 39
   Suprachiasmatic area, median eminence (production), neurohypophysis
   (storage)

10. **Target Tissue**   1, 22, 27, 37, 39
    Anterior pituitary (TSH-producing cells)

11. **Reactive Intermediate**   25, 27, 30, 31, 32, 37, 39
    Cyclic AMP

12. **Unusual Properties**   22, 25, 27
    Destroyed in human serum in 15 min at 37°C
    3-Me-His-TRH analog is 8-10x as potent as TRH. Same molecule active in
    most mammals

PROLACTIN RELEASE-INHIBITING HORMONE (PRIH)

1. **Synonyms**   1, 9, 18
   PIF, RIH, prolactin inhibiting factor (hormone), (PIH)

2. **History**   9, 18, 22, 39
   1963—Meites: showed increased prolactin secretion by pituitaries in tissue
   culture while other hormones decreased
   1962-63—Talwalker;Basteels et al.: reduced prolactin in pituitary culture by
   adding hypothalamic extract

3. **Functions**   1, 9, 22, 30, 25, 27, 37, 39
   Chemical inhibitor: messenger from hypothalamus to prolactin-producing
   cells in anterior pituitary

4. **Structure**   1, 9, 18, 22, 25, 27, 37, 39
   Some similarity to LRH, probably a peptide

5. **Extraction; Purification**   22, 25, 27
   0.1 N HCl extract, concentrate and separate on sephadex G-25

6. **Factors Affecting Release of PIH**   1, 19, 22, 25, 27, 37, 39
   Stimulator—Prolactin
   Inhibitor—Reserpine

7. **Production Sites and Storage Location**   22, 32, 37, 39
   Satiety center, appetite suppressor in hypothalamus

8. **Target Tissues**   1, 22, 27, 37, 39
   Prolactin-producing cells in anterior pituitary

9. **Unusual Features**   22, 25, 27
   Stable to boiling

GROWTH HORMONE-RELEASING HORMONE (GRH)

1. **Synonyms**   1, 9, 18
   GHRH, GRF, somatotrop(h)in-releasing factor (hormone), growth-hormone-releasing factor (hormone), SRF, GHRF

2. **History**   9, 18, 22, 39
   1964—Deuben and Meites: released GH in rat pituitary in tissue culture using rat hypothalamic extracts
   1965—Schally et al.: stimulated release of GH by incubating rat pituitaries with beef, pig, hypothalamic extracts

3. **Functions**   1, 9, 22, 25, 27, 30, 37, 39
   Chemical stimulant; messenger from hypothalamus to STH-producing cells in anterior pituitary

4. **Structure**   1, 9, 18, 22, 25, 27, 37, 39
   Acidic polypeptide—decapeptide;   Val-His-Leu-Ser-Ala-Glu-Glu-Lys-Glu-Ala
   Needs confirmation.

5. **MW**   1, 9, 18, 22, 37, 39
   2500 (approx.) Needs confirmation.

6. **Extraction; Purification**   22, 25, 27
   0.1 N HCl extraction, gel filtration, CMC chromatography

7. **Factors Affecting Release of GRH**   1, 19, 22, 25, 27, 37, 39
   Stimulators—Epinephrine, norepinephrine, dopamine
   Inhibitors—No data

8. **Production Sites and Storage Location**   9, 22, 32, 37, 39
   Hypothalamus, neurohypophysis

9. **Target Tissues**   1, 22, 27, 37, 39
   Anterior pituitary cells producing STH

10. **Reactive Intermediate**   25, 27, 30, 31, 32, 37, 39
    Cyclic AMP

11. **Unusual Features**   22, 25, 27
Biological activity destroyed by trypsin, pepsin and chymotrypsin

MELANOCYTE STIMULATING HORMONE RELEASE-INHIBITING HORMONE (MRIH)

1. **Synonyms**   1, 9, 18
MIF, MSH-inhibiting factor (hormone), (MIH)

2. **History**   9, 18, 22, 39
1962—Etkin: produced frog blackening by repositioning pituitary in other locations in body
1964—Kastin and Ross: produced coloration in albino rat by repositioning pituitary
1971—Nair et al.: determined structure MRIH (rat)
1972—Celis et al.: synthesized MRIH (rat)

3. **Functions**   1, 9, 22, 25, 27, 30, 37, 39
Inhibits release of MSH from intermediate lobe of pituitary

4. **Structure**   1, 9, 18, 22, 25, 27, 37, 39
Tripeptide—Pro-Leu-Gly (NH_2) (derived from oxytocin) (rat only)

5. **Extraction; Purification**   22, 25, 27
2 N acetic acid extraction, gel filtration on sephadex G-25

6. **Production Sites and Storage Location**   9, 22, 32, 37, 39
Hypothalamus (paraventricular nucleus)

7. **Target Tissues**   1, 22, 27, 37, 39
Cells of intermediate pituitary lobe secreting MSH

MELANOCYTE STIMULATING HORMONE-RELEASING HORMONE (MRH)

1. **Synonyms**   1, 19, 18
MSH-releasing factor (hormone)

2. **History**   9, 18, 22, 39
1965—Taliesnik and Orios: found evidence for existence of MRH
1971—Celis et al.: determined structure, synthesized MRH (rat)

3. **Functions**   1, 9, 22, 25, 27, 30, 37, 39
Stimulates release of MSH from intermediate lobe of pituitary

4. **Structure**   1, 9, 18, 22, 25, 27, 37, 39
   Pentapeptide—Cys-Try-Ile-Gln-Asn-OH (derived from oxytocin)

5. **Production Sites and Storage Location**   9, 22, 32, 37, 39
   Paraventricular nucleus

6. **Target Tissues**   1, 22, 27, 37, 39
   Cells of intermediate pituitary lobe secreting MSH

SOMATOSTATIN

1. **Synonyms**   1, 9, 18
   Growth hormone release inhibiting hormone (GH-RIH); somatotrophin release inhibiting factor (SRIF), GHRIF

2. **History**   9, 18, 22, 39
   1973—Brazeau et al.: isolated somatostatin from sheep hypothalami
   1973—Burgus et al.: determined structure of somatostatin
   1973—Rivier et al.: synthesized somatostatin

3. **Functions**   1, 9, 22, 25, 27, 30, 37, 39
   Inhibits release of growth hormone, insulin, glucagon, TSH, secretin, cholecystokinin, gastrin

4. **Structure**   1, 9, 18, 22, 25, 27, 37, 39
   Tetradecapeptide (synthesized)
   Ala-Gly-Cys-Lys-Asn-Phe-Phe-Trp-Lys-Thr-Phe-Thr-Ser
   .
   .... Cys

5. **MW**   1, 9, 18, 22, 37, 39
   1637.9

6. **Extraction; Purification**   22, 25, 27
   Ovine hypothalamus source—Alcohol $CHCl_3$, extraction, ultrafiltration, partitioning, ion exchange chromatography, gel filtration

7. **Production Sites and Storage**   9, 22, 32, 37, 39
   Hypothalamus (median eminence), stomach (?), pancreas (?)

8. **Target Tissues**   1, 22, 27, 37, 39
   Anterior pituitary, pancreas, stomach.

9. **Unusual Features**   22, 25, 27
   Similar activity if reduced or oxydized (linear or cyclic)

Chapter 30.
Growth Hormone (STH)

Growth hormone is a general tissue-controlling hormone and a master hormone (controls insulin); yet it is one of the most mysterious, since its mode of action has defied many investigators. Its chief functions are to stimulate protein, fat, CHO, water, and mineral metabolism, as well as general body growth. Its importance stems from its role as a central hormone in the pituitary as well as its control of body metabolism in the tissues via synergism and antagonism with the other pituitary master hormones. It has been used to treat dwarfism (hypopituitary). Deficiency states are progeria, dwarfism, or hypopituitarism. Its use has been limited because of its species specificity.

Growth hormone is a water-soluble protein with a short half-life in blood (20 min). It is thought to be converted to active forms called somatomedins A, B and C. Toxicity has been reported: the diabetogenic and carcinogenic effect is well known. Excess conditions result in acromegaly and gigantism. Its chief synergists are insulin, testosterone, Mg^{2+}, Zn^{2+}, and K^+, whereas its chief antagonist is cortisol.

Growth hormone is formed in the anterior pituitary gland and is stored there. It is normally released by GHRH, a hypothalamic releasing factor. Releasing factors include: GHRH, sleep, exercise, fasting, hypoglycemia, and arginine. Release-inhibiting factors include: GH-RIH (somatostatin), sleeplessness, glucose hyperglycemia, obesity, and free fatty acids. Because growth hormone controls the nitrogen balance of an organism, it is thought to be involved in the aging process.

Growth hormone acts in the cell via the somatomedins A, B and C, principally to promote RNA synthesis and protein synthesis at the ribosomes, with a resultant increase of proteins and enzymes followed by cell multiplication and differentiation, and hence resulting in growth.

There is some evidence that somatomedins act on C-GMP similarly to insulin.

GENERAL INFORMATION

1. **Synonyms   1, 7, 18**
   Somatotrop(h)in, GH, STH, phyone, (anterior) pituitary growth hormone, adenohypophyseal growth hormone, somatotrophic hormone.

2. **History   9, 18, 28, 36**
   1921—Evans and Long: induced growth in rats with pituitary extract
   1930—Smith: restored growth in hypophysectomized rats with hypophyseal implants
   1945—Li et al.: isolated growth hormone from anterior pituitary (beef)
   1962—Reisfeld et al.: isolated growth hormone from human anterior pituitary
   1964—Glick, Roth, Berson, and Yalow: developed accurate immunoassay of growth hormone in serum
   1966—Li et al.: determined amino acid sequence for human growth hormone, 188 amino acid residues
   1971—Li et al.: synthesized human growth hormone
   1972—Daughaday et al.: proposed name and functions of somatomedin
   1972—Vamasaki et al.: isolated an "active core" fragment from GH

3. **Physiological Forms   9, 26, 37, 39**
   Somatomedins (A, B, C)
   Somatomedin B probably identical with MSA (multiplication stimulating activity) and NSILA (non-suppressible insulin-like activity)

4. **Active Analogs and Related Forms   17, 22, 34, 37, 39**
   Enzyme digests of bovine STH; HPL (human placental lactogen)

5. **Inactive Analogs and Related Forms   17, 22, 37, 39**
   Non-primate GH

6. **Antagonists   9, 17, 37, 39**
   Cortisone, cortisol, insulin (all concentration—dependent), plasma inhibitors of GH and somatomedins

7. **Synergists   9, 17, 37, 39**
   Adrenal corticoids (fat metabolism), ACTH, T4, insulin, testosterone, Mg^{2+}, Zn^{2+}, K^+

8. **Physiological Functions   1, 4, 14, 16, 37, 39**
   General growth of organism

Promotes skeletal growth, protein anabolism, fat metabolism, CHO metabolism, water and mineral metabolism
Controls insulin release and action

9. **Deficiency Diseases and Disorders**   1, 4, 14, 16, 37, 39
Deficiency—Progeria, pituitary dwarf, hypopituitarism
Excess—Acromegaly, gigantism

10. **Essentiality for Life**   1, 9, 38
Absence results in stunted, abnormal growth, with decrease in normal life span

CHEMISTRY

1. **Structure**   1, 8, 9, 15, 18
Growth hormone, structure known and synthesized (human), coiled, unbranched protein, 191 amino acid residues, 2 S-S-bridges, 40% variable amino acid residues among different species

Human—(Phe ———— Phe)

Bovine ⎫
Ovine ⎭ (Ala ———— Phe)

2. **Reactions**   1, 8, 9, 17, 18

Heat—Stable to 100°C, 15 min

Acid (strong)—Unstable

Alkali (strong)—Unstable

Water—Soluble, acidic

Oxidation—Oxidizes S-S bonds (unstable)

Reduction—Reduces S-S bonds

Light—No data

Proteolysis—40% limit of digestion of human growth hormone before loses activity (pepsin)

3. **Properties**   1, 7, 8, 9, 17, 19

MW—21,500 (human)
   22,000 (bovine, ovine, monkey)
Important groups for activity:
   —S—S—
   ϵ—NH$_2$ (lysine)
   Residue fragment #96—133 amino acids ("active core")

Solubility
   H$_2$O—Sol.
   Acet., Alc.—Insol.
   Benz., Chl., Eth.—Insol.
Absn. max.—Approx. 280 mμ
Chemical nature—Simple protein, globulin, α helix content 55%
Miscellaneous—pI = 4.9 (human)
   5.2 (monkey)
   5.9-6.3 (dog, horse, pig, rabbit, rat)
   6.8 (sheep, cattle)

4. **Commercial Production**   9, 18, 22
Not available

5. **Isolation**   22, 25
Sources—Pituitary glands of sheep, ox, pig, monkey
Methods
    Extract with borate buffer, pH 8.8, DEAE chromatography
    Precipitate with $(NH_4)_2SO_4$; column chromatography IRC-50, pH 5.1
    Treat with acetic acid-acetone; precipitate with acetone; column chromatography; precipitate with alcohol
Additional purification—Countercurrent distribution and gel filtration

5. **Determination**   1, 14, 19a, 22, 26, 38
Bioassay
    Tibia test (rat) (5-120 μg)
    Increased weight (rat)
    Increased N retention (rat)
    S^{35} incorporation into cartilage (rat)
Physicochemical
    Immunoassay
    Radioimmunoassay

MEDICAL AND BIOLOGICAL ROLE

1. **Species Occurrence, Specificity and Antigenicity**   1, 9, 38
Occurrence—All vertebrates
Specificity—No crossing of species lines for primates, chickens or guinea pigs; other vertebrates slightly more tolerant
Antigenicity—Monkey, sheep, rat, pig hormones antigenically different

2. **Units**   8, 9, 14
1 USP unit = 1 I.U. = 1 mg = 1000 μg

3. **Normal Blood Levels**   2, 4, 9, 22, 39
0.0-0.3 μg/100 ml, plasma; diurnal rhythm—higher at night (sleep)

4. **Administration**   8, 9, 37, 39
Injection—Preferred route
Topical—Not used
Oral—Not used, inactivated

5. **Factors Affecting Release**   1, 4, 34
Inhibitors—Free fatty acids, obesity, somatostatin, inadequate dietary protein, sleeplessness, hyperglycemia
Stimulators—Plasma amino acids, hypoglycemia, GHRH, vasopressin (fish), ACTH, adequate protein in diet, fasting, exercise, sleep, arginine, levodopa, Ca^{2+}

6. **Deficiency Symptoms**   1, 4, 37, 38, 39
Humans

Dwarfism
Failure of long bones to close
Failure of sexual maturation
Increased fat deposition

7. **Effects of Overdose, Toxicity**   1, 4, 37, 38, 39
Tumors, β-cell destruction (diabetogenic)
Pituitary giants
Bone thickening

METABOLIC ROLE

1. **Biosynthesis**   22, 37, 39
Precursors—Amino acids; all 20 standard
Intermediates—Unknown

2. **Production Sites**   22, 37, 39
Anterior pituitary acidophils

3. **Storage Areas**   8, 9, 16
Anterior pituitary

4. **Blood Carriers**   2, 8, 22, 26
α_2-Macroglobulin, β-lipoprotein

5. **Half-life**   8, 9, 26
20 min

6. **Target Tissues**   1, 22, 37, 39
All except nervous tissue; esp. liver, bone, viscera, muscle, epiphyseal carti-
lage
Converted to somatomedins in liver

7. **Reactions**   4, 5, 22, 25, 34, 38
Reactive forms—somatomedins ⎰ Somatomedin A—cartilage
   (A, B, C) via C-GMP ⎱ Somatomedin B —connective tissue,
                                                   fibroblasts
                                                   insulin activity
                           Somatomedin C—placenta

Organ	Enzyme System	Effect
Most tissues and organs	RNA-polymerase	Activated
	Protein-synthetic	Activated
Blood cells	Alk. phosphatase	Activated

8. **Mode of Action**   1, 4, 5, 8, 9, 16, 31, 37, 39
Cellular

Anabolic
  Increases rate of protein and RNA synthesis
  Increases glycogen deposition (muscles)
Catabolic—Mobilizes unsaturated fatty acids
Other—Increases amino acid permeability of cells; increases salt and H_2O
  transport in kidney
Organismal
  Active form in blood is somatomedin A, B or C
  Increases muscle, skin, viscera, lymph glands, bone, and cartilage size
  Decreases urea formation
  Increases blood sugar
  Increases tissue nitrogen
  Mobilizes fatty acids from adipose tissue
  Increases blood sugar
  Controls insulin release and action

9. **Catabolism**   1, 9, 22, 25, 34
   Intermediates—Liver destruction, to peptides; plasmin in blood inactivates GH
   Excretion products—Small amounts of GH in urine

MISCELLANEOUS

1. **Relationship to Vitamins**   8, 11, 13, 38
   All vitamins—All concerned with growth

2. **Relationship to Other Hormones**   8, 11, 13, 32, 38
   Insulin—Inhibited by GH in certain concentrations; synergist with GH at other
     (low) concentrations
   GHR—GH-releasing factor of hypothalamus
   Vasopressin—A hypothalamic release factor (in fish)
   Cortisol—Antagonist to GH (protein metabolism); also a synergist (fat meta-
     bolism)
   Testosterone—Synergist with GH
   T4—Synergist with GH (differentiation)
   ACTH—Synergist with GH (certain functions); also an antagonist (other
     functions)

3. **Unusual Features**   29, 32, 38
   Guinea pig not sensitive to bovine, primate or own GH
   HGH withstands 15 min at $100°C$
   Increases capacity to form tumors
   Similarity in structure to prolactin

Structural similarity of growth hormones of various species
"Active core" consists of amino acid residues 96-133
Aggregation with increase of GH concentration
Somatomedin exists in 3 forms in blood

4. **Possible Relationships of Deficiency Symptoms to Metabolic Action   11, 13, 37**
   Dwarfism—Lack of protein synthesis due to lack of GH activity
   Failure of long bones to close—Lack of major metabolic action of GH
   Failure of sexual maturation—Lack of synergism of sex hormones and GH
   Increased fat deposition—Lack of catabolic action of GH

5. **Relationships to Minerals   (See references in specific mineral section)**
   Synergists—Mg^{2+}, Zn^{2+}, K^+, PO_4^{3-}, I^- (as T4)
   Excretion of PO_4^{3-} affected by STH ($\downarrow$), also Na^+ ($\uparrow$)
   Release of hormone—Ca^{2+} required
   Absorption—PO_4^{3-} ($\uparrow$) in gut

Chapter 31.
Thyroid Stimulating Hormone (TSH)

TSH is an anterior pituitary hormone occupying a master position controlling another endocrine gland, the thyroid gland. Its chief functions are to control synthesis and release of thyroxine (T4) and to stimulate iodine uptake by the thyroid gland. Its main importance stems from its control of body metabolism and temperature via T4. Deficiencies include Sheehan's syndrome and goiter.

TSH is a water-soluble glycoprotein containing two subunits with a short half-life in blood (1 hour). An excess of TSH results in toxic effects: exophthalmos, increased basal metabolic rate, and goiter. Its chief synergists are the pituitary hormones, whereas the chief antagonists are thiourea, thiouracil, thiocyanate, and perchlorate.

TSH is formed in the anterior pituitary with no known storage. It is normally released by TRH, a hypothalamic releasing factor. Releasing factors include *TRH*, epinephrine, decreased blood levels of T4, and low temperature. Release-inhibiting factors include high temperature, T4 (feedback), high vitamin A, and serum iodine. TSH controls thyroid cell membrane uptake of iodine and release of T4. On the cellular level TSH stimulates cyclic AMP production by adenyl cyclase in the cell membranes, followed by release of T4.

GENERAL INFORMATION

1. **Synonyms**   1, 7, 18

    Thyroid-stimulating hormone, thyr(e)otrop(h)ic hormone, TTH, thyrotrop(h)in

2. **History**   9, 18, 28, 36
   1921—Evans and Long: first noted effects of pituitary extracts on growth
   1927-30—Smith: reported that hypophysectomy in rat causes atrophy of thyroids (and other organs) correctable by hypophyseal implants
   1929—Basset, Aron and Loeb: defined properties of a thyrotrophic hormone
   1945—Ciereszko: isolated crude TSH from beef pituitaries
   1960—Wynston et al.: obtained purified TSH from beef, sheep, and whale pituitaries
   1963—Carsten et al.: determined amino acid composition of beef TSH
   1973—Sairam and Li: Determined amino acid sequences of α and β human TSH

3. **Physiological Forms**
   TSH

4. **Active Analogs and Related Compounds**   17, 22, 37, 39
   LATS (long-acting thyroid stimulator)

5. **Inactive Analogs and Related Compounds**   17, 22, 37, 39
   TSH minus CHO moeity, oxidized TSH

6. **Antagonists**   9, 17, 37, 39
   Acetylated TSH, p-aminosalicylic acid, perchlorate, sulfathiazole, thiocyanate, thiouracil, thiourea

7. **Synergists**   9, 17, 37, 39
   STH, ACTH, MSH, T4, I (as T4), Ca^{2+}

8. **Physiological Functions**   1, 4, 14, 16, 37, 39
   Regulation of body temperature via T4
   Maintains thyroid gland and its secretory activity (colloid discharge)
   Maintains iodine uptake by thyroid gland
   Promotes differentiation in embryo during development (via T4)
   Stimulates coupling of diiodotyrosine to form thyroxine (T4)

9. **Deficiency Diseases, Disorders**   1, 4, 14, 16, 37, 39
   Thyrotoxicosis (excess), goiter (excess of deficiency), exophthalmos (excess), Sheehan's syndrome (deficiency)

10. **Essentiality for Life**   1, 9, 38
    Required by all vertebrates for proper development; possible shortening of life span in absence of TSH

CHEMISTRY

1. **Structure**   1, 8, 9, 15, 18
   Glycoprotein—Two subunits α and β—both contain CHO (14%), are straight chains

   α—89 amino acids identical to LH α ⎫ CHOs are fucose, galactose,
   β—112 amino acids hormone-specific ⎬ mannose, glucosamine,
   Both α and β needed for activity ⎭ galactosamine, sialic acid

2. **Reactions**   1, 8, 9, 17, 18
   Heat—Inactivates
   Acid—Easily inactivates
   Alkali—Inactivates
   Water—Basic

   Oxidation—Inactivates using bromine, iodine, and permanganate
   Reduction—May potentiate effects of TSH
   Light—No data
   Proteolysis—Inactivates with pepsin or trypsin

3. **Properties**   1, 7, 8, 9, 17, 19
   MW—26,000-28,000 (human)
   Important groups for activity
      α-NH$_2$, tyrosine, CHO moiety
      —S—S—, α and β subunits

   Solubility
      H$_2$O—Sol.
      Acet., Alc.—Insol.
      Benz., Chl., Eth.—Insol.
   Absn. max.—Approx 280 mμ
   Chemical nature—Basic glycoprotein, globulin
   Miscellaneous—pI = 7.8

4. **Commercial Production**   9, 18, 22
   Extract bovine pituitary glands

5. **Isolation**   22, 25
   Sources—Bovine pituitary glands
   Methods
      Extract pituitary (frozen-dried) in 2% NaCl, pH 7.6; precipitate at pI with acetone (1 I.U./mg)
      Precipitate from 3.6 M ammonium sulfate
   Purification
      Chromatography on IRC-50; elute with 1 M NaCl
      Chromatography on CM cell: elute with 0.2 M NaCl 0.05 M formate, pH 3-4
      Gel filtration on sephadex G-50, G-100
      Chromatography on IRC-50 in urea (60 I.U./mg)

6. **Determination**   1, 14, 19a, 22, 26, 38
   Bioassay
      Height of secretory epithelium in thyroid—guinea pig
      Number colloid droplets in guinea pig thyroid
      I_2 depletion of 1-day chick
      Uptake I^{131} by thyroid of rats
      In vitro assay, slice uptake of I^{131}
   Physicochemical—Radioimmunoassay

MEDICAL AND BIOLOGICAL ROLE

1. **Species Occurrence, Specificity, and Antigenicity**   1, 9, 38
   Occurrence—All vertebrates
   Specificity—Incomplete; bovine TSH active in all species (chick and guinea pig most sensitive)
   Antigenicity—High; bovine TSH antigenic in rabbits

2. **Units**   8, 9, 14
   1 I.U. = 13.5 mg of standard = 1 USP unit

3. **Normal Blood Levels (Man)**   2, 4, 9, 22, 39
   .04-.30 milliunits/100 ml plasma

4. **Administration**   8, 9, 37, 39
   Injection—Preferred route
   Topical—Inactive
   Oral—Inactive

5. **Factors Affecting Release**   1, 4, 34
   Inhibitors
      Somatostatin
      Feedback via hypothalamus from high serum T4
      High serum iodide, massive doses vitamin A
      High temperature
      Inhibition of hypothalamus
      Nerve stimuli

Stimulators
    Release factor of hypothalamus (TRH)
    Decreased serum T4 via hypothalamus
    Low temperature
    Stimulation of hypothalamus
    Nerve stimuli
    Epinephrine
    Ca^{2+}

6. **Deficiency Symptoms**   1, 4, 37, 38, 39
    Decreased synthesis of thyroid hormones
    Low serum protein-bound iodine (PBI)
    Decreased iodine uptake by thyroid
    Secondary symptoms of thyroxine deficiency

7. **Effects of Overdose, Toxicity**   1, 4, 37, 38, 39
    Exophthalmic effect
    Increased synthesis of thyroid hormones
    Increased PBI
    Increased iodide uptake by thyroid
    Increased basal metabolic rate
    Decreased thyroid iodine
    Decreased blood cholesterol
    Goiter

METABOLIC ROLE

1. **Biosynthesis**   22, 37, 39
    Precursors—17 of 20 standard amino acids; no glutamine, asparagine, trypto-
        phan
    Intermediates—Unknown
    Site(s) in cell—Basophilic cytoplasm

2. **Production Sites**   22, 37, 39
    S^2 type cell, anterior pituitary

3. **Storage Areas**   8, 9, 16
    Not stored

4. **Blood Carriers**   2, 8, 22, 26
   β-globulins

5. **Half-life**   8, 9, 26
   54 min

6. **Target Tissues**   1, 22, 37, 39
   Thyroid, reproductive glands, liver, probably muscles

7. **Reactions**   4, 5, 22, 25, 34, 38
   Reactive intermediates—Cyclic AMP (secondary messenger) and Ca^{2+}

Organ	Enzyme System	Effect
Thyroid	Proteolytic enzymes (on colloid)	Activated
Thyroid	Synthetic enzymes for T4	Activated
Thyroid	Adenyl cyclase	Activated
Thyroid	DPN kinase	Activated
Thyroid	HMP enzymes (hexose mono-PO_4 shunt)	Activated

8. **Mode of Action**   1, 4, 5, 8, 9, 16, 31, 37, 39
   Cellular
   Anabolic
   RNA and protein synthesis (thyroid)
   Thyroid hormone synthesis (thyroid)
   Catabolic
   Lipolytic activity increased
   Proteolytic activity increased (thyroid)
   Glucose oxidation increased via TCA, HMP, and glycolysis
   Other
   Activates thyroid cell membrane enzymes
   Increases oxidase granules (thyroid), and O_2 consumption by thyroid
   cells
   Increases glucose and iodine entry into cells
   No increase in $NADP^+$
   Organismal
   Mobilization of thyroid hormones
   Increases serum-bound iodine
   Maintains body temperature via T4

9. **Catabolism**   1, 9, 22, 25, 34
   Intermediates—Hydrolyzed in liver
   Excretion products—Present in urine

MISCELLANEOUS

1. **Relationship to Vitamins**   8, 11, 13, 38
   Vitamin A—Massive doses of vitamin A inhibit secretion of TSH; thyroid hormones required for carotene and retinene conversions
   Vitamins B_1, B_2, B_{12}, C—Requirements increased in hyperthyroidism; tissue concentrations reduced
   Vitamin B_6, nicotinic acid—Conversion to phosphorylated reactive forms impaired in hyperthyroidism
   Vitamins A, D, E, K—Requirements increased in hyperthyroidism; tissue concentrations reduced in hyperthyroidism

2. **Relationship to Other Hormones**   8, 11, 13, 32, 38
   T4—TSH stimulates production of T4; synergist in lactation
   LH—Contained frequently as a contaminant in TSH
   LH—α LH subunit identical to α TSH subunit

3. **Unusual Features**   29, 32, 38
   Not inactivated by neuraminidase (sialic acid not active group)
   CHO moiety needed for activity
   Different functions in lower species
   Rapid loss of potency in solution
   Inactivation by freeze-drying
   Reduction may potentiate activity
   High cystine content
   Phospholipase activity of TSH reported
   α subunit identical to α subunit of LH

4. **Possible Relationships of Deficiency Symptoms to Metabolic Action**   11, 13, 37
   Decreased synthesis of thyroid hormones—Insufficient activation of thyroid cell membrane enzymes
   Low serum PBI—Reduction of T4 output due to decreased TSH
   Decreased iodide uptake by thyroid—Decreased reactivity of thyroid gland

5. **Relationship to Minerals**   (See references in specific mineral section)
   Synergist—I^- (as T4), PO_4^{3-} (as cyclic AMP), Ca^{2+}
   Release of hormone—Ca^{2+} required

Chapter 32.
Luteinizing Hormone (LH)

LH is an anterior pituitary hormone, a master hormone controlling sex hormone output by the ovary in females and testes in the male. Its chief functions are to synergize FSH and: *in the female*—promote ovulation, corpus luteum formation, and estrogen and progesterone secretion; and *in the male*—stimulate testosterone secretion (Leydig cells) and promote growth of sex organs. Deficiencies include hypogonadism and irregular sexual development.

LH is a water-soluble glycoprotein with two half-lives (20 min and 4 hr) (i.e., two active components in blood).

An excess of LH causes: *in the male*—increased androgen synthesis, hypertrophy, then atrophy of Leydig cells (testes), and *in the female*—increased estrogen secrection, then precocious ovulation. The chief synergist to LH is FSH; its chief antagonist is prolactin.

LH is formed in the anterior pituitary with some storage in the pituitary, and released normally by LRH (GonRH), a hypothalamic releasing hormone. Releasing factors include LRH, low sex hormone levels, and external stimuli. Release-inhibiting factors are cortisol, stress, hyperthyroidism, high levels of sex hormones, and decreased LRH from hypothalamus. On the cellular level, LH stimulates enzymes in gonadal cells to produce cyclic AMP followed by production of steroid hormones.

GENERAL INFORMATION

1. **Synonyms**   1, 7, 18
    Luteotrop(h)in, interstitial cell-stimulating hormone, ICSH, Prolan B, gonadotrop(h)in II, Metakentrin, corpus luteum-ripening hormone

2. **History**   9, 18, 28, 36
   1921—Evans and Long: first noted gonadotropic effect of pituitary extracts on rats
   1927-30—Smith: noted hypophysectomy in rat caused atrophy of gonads (and other organs) correctable by hypophyseal implants
   1933—Fevold et al.: identified a separate luteinizing hormone in pituitaries
   1940—Li, Simpson, and Evans isolated LH from sheep pituitaries
   1940—Shedlovsky et al. ⎫
   1942—Chow et al.   ⎬ Isolated LH from pig pituitaries
   1962—Squire et al.: isolated a purified LH from human pituitaries
   1973—Shome and Parlow: determined amino acid sequences of α and β subunits, human LH

3. **Physiological Forms**   9, 26, 37, 39
   Two components with different half-lives

4. **Active Analogs and Related Compounds**   17, 22, 24, 37, 39
   HCG, HMG (mixture of FSH and LH) ⎧ Human chorionic gonadotropin
                                    ⎨ Human menopausal gonadotropin
   PMSG (properties of FSH and LH) (Pregnant more serum gonadotropin)

5. **Inactive Analogs and Related Compounds**   17, 22, 37, 39
   LH minus CHO moiety, α and β units separately

6. **Antagonists**   9, 17, 37, 39
   Prolactin, insulin (both concentration-dependent)

7. **Synergists**   9, 17, 37, 39
   FSH, prolactin, T4, insulin, Ca^{2+}

8. **Physiological Functions**   1, 4, 14, 16, 37, 39
   Female
      Promotes estrogen and progesterone secretion, ovulation, maintains ovarian tissues
      Stimulates rupture of follicles and formation of corpora lutea
   Male
      Stimulates Leydig cells to secrete testosterone, gametogenic with FSH
      Promotes growth of seminal tubules and accessory sex organs

9. **Deficiency Diseases, Disorders**   1, 4, 14, 16, 37, 39
   Hypogonadism; irregular sexual development

10. **Essentiality for Life**   1, 9, 38
   Not required for life of organism, but required for reproduction by all analyzed vertebrates

CHEMISTRY

1. **Structure**   1, 8, 9, 15, 18
   Glycoprotein—Two subunits α and β structures known—both contain CHO
   (14%)—both straight chain

   α—89 amino acids (identical to FSH α subunit)   ⎰ CHO's are fucose, galactose,
   β—115 amino acids (hormone-specific)   ⎱ galactosamine, glucose, glucosamine, mannose, sialic acid

   Both α and β subunits needed for activity

2. **Reactions**   1, 8, 9, 17, 18
   Heat—Inactivates
   Acid—Picric, TCA, picrolonic,
      and flavianic acids precipitate
      LH without loss of activity
   Alkali—No data
   Water—Sol., acidic

   Oxidation—H_2O_2, periodate, performic acid—inactivate
   Reduction—Cysteine, ketene—inactivate
   Light—No data
   Proteolysis—Inactivates
   Urea—Unstable in 6 M urea

3. **Properties**   1, 7, 8, 9, 17, 19
   Appearance—White powder
   MW—26,000 (human); 30,000
      (sheep)
   Solubility
      H_2O—soluble
      Alc.—Sol. 4% alc.
      Acet., Benz., Chl., Eth.—Insol.
   Absn. max.—Approx 280 mμ

   Important groups for activity
      Cys., Pro.
      CHO moiety
      —S—S—
      α and β subunits linked together
   Chemical nature—Acidic, globular
      glycoprotein
   Miscellaneous—pI = 5.4 (human);
      pI = 4.6 (sheep); pI = 7.45 (pig)

4. **Commercial Production**   9, 18, 22
   Extraction of human or sheep pituitaries

5. **Isolation**   22, 25
   Sources—Pituitary of human, sheep, swine, and beef
   Method
      Aqueous extract at pH 5.5
      Ammonium sulfate precipitation
      Metaphosphoric acid precipitation
      Ethanol fractionation
      IRC-50; sephadex G-100

6. **Determination**   1, 14, 14a, 22, 26, 38
Bioassay
   Vitamin C depletion of rat ovary
   Increased hyperemia in immature rat ovary
   Increased weight in male sex accessory organs
   Weaver-Finch test
Physicochemical—Radioimmunoassay

MEDICAL AND BIOLOGICAL ROLE

1. **Species Occurrence, Specificity, and Antigenicity**   1, 9, 38
Occurrence—Found in all vertebrate species studied
Specificity—Sight species specificity
Antigenicity—Definite

2. **Units**   8, 9, 14
1 mg = 577 I.U. (NIH—LS—SI) sheep standard

3. **Normal Blood Levels (Man)**   2, 4, 9, 22, 39
0.1-0.2 μg/100 ml plasma (males and females), cyclic during 28-day period in
   females; preovulatory and menopausal women 0.5-1.0 μg/100 ml plasma

4. **Administration**   8, 9, 37, 39
Injection—Preferred route
Topical—Inactive
Oral—Inactive

5. **Factors Affecting Release**   1, 4, 34
Inhibitors
   Cortisol
   Stress
   High sex hormone levels
   Feedback to hypothalamus by sex hormones
   Hyperthyroidism
   Serotonin
Stimulators
   Low sex hormone levels
   External stimuli
   Male—Continuous LRH from hypothalamus
   Female—Continuous LRH (hypothalamus) in induced ovulators—rabbit
         Cyclic LRH (hypothalamus) in spontaneous ovulators—human
           and dog

6. **Deficiency Symptoms**   1, 4, 37, 38, 39
   Estrogen or androgen secretion inhibited
   Atrophy of interstitial tissue in ovary or testis
   Lack of ovulation, luteinization in female

7. **Effects of Overdose, Toxicity**   1, 4, 37, 38, 39
   Hypertrophy, then atrophy of Leydig cells in male
   Increases estrogen or androgen secretion (with FSH)
   Precocious ovulation and luteinization of prepared follicles

METABOLIC ROLE

1. **Biosynthesis**   22, 37, 39
   Precursors—19 of 20 standard amino acids, tryptophan missing
   Intermediates—Unknown

2. **Production Sites**   22, 37, 39
   Anterior pituitary, central cells, basophilic cells

3. **Storage Areas**   8, 9, 16
   Stored in pituitary prior to ovulation in female

4. **Blood Carriers**   2, 8, 22, 26
   Complex with inactive protein

5. **Half-life**   8, 9, 26
   Approx. 20 min, 4 hr (two components)

6. **Target Tissues**   1, 22, 37, 39
   Gonads

7. **Reactions**   4, 5, 22, 25, 34, 38
   Reactive intermediates—Cyclic AMP (secondary messenger) and Ca^{2+}

Organ	Enzyme System	Effect
Gonads	Adenyl cyclase	Activated
	Enzymes incorporating acetate into squalene	Activated

8. **Mode of Action**   1, 4, 5, 8, 9, 16, 31, 37, 39
   Cellular
       Anabolic—Increased synthesis of steroid hormones
           Female—Interstitial ovarian cells synthesize estradiol
           Male—Leydig cells synthesize testosterone
       Catabolic—Increased CHO catabolism to produce NADH, NADP
   Organismal
       Promotes gametogenesis
       Promotes growth of accessory sex organs
       Stimulates rupture of follicles in ovary

9. **Catabolism**   1, 9, 22, 25, 34
   Intermediates—Hydrolysis in liver
   Excretion products—Active hormone in urine

MISCELLANEOUS

1. **Relationship to Vitamins**   8, 11, 13, 38
   Vitamin C—Ovarian depletion on LH stimulation
   Vitamin E—Involved in spermatogenesis

2. **Relationship to Other Hormones**   8, 11, 13, 32, 38
   FSH—Synergist to LH
   Prolactin—Synergist to LH
   HMG—Mixture of FSH and LH
   PMSG—Properties of FSH and LH
   HCG—Analog to LH

3. **Unusual Features**   29, 32, 38
   More stable on freeze-drying than FSH
   LH causes multiple ovulation in birds
   Insensitive to neuraminidase
   Inactivated by trypsin and carboxypeptidase, pepsin, chymotrypsin
   Not inactivated by CHO splitting enzymes; CHO moiety unharmed
   CHO moiety needed for activity
   Cyclic release in certain females (spontaneous ovulators)

4. **Possible Relationships of Deficiency Symptoms to Metabolic Action**   11, 13, 37
   Estrogen or androgen secretion inhibited—Lack of cyclic AMP to stimulate
   ovary or testis production

Atrophy of interstitial tissue in ovary or testis—Lack of stimulus by cyclic AMP

Lack of ovulation or luteinization in female—Lack of cyclic AMP to initiate events leading to ovulation

5. **Relationship to Minerals   (See references in specific mineral section)**

Synergists—I^- (as T4), PO_4^{3-} (as cyclic AMP), Ca^{2+}

Chapter 33. Follicle Stimulating Hormone (FSH)

FSH is an anterior pituitary hormone occupying a central position controlling the development of the sex glands. Its chief functions are to stimulate growth and development of the ovary in females, and the testes in the male. Its main importance stems from its effects on its control of development of the gonads during puberty and consequent synergistic action with LH during pregnancy. FSH primes the ovary and testes for LH action.

Deficiency conditions include Klinefelter's syndrome, Turner's syndrome, and hypogonadotropic eunuchoidism.

FSH is a water-soluble glycoprotein with two long half-lives in blood (4 hr and 20 hr). An excess of FSH causes hypertrophy of sex organs, increased follicular growth, and ovarian cyst formation. Its chief synergists are LH, STH, and T4. No antagonists have been reported.

FSH is formed in the anterior pituitary with some storage in the anterior pituitary and normally released by LRH (Gon RH), a hypothalamic releasing factor. Releasing factors include: LRH (Gon RH), castration, menopause, low sex hormone levels, clomiphene. Release-inhibiting factors are: estradiol, cortisol, stress, hyperthyroidism, negative feedback from the hypothalamus (low LRH).

On the cellular level FSH stimulates production of RNA and cyclic AMP in the gonadal cells.

GENERAL INFORMATION

1. **Synonyms**   1, 7, 18
   Follotropin, Luteoantine, Thylakentrin, Prolan A, gonadotropin I, gametogenic hormone, follicle ripening hormone, gametokinetic hormone

2. **History**   9, 18, 28, 36
   1921—Evans and Long: first noted gonadotropic effect of pituitary extracts on rats
   1927-30—Smith: reported that hypophysectomy in rat causes atrophy of gonads (and other organs) correctable by hypophyseal implants
   1928—Aschheim and Zondek: discovered a follicle-stimulating gonadotropin in menopausal urine
   1933—Fevold et al.: identified a separate follicle-stimulating hormone in the pituitary
   1939—Chow et al.: demonstrated FSH to be resistant to inactivation by proteolytic enzymes
   1940—Fevold et al.　　　⎱ Described isolation procedures
   1949—Li, Simpson and Evans ⎰ for animal FSH
   1965—Roos and Gemzell: prepared human FSH from menopausal urine
   1974—Shome and Parlow: determined amino acid sequences for α and β subunits, human FSH

3. **Physiological Forms**   9, 26, 37, 39
   Unknown (two components in plasma)

4. **Active Analogs and Related Forms**   17, 22, 34, 37, 39
   PMSG, HMG (mixture of FSH and LH)

5. **Inactive Analogs and Related Forms**   17, 22, 37, 39
   FSH without sialic acid moiety

6. **Antagonists**
   No data

7. **Synergists**   9, 17, 37, 39
   LH, STH, T4, Ca^{2+}

8. **Physiological Functions: Gametogenic**   1, 4, 14, 16, 37, 39
   Female—Stimulates ovarian follicles to grow and to develop, forming multiple layers and antra
   Male—Stimulates seminiferous tubules; stimulates spermatogenesis

9. **Deficiency Diseases, Disorders**   1, 4, 14, 16, 37, 39
   Klinefelter's syndrome (deficiency), Turner's syndrome (deficiency), hypogonadotropic eunuchoidism (deficiency)

10. **Essentiality for Life**   1, 9, 38
    Not required for life of organism, but required for reproduction by all vertebrates analyzed

CHEMISTRY

1. **Structure**   1, 8, 9, 15, 18
   Glycoprotein—Two subunits α and β structures known—both contain carbohydrate (18%)

   α—89 amino acids (identical to LH α subunit) $\Big\}$ Carbohydrates are hexose,
   β—111-115 amino acids (hormone-specific) $\Big\}$ hexosamine, fucose, sialic acid

   Both α and β needed for activity

2. **Reactions**   1, 8, 9, 17, 18

   Heat—No data

   Acid—Stable

   Alkali—Stable

   Water—Acidic

   Oxidation—H_2O_2, periodate—inactivate

   Reduction—Cysteine, ketene—inactivate

   Light—No data

   Proteolysis—Resistant to digestion with
   trypsin or chymotrypsin; inactivated
   by pronase, ptyalin and neuramini-
   dose

   Urea—Stable in 6 M urea

3. **Properties**   1, 7, 8, 9, 17, 19

   MW—30,000 (pig); 28,000 (sheep);
   27,000 (human)

   Miscellaneous—pI = 5.1 (pig);
   4.5 (sheep), 4.5-5.0 (human)

   Important groups for activity

   Sialic acid (complex), α and β subunits linked together

   —S–S—, terminal NH_2

   Solubility

   H_2O—soluble

   Acet., Alc.—Insol.

   Sol. 50% Acet.

   Sol. 70% Alc.

   Benz., Chl., Eth.—Insol.

   Absn. max.—Approx 280 mμ

   Chemical nature—Acidic glycoprotein

4. **Commercial Production**   9, 18, 22
   Extracted from human and sheep pituitaries

5. **Isolation**   22, 25
   Sources—Human, horse, sheep, swine, pituitary
   Method—Extract frozen pituitaries in aqueous salts; fractional precipitation
   from ammonium sulfate; DEAE cellulose; sephadex G-100; polyacrylamide
   gel electrophoresis

6. **Determination**   1, 14, 14a, 22, 26, 38
   Bioassay—Problems with LH contamination
   Ovarian weight change

Stimulation of young ovarian follicles (rabbit)
Increase in weight of testes
Physiochemical
Immunoassay
Radioimmunassay

MEDICAL AND BIOLOGICAL ROLE

1. **Species, Occurrence, Specificity, and Antigenicity**   1, 9, 38
   Occurrence—Found in all species of vertebrates studied
   Specificity—Strong species specificity (fish FSH inactive in mammals)
   Antigenicity—Moderately antigenic

2. **Units**   8, 9, 14
   1 mg = 25 I.U. (NIH-FSH-SI)—Sheep standard

3. **Normal Blood Levels (Man)**   2, 4, 9, 22, 39
   0.2-0.5 μg/100 ml plasma, females and males, cyclic during 28-day period in
      females; (Menopausal female 1.0-1.7 μg/100 ml)

4. **Administration**   8, 9, 37, 39
   Injection—Preferred route
   Topical—Inactive
   Oral—Inactive

5. **Factors Affecting Release**   1, 4, 34
   Inhibitors—Estradiol, cortisol, stress, hyperthyroidism, feedback by sex hor-
      mones via hypothalamus, serotonin
   Stimulators—LRH from hypothalamus, castration, menopause, low sex hor-
      mone levels; female—rhythmic control by hypothalamus via LRH secre-
      tion; male—continuous secretion of LRH by hypothalamus

6. **Deficiency Symptoms**   1, 4, 37, 38, 39
   Decreased gametogenic function and development (nonfunctional)
   Atrophy of gonads
   No maturation of ova, sperm
   Obesity
   Decreased libido, potency, hair growth
   Decreased blood levels of estrogen

7. **Effects of Overdose, Toxicity**   1, 4, 37, 38, 39
   Hypertrophy of secondary sex organs
   Increased growth and maturation of numerous follicles

Increased estrogen secretion (with LH)
Follicular cysts

METABOLIC ROLE

1. **Biosynthesis**   22, 37, 39
   Precursors—All 20 standard amino acids except methionine
   Intermediates—Unknown

2. **Production Sites**   22, 37, 39
   Anterior pituitary—basophilic cells (peripheral)

3. **Storage Areas**   8, 9, 16
   Anterior pituitary

4. **Blood Carriers**   2, 8, 22, 26
   α, β-Plasma proteins

5. **Half-life**   8, 9, 26
   Approx. 4 hr, 70 hr (two components)

6. **Target Tissues**   1, 22, 37, 39
   Ovary, testis

7. **Reactions**   4, 5, 22, 25, 34, 38
   Reactive intermediate—Cyclic AMP (secondary messenger) and Ca^{2+}
   Enzyme systems—Adenyl cyclase in ovary and testis activates various enzymes
      in gonads

8. **Mode of Action**   1, 4, 5, 8, 9, 16, 31, 37, 39
   Cellular
      Anabolic—Promotes luteinization (with LH), increases DNA synthesis in
         ovary, RNA synthesis in testis
      Catabolic—Unknown
      Other—Stimulates incorporation of glucose and α-aminoisobutyric acid
         into rat ovaries
   Organismal
      Promotes growth of ovarian follicles
      Promotes development of ovarian follicle
      Promotes growth of seminiferous tubules
      Promotes spermatogensis
      Promotes steroid secretion (with LH)

9. **Catabolism**   1, 9, 22, 25, 34
   Intermediates—Liver hydrolysis
   Excretion products—Free in urine (active)—small amounts

MISCELLANEOUS

1. **Relationship to Vitamins   8, 11, 13, 38**
   Vitamin C—Depletion in ovary due to LH and FSH action
   Vitamin E—Needed for maintenance of membranes in sex organs

2. **Relationship to Other Hormones   8, 11, 13, 32, 38**
   STH, LH—Synergists to FSH
   PMSG, HMG—Active analogs to FSH
   ACTH—Inhibitor of FSH
   T4—Inhibitor of FSH

3. **Unusual Features   29, 32, 38**
   Increased instability with purer preparations
   The only pituitary hormone not precipitated with 50% saturated $(NH_4)_2SO_4$
   Bird migration, ovulation, sex behavior controlled by FSH via light and
     temperature
   Gonadotropins of mammals stimulate thyroids of fish
   CHO groups needed for activity—Neuraminidase inactivates
   Cyclic release in females (spontaneous ovulators)
   Very high cysteine content

4. **Possible Relationships of Deficiency Symptoms to Metabolic Action   11,
      13, 37**
   Decreased gametogenesis and development of gonads, atrophy of gonads, no
     maturation of ova or sperm, decreased potency—Decreased FSH stimulus
     to sex tissues and synergism with LH
   Obesity—Decreased synergism with TSH (lower T4)
   Decreased libido—Decreased synergism with testosterone and LH
   Decreased hair growth—Decreased synergism with sex hormones and LH
   Decreased blood levels of estrogen—Decreased synergism with LH

5. **Relationship to Minerals   (See references in specific mineral section)**
   Synergists—I^- (as T4), PO_4^{3-} (as cyclic AMP), Ca^{2+}
   Release of hormone—K^+ increases

Chapter 34.   Prolactin

Prolactin is mainly a female hormone in humans. It is an anterior pituitary hormone, as mysterious as STH in its range of activities and a tissue controller of development and functioning of mammary glands in the female. Its chief functions are to initiate lactation and promote female breast development and maternal behavior. It has no known specific functions in the male, although it has some growth hormone activity. Deficiencies include galactorrhea and failure of lactation. Its chief importance is in the functions of lactation.

Prolactin is a water-soluble protein with a very short half-life in blood. An excess of prolactin causes precocious lactation, and longer maintenance of the corpus luteum in the ovary. No toxicity has been reported. Its chief synergists are STH, LH, estrogen, and progesterone; its antagonists are the same, but at different concentrations from the synergistic ones, usually higher.

Prolactin is formed in the anterior pituitary and stored there. Prolactin is unique among the pituitary hormones in being normally controlled by an inhibitor (PIF) rather than by a releasing hormone from the hypothalamus, as are the other pituitary hormones. Releasing factors include: tranquilizers, oxytocin, external stimuli, TRH, estrogen, T4, serotonin, exercise, tryptophan. Release-inhibiting factors are: PIF, L-dopa, progesterone. Prolactin apparently acts on the cell membranes, but no other details are available.

GENERAL INFORMATION

1. **Synonyms**   1, 7, 18
   Lactogenic hormone, luteotrop(h)ic hormone, LTH, luteotrop(h)in, lactogen, galactin, mammotropin

2. **History**   9, 18, 28, 36
   1928—Stricker and Grüter: discovered prolactin
   1933—Riddle et al.: coined term prolactin
   1937—Lyons: isolated prolactin from pituitary glands of ox, sheep, and pig
   1939—Astwood, Fevold: suggested luteotropin distinct from LH
   1941—Evans, Simpson, Lyons: suggested identity of prolactin and luteotropin
     in rat
   1942—Li: crystallized prolactin (first pituitary hormone to be crystallized)
   1970—Franz and Kleinberg: demonstrated human prolactin a separate entity
     from STH
   1970—Li et al.: determined structure of ovine prolactin

3. **Physiological Forms**   9, 26, 37, 39
   Human prolactin

4. **Active Analogs and Related Forms**   17, 22, 37, 39
   50% digested residue—"active core", HPL (human placental lactogen)

5. **Inactive Analogs and Related Forms**   17, 22, 37, 39
   Reduced molecule (with cysteine)
   Acetylated molecule (on lysine residues)
   Iodinated molecule (tyrosine residues iodinated)

6. **Antagonists**   9, 17, 37, 39
   Progesterone, testosterone, estradiol, LH (all concentration-dependent)

7. **Synergists**   9, 17, 37, 39
   STH, T4, prednisone, estradiol, progesterone, cortisol, oxytocin, PTH, LH

8. **Physiological Functions**   1, 4, 14, 16, 37, 39
   Initiation of lactation
   Development of mammary glands in female
   Increases weight and growth (similar to somatotropin) (some species)
   Nidation of zygote
   Protein anabolism (some species)
   Growth and secretion of crop gland (birds)
   Luteotropic (only in mouse and rat)
   Promotes maternal behavior

9. **Deficiency Diseases, Disorders**   1, 4, 14, 16, 37, 39
   Mammary carcinoma, galactorrhea, failure of lactation

10. Essentiality for Life   1, 9, 38

Not essential except where it functions as a growth hormone in certain species (birds, reptiles)

CHEMISTRY

1. Structure   1, 8, 9, 15, 18

Single-chain protein
Pig: Ala.———Cys—Tyr—Leu—Asn—Cys (205 amino acids)
Sheep: Thr.———Cys—Tyr—Leu—Asn—Cys (198 amino acids)
Human: Leu———first 50 amino acids known, similar to STH

2. Reactions   1, 8, 9, 17, 18

Heat—Stable (20 minutes at 100°C)
Acid—Precipitation with 0.5% TCA
Alkali—Unstable
Water—Soluble, acidic

Oxidation—Inactivates
Reduction—Inactivates
Light—Not reported
Proteolysis: 50% digestion leaves
active core

3. Properties   1, 7, 8, 9, 17, 19

Appearance—Crystalline powder
MW—25,000 (pig); 23,000 (sheep);
22,000 (human) approx.
Solubility
H_2O—Insoluble
Alc.—Soluble
Acet., Benz., Chl., Ether—Insol.
Absn. max.—Approx. 290 mμ

Important groups for activity
Tyr, Lys, Cys (S—S bridges)
Chemical nature—Single-chain
simple acidic protein
$\alpha_D^{25} = -40.5°$ (H_2O)
Miscellaneous—pI = 4.97 (pig);
5.74 (sheep), 4.9 (human)

4. Commercial Production   9, 18, 22

Extraction of pituitary glands of ox, sheep, swine

5. Isolation   22, 25

Sources—Pituitary glands of sheep
Methods
Ovine acetone powder extracted with pH 3 buffer
Precipitate prolactin with 0.06 saturated NaCl
Fractional precipitation, pH 5.6
Probability of protease contamination
Purify by: Countercurrent distribution; DEAE chromatography

6. **Determination** 1, 14, 14a, 22, 26, 38
   Bioassay
       Crop sac thickening (pigeons)
       Mammary gland growth in pseudopregnant rabbit
       Luteotropic, inhibition of estrus (mice)
   Physicochemical assay
       Immunoassay
       Radioimmunoassay

MEDICAL AND BIOLOGICAL ROLE

1. **Species Occurrence, Specificity, and Antigenicity** 1, 9, 38
   Occurrence—Found in all vertebrates
   Specificity—Some tolerance in crossing species lines
   Antigenicity—Moderate; bovine X rabbit no antigenicity
                 Human prolactin antigenically distinct from human GH

2. **Units** 8, 9, 14
   1 mg = 22 I.U., international standard II (sheep); 1 microgram = .001 mg

3. **Normal Blood Levels (Man)** 2, 4, 9, 22, 39
   Plasma: 0.5-1.0 μg/100 ml (male and female); diurnal rhythm—higher during
      sleep

4. **Administration** 8, 9, 37, 39
   Injection—Currently used
   Topical—Not active
   Oral—Not active

5. **Factors Affecting Release** 1, 4, 34
   Inhibitors—Hypothalamus (PIF factor), CNS, progesterone, L-dopa, dopa-
      mine
   Stimulators—CNS, suckling stimulus, oxytocin, tranquilizers, PRH (in birds),
      TRH, tryptophane, exercise, serotonin, T4, estrogen

6. **Deficiency Symptoms** 1, 4, 37, 38, 39
   Lactation not maintained
   Growth inhibited (some species)

7. **Effects of Overdose, Toxicity** 1, 4, 37, 38, 39
   Corpus luteum maintained past normal regression time
   Precocious lactation

METABOLIC ROLE

1. **Biosynthesis**   22, 37, 39
   Precursors—Amino acids, 20 standard
   Intermediates—Unknown

2. **Production Sites**   22, 37, 39
   Anterior pituitary—acidophils, E cells
   Placenta

3. **Storage Areas**   8, 9, 16
   Pituitary

4. **Blood Carriers**   2, 8, 22, 26
   Free and combined with blood proteins

5. **Half-life**   8, 9, 26
   20 min

6. **Target Tissues**   1, 22, 37, 39
   Mammary gland, ovary, crop sac (pigeons)

7. **Reactions**   4, 5, 22, 25, 33, 34, 38
   Reactive form—No data
   Enzyme systems—No data

8. **Mode of Action**   1, 4, 5, 8, 9, 16, 31, 37, 39
   Cellular
       Anabolic—Protein synthesis (some species)
       Catabolic—Unknown
       Other—Membrane effects
   Organismal
       Initiates and maintains lactation
       Increases life of corpus luteum
       Increases weight and growth
       Releases progesterone (in mouse and rat)

9. **Catabolism**   1, 9, 22, 25, 34
   Intermediates—Unknown
   Excretion products—Free in urine

MISCELLANEOUS

1. **Relationship to Vitamins** 8, 11, 13, 38
   None specifically, all indirectly via growth action in species where acts as growth hormone

2. **Relationship to Other Hormones** 8, 11, 13, 32, 38
   Progesterone, STH, T4, PTH, estradiol, cortisol, oxytocin—Synergists in lactation [STH, prolactin, ACTH (or adrenal steroids) needed for lactation in rats]
   LH—Synergism to maintain functional corpus luteum

3. **Unusual Features** 29, 32, 38
   Release not stimulated, but is inhibited, by hypothalamus (PIF) (except in birds) (negative controls)
   The only anterior pituitary hormone precipitated with 0.5% TCA
   Present in male pituitary (human) and in blood of male with unknown function
   Antigonadal in male bird; otherwise no known functions in male
   Terminal ring similar to oxytocin ring structure
   Different functions in various species
   Human prolactin more difficult to purify than sheep prolactin
   Gonadotropic effects in some mammals

4. **Possible Relationships of Deficiency Symptoms to Metabolic Action** 11, 13, 37
   Lactation not maintained—Metabolic functions of prolactin absent
   Growth inhibited—Prolactin needed to synergize growth hormone in certain species

5. **Relationship to Minerals** (See references in specific mineral section)
   Synergism—I^- (as T4)

Chapter 35.
ACTH

ACTH is an anterior pituitary hormone of the master type, since it controls another endocrine gland, the adrenal cortex. Its chief functions are to maintain and control secretion by the adrenal cortex, plus fat mobilization and promotion of gluconeogenesis in the liver. Its chief importance is its role in stress reactions and its antagonism to STH. Deficiency conditions are Simmonds' and Addison's diseases, adrenal insufficiency, and hypopituitarism.

ACTH is a water-soluble polypeptide (30 amino acids) with a short half-life (15 min). The hormone has been synthesized. Toxicity is known for excess ACTH, the effects including pigmentation, hypersensitivity, and hypertrophy of adrenal cortex. Its chief synergists are: epinephrine, cortisol, and corticosterone. Its chief antagonists are: STH and insulin.

ACTH is formed in the anterior pituitary and stored there. It is normally released by CRH. Releasing factors are: CRH, vasopressin, epinephrine, histamine, low glucocorticoids, and psychic trauma. Release-inhibiting factors are: high glucocorticoids. Apparently ACTH acts by stimulating protein synthesis in the liver and steroid syntheses in the adrenal, via cyclic AMP.

GENERAL INFORMATION

1. **Synonyms**   1, 7, 18
   Adrenocorticotrop(h)in, corticotrop(h)ic hormone, adrenocorticotrop(h)ic hormone

2. **History**   9, 18, 28, 36
   1930—Smith, P.E.: first observed direct relationship between the pituitary and the adrenal cortex
   1933—Collip et al.; Evans; Houssay et al.: noted that cell-free extracts of anterior pituitary stimulate adrenal cortex of hypophysectomized animal
   1943—Li et al.; Sayers et al.: isolated protein hormones from anterior pituitary that stimulate adrenal cortex
   1954—Bell: analyzed amino acid sequence of ACTH
   1961—Hofmann
   1963—Li   } Synthesized ACTH

3. **Physiological Forms**   9, 26, 37, 39
   No data

4. **Active Analogs and Related Compounds**   17, 22, 34, 37, 39
   ACTH sequence 1-20 (100% active)
   ACTH sequence 1-29 (30% active)
   ACTH sequence 1-19 with substitutions on #1, 11, 18 (>100% active as ACTH)
   β-Lipotropin (sheep, pig, beef)

5. **Inactive Analogs and Related Compounds**   17, 22, 37, 39
   α-MSH, β-MSH, ACTH sequence 2-39

6. **Antagonists**   9, 17, 37, 39
   Insulin; concentration—dependent for corticosterone, cortisol; STH (protein metabolism)

7. **Synergists**   9, 17, 37, 39
   Epinephrine, cortisol, corticosterone, STH (fat metabolism), Ca^{2+}

8. **Physiological Functions**   1, 4, 14, 16, 37, 39
   Maintenance of adrenal cortex
   Promotes secretion of steroids, oxidative phosphorylation in adrenal cortex
   Mobilizes and increases oxidation of free fatty acids in adipose tissue
   Increases gluconeogenesis in liver; increases cyclic AMP in adrenal cortex
   Decreases urea formation in liver
   Stimulates growth hormone release

9. **Deficiency Diseases, Disorders**   1, 4, 14, 16, 37, 39
   Adrenal insufficiency; hypopituitarism; Addison's disease (excess); Cushing's syndrome (excess); Simmonds' disease (deficiency)

10. **Essentiality for Life**   1, 9, 38
    One of the most essential hormones—Absence causes notable shortening of normal life span

CHEMISTRY

1. **Structure**   1, 8, 9, 15, 18
   Straight chain, simple polypeptide, 39 amino acids, $C_{214}H_{386}O_{93}N_{56}S$
   Structure known and synthesized; human ACTH: Ser—Tyr—Ser—Met—
   Glu—His—Phe—Arg—Try—Gly—Lys—Pro—Val—Gly—Lys—Lys—Arg—
   Arg—Pro—Val—Lys—Val—Tyr—Pro—Asp—Ala—Gly—Glu—Asp—Glu—
   Ser—Ala—Glu—Ala—Phe—Pro—Leu—Glu—Phe
   No S—S bridges
   Amino acids #1-20 essential, same in all species

2. **Reactions**   1, 8, 9, 17, 18

   Heat—Stable

   Acid

      Weak—Stable

      Strong—Hydrolysis

   Oxidation

      Irreversibly inactivates using
        periodate

      Reversibly inactivates using H_2O_2

   Reduction—Stable

   Alkali

      Inactivates

      Hydrolysis

   Water—Soluble, acidic

   Light—Stable

   Proteolysis—50% digestion of C-termi-
      nal end leaves active core

3. **Properties**   1, 7, 8, 9, 17, 19

   Appearance—White powder

   MW—4500 (39 amino acids)

   Important groups for activity

      Methionine—redox center—
        reacts with thiol; if change
        proline at #12, 19, 24 or
        serine #1, lose activity;
        1-20 essential

   Solubility

      H_2O—Freely sol.

      Acet., Alc.—Sol. in 60% alc.

      Benz., Chl., Eth.—Insol.

   Absn. max.—Approx. 280 mμ

   Chemical nature—Acidic polypeptide

   Miscellaneous—pI = 4.65-4.80

4. **Commercial Production**   9, 18, 22
   Extract pig, cattle, sheep, whale pituitaries
   Synthetic production possible

5. **Isolation**   22, 25
   Sources—Pituitaries of various animals
   Method
      Extract with 1 N acetic acid; precipitate with ethanol
      Adsorb on and elute from oxycellulose; freeze-dry
      Countercurrent distribution—500X purification using s-butanol—0.2%
        TCA
      Zone electrophoresis, end group analysis, analytical ultracentrifugation

6. Determination   1, 14, 14a, 22, 26, 38
   Bioassay
      Maintenance of weight of adrenal gland in hypophysectomized rats
      Depletion of vitamin C in adrenals of hypophysectomized rats
      Involution of thymus
   Physicochemical
      Immunoassay
      Radioimmunoassay

MEDICAL AND BIOLOGICAL ROLE

1. Species Occurrence, Specificity, Antigenicity   1, 9, 38
   Occurrence—All vertebrates
   Specificity—Slight biological differences, species differences located in
      sequence of amino acids 25-34
   Antigenicity—Slight

2. Units   8, 9, 14
   1 USP unit = 1 I.U. = 1.14 mg; 1 m I.U. = .001 I.U.

3. Normal Blood Levels (Man)   2, 4, 9, 22, 39
   0.1-1.0 m I.U./100 ml, plasma; diurnal fluctuation (high A.M.)

4. Administration   8, 9, 37, 39
   Injection—Intravenous, intramuscular, subcutaneous
   Topical—No data
   Oral—Active (stimulates release of cortisol)

5. Factors Affecting Release   1, 4, 34
   Inhibitors—Increased plasma level glucocorticoids (feedback)
   Stimulators
      Cortical release factors (CRH)—Diurnal rhythm
      Vasopressin, increased hepatic inactivation
      Epinephrine, histamine
      Stimulation of median eminence
      Psychic trauma (via hypothalamus)
      Decreased level of glucocorticoids

6. Deficiency Symptoms   1, 4, 37, 38, 39
   Decreased weight of adrenal (atrophy)
   Decreased mobilization of free fatty acids
   Decreased steroids in blood, urine (17-hydroxy and 17-keto)
   Fasting hypoglycemia
   Increased insulin sensitivity

7. **Effects of Overdose, Toxicity   1, 4, 37, 38, 39**
   Increased cortical secretions → hypertrophy and hyperplasia → destruction
   Increased pigmentation
   Death
   Hypersensitivity

METABOLIC ROLE

1. **Biosynthesis   22, 37, 39**
   Precursors—16 of 20 standard amino acids; no Cys, Thr. Ile, or Asn
   Intermediates—MSH (?)

2. **Production Sites   22, 37, 39**
   Anterior pituitary—basophilic cells; placenta

3. **Storage Areas   8, 9, 16**
   Anterior pituitary

4. **Blood Carriers   2, 8, 22, 26**
   Free and combined with plasma proteins

5. **Half-life   8, 9, 26**
   15-25 min

6. **Target Tissues   1, 26, 37, 39**
   Adrenal cortex, perirenal cells, embryonic rest cells

7. **Reactions   4, 5, 22, 25, 34, 38**
   Reactive intermediates: cyclic AMP—Secondary messenger and Ca^{2+}

Organ	Enzyme System	Effect
Adrenal cortex	Adenyl cyclase	Activated
	Phosphorylase b	Activated
	Cholesterol 20-Hydroxylase	Activated

8. **Mode of Action   1, 4, 5, 8, 9, 16, 31, 37, 39**
   Cellular—
      Anabolic—
         Increases melanin synthesis in skin
         Increases steroid synthesis in adrenal
         Increases protein synthesis in liver (via cortisol)

Catabolic
   Increases glycogenolysis (adrenal cortex)
   Increases gluconeogenesis (liver) (via cortisol)
   Increases lipolysis and oxidation of fatty acids in adipose tissue
Other:
   Increases oxidative phosphorylation in adrenal cortex
   Increases production of cyclic AMP to produce $NADPH_2$ in adrenal
      cortex
   Decreases cholesterol in adrenal cortex
Organismal
   Increases weight of adrenals, depletes cortex of vitamin C
   Mobilizes free fatty acids from adipose tissue
   Hypoglycemic, reduces urea formation
   Increases iodine uptake by thyroid
   Stimulates secretion of gluco- and mineralocorticoids by adrenal cortex
   Stimulates melanophores, darkening of skin

9. **Catabolism**   1, 9, 22, 25, 34
   Intermediates—Liver destruction
   Excretion Products—Free in urine (very little)

MISCELLANEOUS

1. **Relationship to Vitamins**   8, 11, 13, 38
   Vitamin C—Depleted in adrenal cortex on stimulation by ACTH
   Niacin—Production of $NADPH_2$ by ACTH via cyclic AMP
   Vitamin D—Antagonized indirectly by ACTH via cortisol action
   Biotin and vitamin A—Adrenocortical insufficiency noted in biotin and vita-
      min A deficiency
   Pantothenic acid, niacin—Synergistic with ACTH in steroid hormone syn-
      thesis

2. **Relationship to Other Hormones**   8, 11, 13, 32, 38
   Epinephrine—Synergist, stimulates release of ACTH
   Cortisol, corticosterone—Synergists or antagonists depending on concentra-
      tion; production stimulated by ACTH
   CRH—Stimulates release of ACTH
   Vasopressin—Similar to CRH, in action
   T4 and TSH—ACTH stimulates iodine uptake by thyroid
   MSH—MSH is a part of ACTH molecule
   Insulin—Antagonist to ACTH
   STH—Antagonist (protein metabolism) synergist (fat metabolism) releases
      ACTH

3. **Unusual Features   29, 32, 38**
   Reversible loss of activity on oxidation with H_2O_2
   Reacts with thiols
   Irreversible deactivation by periodate
   First 13 amino acids essential for corticotropic activity
   Full activity at first 20 amino acids
   MSH, a part of ACTH, and its activity increased by *N*-acetylation
   Second messenger (cyclic AMP) involved in adrenal cortex

4. **Possible Relationships of Deficiency to Metabolis Action   11, 13, 37**
   Atrophy of adrenal cortex—Lack of stimulus from ACTH
   Decreased mobilization of fatty acids—Decreased glucocorticoids, increased
     insulin activity
   Decreased steroids in blood and urine—Decreased production of adrenal cor-
     ticoids
   Fasting hypoglycemia—Decreased gluconeogenesis
   Increased insulin sensitivity—Insulin antagonism to ACTH and cortisol

5. **Relationship to Minerals   (See references in specific mineral section)**
   Synergism—PO_4^{3-} (as cyclic AMP), Ca^{2+}
   Absorption—I^- uptake by thyroid increased
   Excretion of Na^+, K^+ via mineralocorticoid release (↑)
   Regulates serum levels—Cu^{2+} (↓)

Chapter 36.
MSH

MSH is not presently recognized as a functioning hormone in humans. It is an intermediate lobe pituitary hormone of the tissue-controlling type. Its chief functions are not all known, but mainly they have to do with skin pigmentation. Its chief importance is in mediating reactions to light in lower vertebrates. MSH can cause slow increase in pigmentation in man, but no other functions in man are known. A deficiency is hypopituitarism (in animals).

MSH is a water-soluble peptide, a fragment of ACTH with a very short half-life. It has been synthesized. Excess dosages result in skin darkening and hypoglycemia. Its chief synergists are: STH, TSH, and caffeine. Its chief antagonists are: cortisone and melatonin.

MSH is formed in the intermediate lobe of the pituitary and is stored there. Releasing factors include: MRH, nerve stimuli, metabolic factors. Release-inhibitors include: MIF, epinephrine, melatonin, nerve stimuli. MSH apparently acts by stimulating melanin enzymes and increasing cellular permeability, via cyclic AMP.

GENERAL INFORMATION

1. **Synonyms**   1, 7, 18

    Melanophore (affecting) hormone, melanophore-stimulating hormone, melanotrophin, melanotrophic hormone, chromatophorotropic hormone, melanosome-dispersing hormone, pigmentation hormone, β-hormone melanotropin

2. **History**   9, 18, 28, 36
   1932—Zondek and Krohn: noted factor in intermediate lobe mediating pigmentary responses in lower vertebrates
   1954—Lerner: proposed term melanocyte-stimulating hormone for above factor
   1956—Geschwind et al.: isolated β-MSH from pit pituitary
   1957—Harris and Lerner: isolated α-MSH from pig pituitary tissue
   1959—Harris and Roos: isolated β-MSH from bovine pituitary
   1960—Dixon: isolated β-MSH from human pituitary
   1960—Hofmann et al.: synthesized derivatives of β-MSH
   1960—Li, Dixon: isolated α-MSH from horse pituitary
   1960—Lee et al.: determined structure of α-MSH
   1963—Schwyzer et al.: synthesized α-MSH and β-MSH

3. **Physiological Forms**   9, 26, 37, 39
   l-α-MSH, l-β-MSH (intermedin) (approx. equal biological activity)

4. **Active Analogs and Related Compounds**   17, 22, 37, 39
   Acetylated N-terminal (β-MSH and ACTH)
   Common heptapeptide (Met—Glu—His—Phe—Arg—Try—Gly) of α,β-MSH and ACTH

5. **Inactive Analogs and Related Compounds**   17, 22, 37, 39
   ACTH (1% of MSH activity)
   Hydrolyzed fragments

6. **Antagonists**   9, 17, 37, 39
   Cortisone, d-amino acid analogs (competitive inhibitors), melatonin

7. **Synergists**   9, 17, 37, 39
   STH, TSH (amphibians), caffeine, theophylline, Ca^{2+}

8. **Physiological Functions**   1, 4, 14, 16, 37, 39
   Function in mammals is obscure (protection from sunlight?), small effect on skin pigmentation
   Expands or contracts pigments in various chromatophores
   Expands melanophore pigments with color changes in amphibians (adaptation to environment); weak ACTH activity; adipokinetic effect, stimulates T4 secretion
   Increases sensitivity to light, decreases dark adaptation time (lower vertebrates)

9. **Deficiency Diseases, Disorders**   1, 4, 14, 16, 37, 39
   Excess—Addison's disease, adrenal insufficiency (darkening)
   Deficiency—Hypopituitarism (light)

10. **Essentiality for Life** 1, 9, 38

Not required; present in all vertebrates with differing functions

CHEMISTRY

1. **Structure**   1, 8, 9, 15, 18

Polypeptide—purified, synthesized, α and β-forms, straight chains

α, 13 amino acids: Ser—Tyr—Ser—[Met—Glu—His—Phe—Arg—Try—Gly]—Lys—Pro—Val

N-terminal = $CH_3CO—$, C-terminal = $—NH_2$ similar all species

β, 18 amino acids in most species except 22 in human: Ala—Glu—Lys—Lys—Asp—Glu—Gly—Pro—Tyr—Arg [Met—Glu—His—Phe—Arg—Try—Gly] Ser—Pro—Pro—Lys—Asp

No S—S bridges, [   ] = common heptapeptide

α and β forms equally active

2. **Reactions**   1, 8, 9, 17, 18

Heat—Stable	Oxidation—H_2O_2 reversibly inactivates
Acid—Stable	Reduction—Thiols reversibly inactivate
Alkali—Stable (potentiates)	Light—No effect
Water—Sol., basic	Proteolysis—Decreases activity

3. **Properties**   1, 7, 8, 9, 17, 19

Appearance—White powder

MW—α 1500 (13 amino acids); β 2100-2600 (18-22 amino acids)

Important groups for activity
Met (redox center)
Tyr
Common hepapeptide in all α's, β's, and ACTH (Met———Gly)

Solubility
H_2O—Sol.
Acet., Alc.—Insol.
Benz., Chl., Eth.—Insol.

Absn. max.—Approx. 280 mμ

Chemical nature
Simple, peptides (α—acidic, β—basic)
α-MSH: α_D^{25} = 58.5°C (10% acetic acid)

Miscellaneous—pI = α 5.5-7.0, β 11.0

4. **Commercial Production**   9, 18, 22, 24, 35

Synthetic

5. **Isolation**   22, 25

Sources—Human, pig, bovine, pituitary glands, urine, blood

Methods

β-MSH

Extract with KCl at pH 5.5; precipitate with salt; adsorb on oxycellulose

Purify via carboxylic acid resin

Countercurrent distribution (1.2 M urea, 0.2 M ethylenediamine, 0.1 N HCl)

6. **Determination**   1, 14, 14a, 22, 26, 38
   Bioassay—Darkening of frog skin ($\alpha > \beta$)
   Physicochemical
       Photoelectric reflectance assay
       Immunoassay
       Radioimmunoassay

MEDICAL AND BIOLOGICAL ROLE

1. **Species Occurrence, Specificity, and Antigenicity**   1, 9, 38
   Occurrence: All vertebrates (α-MSH, β-MSH); all preparations similar in
       activity from all animals
   Specificity
       α-MSH—Slight species differences in activity
       β-MSH—Definite species differences in activity
   Antigenicity: α—none; β—slight

2. **Units**   8, 9, 14
   Relative to posterior pituitary standard or by weight (1 μg = 1 microgram)

3. **Normal Blood Levels (Man)**   2, 4, 9, 22, 39
   .01 μg/100 ml, plasma

4. **Administration**   8, 9, 37, 39
   Injection—Subcutaneous
   Topical—Active, used in amphibian experiments
   Oral—Active, used in amphibian experiments

5. **Factors Affecting Release**   1, 4, 34
   Inhibitors—MIF via hypothalamus, epinephrine, nervous controls, melatonin
   Stimulators—Metabolic, nervous controls, MRH via hypothalamus

6. **Deficiency Symptoms**   1, 4, 37, 38, 39
   Lightened skin color (amphibians)
   Chromatophore contraction
   Guanophore expansion

7. **Effects of Overdose, Toxicity**   1, 4, 37, 38, 39
   Darkening of skin (amphibians and humans), temporary
   Hyperglycemia

METABOLIC ROLE

1. **Biosynthesis**   22, 37, 39
   Precursors—13-14 of 20 standard amino acids (missing: Cys, Asn, Gln, Leu, Ile, Thr, Val)
   Intermediates—Unknown

2. **Production Sites**   22, 37, 39
   Intermediate lobe of pituitary, except in birds, whales, elephants, armadillos, where it is in anterior lobe
   Also in posterior lobes

3. **Storage Areas**   8, 9, 16
   In intermediate lobe of pituitary

4. **Blood Carriers**   2, 8, 22, 26
   Free and combined with plasma proteins

5. **Half-life**   8, 9, 26
   Est. 10 min

6. **Target Tissues**   22, 37, 39
   Skin (melanophores) (amphibians)

7. **Reactions**   4, 5, 22, 25, 34, 38
   Reactive intermediates: Cyclic AMP (secondary messenger), Ca^{2+}

Organ	Enzyme System	Effect
Skin	Adenyl cyclase	Activated
	Tyrosinase; see ACTH enzymes	Activated

8. **Mode of Action**   1, 4, 5, 8, 9, 16, 31, 37, 39
   Cellular
      Anabolic—Melanin formation
      Catabolic—Blocks glycolytic pathways
      Other—Increases permeability to Na^+, changes protoplasmic viscosity, expands pigments in melanophores
   Organismal
      ACTH function (weak)
      Blocks action of melatonin
      Regulates skin color changes, light adaptations

9. **Catabolism**   1, 9, 22, 25, 34
Intermediates—Unknown
Excretion products—Free in urine; also breakdown products

MISCELLANEOUS

1. **Relationship to Vitamins**   8, 11, 13, 38
Vitamin C—Adrenal cortex depleted on ACTH and MSH activity
Vitamin A—MSH decreases dark adaptation time

2. **Relationship to Other Hormones**   8, 11, 13, 32, 38
STH, TSH—Synergists to MSH
T4—Secretion stimulated by MSH
Cortisone, melatonin—Antagonist to MSH
Epinephrine—Inhibitor of MSH release

3. **Unusual Features**   29, 32, 38
Very resistant to degradation or inactivation
Reversibly inactivated by oxidation (H_2O_2)
Reduced with thiols
Heptapeptide 4-10 similar to ACTH
α and β forms with similar activity but different amino acid contents

4. **Possible Relationships of Deficiency to Metabolic Action**   11, 13, 37
Lightened skin color (amphibians)—No MSH available to promote melanin
    dispersion

5. **Relationship to Minerals**   (See references in specific mineral section)
Synergism—PO_4^{3-} (as cyclic AMP), Ca^{2+}
Absorption by kidney of Na^+ ($\uparrow$) (increased permeability)

Chapter 37.
Oxytocin

Oxytocin, which is primarily a female sex hormone, is a posterior pituitary hormone of the tissue-controlling variety. Its chief functions are: to promote uterine contractions, and milk ejection; and to increase blood sugar, and urinary sodium and potassium. Its chief importance is to expedite processes of child-birth and lactation. Deficiencies result in insufficiency of labor and atonic uterine bleeding.

Oxytocin is small water-soluble peptide (octapeptide) with a short half-life (9 min) in blood. It has been synthesized. Excess dosages result in tetanic con-traction of a pregnant uterus and an increase in milk flow. Its chief synergists are prolactin, relaxin, and estradiol, whereas its antagonist is $2'$-o-methyltyro-sine oxytocin.

Oxytocin is formed in the hypothalamus and is stored in the posterior pi-tuitary. Releasing factors include: relaxin, nerve impulses. Oxytocin acts mainly by effects on membranes, especially of uterine muscle, which contracts strongly in response, via cyclic AMP.

GENERAL INFORMATION

1. **Synonyms**   1, 7, 18
   Oxytocic hormone, postlobin-O, posterior-lobe principle, Pitocin, lactogogin, uteracon, α-hypophamine

2. **History**   9, 18, 28, 36

1906—Dale: noted effect of posterior pituitary factor in stimulating uterine contraction

1928—Kamin et al.: separated two active fractions from neural lobe; one was active in raising blood pressure in mammals; the other promoted uterine contractions

1952—Pierce et al.: isolated oxytocin

1953—du Vigneaud et al.: synthesized oxytocin

1965—Flouret et al.: synthesized d-oxytocin

3. **Physiological Forms**   9, 26, 37, 39

l-Oxytocin

4. **Active Analogs and Related Compounds**   17, 22, 37, 39

Vasopressin

Isotocin (some fish)

8-Isoleucine oxytocin (other fish, amphibians)

Arginine vasotocin (all vertebrates, except mammals)

5. **Inactive Analogs and Related Compounds**   7, 22, 37, 39

Reduced form of oxytocin, enlarged or smaller ring forms, forms with side chains removed

6. **Antagonists**   9, 17, 37, 39

2'-o-methyltyrosine oxytocin

7. **Synergists**   9, 17, 37, 39

Uterus—Prolactin, relaxin, estradiol

Mammary gland—STH, progesterone, estradiol, T4, cortisol

8. **Physiological Functions**   1, 4, 14, 16, 37, 39

Uterine contraction; milk ejection; facilitates sperm ascent in female tract

Decreases: Membrane potential of myometrium; BMR, liver glycogen

Stimulates oviposition in hen, releases LH

Increases: Blood sugar, urinary Na and K

9. **Deficiency Diseases, Disorders**   1, 4, 14, 16, 37, 39

Insufficiency of labor, atonic uterine bleeding

10. **Essentiality for Life**   1, 9, 38

Not essential

CHEMISTRY

1. Structure   1, 8, 9, 15, 18
Octapeptide—synthesized

Cys—Tyr—Ile—Gln—Asn—Cys—Pro—Leu—Gly—(NH$_2$)
Oxytocin—C$_{43}$H$_{66}$N$_{12}$O$_{12}$S$_2$

2. Reactions   1, 8, 9, 17, 18
Heat—No data
Acid—Stable (weak), unstable
    (strong)
Alkali—Unstable
Water—Sol., basic

Oxidation—Stable
Reduction—Inactivates (ring opens)
Light—No data
Proteolysis by chymotrypsin, tryp-
    sin or tyrosinase inactivates

3. Properties   1, 7, 8, 9, 17, 19
Appearance—Amorphous white
    powder
MW—1007
Salts—Citrate, flavianate
Important groups for activity
    Ile, Glu, Asp, Leu, Gly, Cys
    Ring (opening inactivates)

Solubility
    H$_2$O—Soluble
    Acet., Alc.—Sl. Sol., Sol.
    Benz., Chl., Ether—Insol.
Absn. max.—Approx. 280 mμ
Chemical nature—Basic octapeptide
α_D^{22} = —26.2°
Miscellaneous—pI = 7.7

4. Commercial Production   9, 18, 22
Synthetic, from amino acids
Posterior pituitary lobe of cattle, sheep (extraction)

5. Isolation   22, 25
Sources—Posterior lobe of pituitary, cattle
Methods
    Dissociate from protein with acid hydrolysis
    Electrodialysis, precipitation
    DEAE cellulose, pH 5.5

6. Determination   1, 14, 19a, 22, 26, 38
Bioassay
    Blood pressure drop in chick
    Milk ejection in rat
    Contraction of isolated uterus of virgin guinea pig
Physicochemical—No information

MEDICAL AND BIOLOGICAL ROLE

1. **Species Occurrence, Specificity, and Antigenicity**   1, 9, 38
   Occurrence: Found in most vertebrates, in slightly different forms
   Specificity: Interspecies reactivity—Decrease in action in lower forms
   Antigenicity: Low

2. **Units**   8, 9, 14
   1 USP unit = approx. 2 μg of pure hormone; 1 mμg = .001 μg; 1 μg = microgram

3. **Normal Blood Levels (Man)**   2, 4, 9, 22, 39
   0.03 mμg-0.3 mμg/100 ml plasma

4. **Administration**   8, 9, 37, 39
   Injection—Intramuscular, subcutaneous, I.V. drip
   Topical—Nasal spray
   Oral—Inactivated by chymotrypsin in intestine

5. **Factors Affecting Release**   1, 4, 34
   Inhibitors: No data
   Stimulants: Reflex arcs—Chemical and neural reflexes from suckling, milking,
      from cervix, vagina (dilatation of birth canal); psychic events; relaxin

6. **Deficiency Symptoms**   1, 4, 37, 38, 39
   Delayed uterine contraction in pregnancy
   Decreased milk flow

7. **Effects of Overdose, Toxicity**   1, 4, 37, 38, 39
   Tetanic contraction of pregnant uterus
   Increase in milk flow

METABOLIC ROLE

1. **Biosynthesis**   22, 37, 39
   Precursors—8 of 20 standard amino acids; missing are Glu, Asp, Met, Arg,
      Lys, His, Pro, Try, Phe, Ala, Thr, Ser
   Intermediates: Neurophysin—Peptide complex

2. **Production Sites**   22, 37, 39
   Hypothalamus (paraventricular nuclei?)

3. **Storage Areas**   8, 9, 16
Posterior pituitary and hypothalamus

4. **Blood Carriers**   2, 8, 22, 26
Unbound and in loose association with plasma proteins

5. **Half-life**   8, 9, 26
1-6 min in pregnant women

6. **Target Tissues**   1, 22, 37, 39
Uterus (pregnant), mammary gland, other smooth muscle

7. **Reactions**   4, 5, 22, 25
Reactive intermediate—Probably cyclic AMP, Ca^{2+}

8. **Mode of Action**   1, 4, 5, 8, 9, 16, 31, 37, 39
Cellular
    Anabolic—No data
    Catabolic—No data
    Other—Contraction of myoepithelial cells around mammary alveoli
        Contraction of uterine smooth muscle
Organismal
    Uterine contraction
    Milk ejection
    Vasodilator ⎫
    Antidiuretic ⎭ in large doses only

9. **Catabolism**   1, 9, 22, 25, 34
Intermediates
    In pregnancy, plasma oxytocinase inactivates
    Oxytocinase formed in placenta breaks down oxytocin
    Removed from plasma by liver, *kidney*, and mammary gland
Excretion products: A little, free in urine

MISCELLANEOUS

1. **Relationship to Vitamins**
No data

2. **Relationship to Hormones**   8, 11, 13, 32, 38
Vasopressin (ADH)—structurally similar to vasopressin; always secreted with
    vasopressin irrespective of stimulus
Prolactin—Oxytocin may stimulate release of prolactin

STH, TSH, ACTH, LH, FSH, PROL—Anterior pituitary hormones; related in
     milk production
Estradiol—Uterine effect dependent on estrogen presence
LH—Oxytocin stimulates LH release
Norepinephrine ⎱
                   ⎰ Occur with oxytocin in posterior pituitary
Serotonin
CRH—Structural similarity to oxytocin
Relaxin—Stimulates oxytocin release

3. **Unusual Features**   29, 32, 38
   Very similar structurally to vasopressin but main physiological actions very
        different (only two amino acids differ)
   No known function in male mammal
   Protein, neurophysin, binds neurohypophysial hormones specifically
   Always secreted with vasopressin irrespective of nature of stimulus
   Nonpregnant uterus is more sensitive to ADH than to oxytocin
   Vasodilator effect of oxytocin is blocked by ADH
   Releases anterior pituitary hormones in fish
   Increases oviposition in birds and reptiles
   Increases spawning reflex in fish

4. **Possible Relationships of Deficiency Symptoms to Metabolic Action**   11,
        13, 37
   No data

5. **Relationships to Minerals**   (See references in specific mineral section)
   Synergism—I^- (as T4), PO_4^{3-} (as cyclic AMP)
   Excretion of Na^+, K^+

Chapter 38.
Vasopressin (ADH)

ADH is a posterior pituitary hormone of the tissue-controlling type. Its chief functions are to elevate blood pressure and to regulate water and sodium balance. Its chief importance lies in its removal of sodium and maintenance of water balance. A deficiency disease is diabetes insipidus.

ADH is a water-soluble octapeptide with a short half-life in blood. It has been synthesized. Excess dosages result in increased water absorption and blood pressure, gastrointestinal disturbances, uterine cramps, urinary circulation problems, and release of anterior pituitary hormones. Its chief synergists are aldosterone, epinephrine, and T4, whereas its chief antagonists are norepinephrine and some prostaglandins.

ADH is formed in the hypothalamus and is stored in the posterior pituitary. Releasing agents include: Ca^{2+}, excess Na^+, stress, exercise, some sedatives and anesthetics; while release inhibitors include: alcohol, low Na^+, high extracellular fluid volume. ADH acts by increasing kidney water reabsorption by changing permeability of certain kidney cells, via cyclic AMP.

GENERAL INFORMATION

1. **Synonyms**   1, 7, 18
   (Arginine) vasopressin, ADH (antidiuretic hormone), antidiuretin, Pitressin, β-hypophamine, Tonephin, Vasophysin

2. **History**   9, 18, 28, 36

   1895—Oliver and Schafer: noted effect of posterior pituitary factor on rise in blood pressure

   1937—Gilman and Goodman: showed dehydration increased plasma and urine levels of vasopressin

   1942—Van Dyke: isolated crude protein fraction possessing oxytocin and vasopressin activities from oxen pituitaries

   1953-54—DuVigneaud et al.: determined structure and synthesized ADH

3. **Physiological Forms**   9, 26, 37, 39

   l-vasopressin, *l*-ADH

4. **Active Analogs and Related Compounds**   17, 22, 37, 39

   Arginine vasopressin (most mammals)

   Lysine vasopressin (pig)

   Vasotocin (birds, amphibians, fish)

5. **Inactive Analogs and Related Compounds**   17, 22, 37, 39

   Opening of ring; removal of side chain

   Change in size of ring

6. **Antagonists**   9, 17, 37, 39

   Norepinephrine, prostaglandins

7. **Synergists**   9, 17, 37, 39

   Aldosterone, STH, prolactin, corticosterone, T4, testosterone, epinephrine

8. **Physiological Functions**   1, 4, 14, 16, 37, 39

   Elevates blood pressure (mammals) (reverse effect in birds)

   Decreases kidney blood flow

   Antidiuretic; acts as CRH; releases ACTH

   Increases NaCl concentration in urine

   Regulates water balance

   Stimulates contraction of smooth muscles

   Increases renal tubular H_2O reabsorption

   Releases anterior pituitary hormones

9. **Deficiency Diseases, Disorders**   1, 4, 14, 16, 37, 39

   Deficiency—Diabetes insipidus

   Excess—Schwartz-Bartter syndrome (oat-cell carcinoma)

10. **Essentiality for Life**   1, 9, 38

    Not essential

CHEMISTRY

1. **Structure**   1, 8, 9, 15, 18
   Octapeptide—Synthesized

   Cys—Tyr—Phe—Gln—Asn—Cys—Pro—Arg—Gly(NH$_2$)
   Arginine vasopressin, $C_{46}H_{65}N_{15}O_{12}S_2$

2. **Reactions**   1, 8, 9, 17, 18

   Heat—Degrades in solution
   Acid—Stable
   Alkali—Unstable
   Water—Soluble, basic

   Oxidation—Stable
   Reduction—Inactivates (ring opens)
   Light—Unstable
   Proteolysis inactivates (by trypsin, which removes terminal glycine amide group, but not by pepsin)

3. **Properties**   1, 7, 8, 9, 17, 19

   Appearance—Amorphous white powder
   MW—1084 (arginine vasopressin)
   Salts, esters—Tannate
   Solubility
     H$_2$O—Soluble
     Alc.—Sol.
     Acet., Benz., Chl., Eth.—Insol.

   Important groups for activity
     Cyclic pentapeptide (opening inactivates)
     Tripeptide side chain
     Cys-Cys
   Absn. max.—Approx. 280 mμ
   Chemical nature—Basic peptide
   Miscellaneous—p/ = 10.9

4. **Commercial Production**   9, 18, 22
   Synthesized from amino acids
   Posterior lobe of pituitary of domestic animals (hog, beef)

5. **Isolation**   22, 25
   Sources: Posterior pituitary glands (hog, beef)
   Methods:
     Acetic acid extraction of posterior pituitary powder
     Percolation through Celite using 70% ethanol and gradually increasing concentrations of water and acetic acid
     Or the neurophysin peptide complex is extracted with acetic acid and the protein precipitated with NaCl; treatment with trichloroacetic acid then dissociates the complex and precipitates the protein

6. **Determination**   1, 14, 19a, 22, 26, 38
   Bioassay
     Blood pressure measurements on cats, dogs, or chickens
     Diuretic studies on dogs, rats, and rabbits
     Weight gain in frogs
   Physicochemical: Radioimmunoassay

MEDICAL AND BIOLOGICAL ROLE

1. **Species Occurrence, Specificity, and Antigenicity**   1, 9, 38
   Occurrence
   > Vasopressin-like substances found in vertebrates from cyclostomes through mammals
   > Loss of activity as go to amphibians and fish
   Specificity—Decreasing interspecies reactivity in lower vertebrates
   Antigenicity—Low

2. **Units**   8, 9, 14
   1 USP posterior pituitary unit = 1 international posterior pituitary unit = 0.5 mg of the international standard oxytocic, vasopressor, and antidiuretic substances (ox posterior pituitary)
   1 mμg = .001 μg; 1 μg = 1 microgram

3. **Normal Blood Levels (Man)**   2, 4, 9, 22, 37
   .05-.70 mμg/100 ml, plasma

4. **Administration**   8, 9, 37, 39
   Injection—Intravenous, intramuscular, or subcutaneous
   Topical—Inhalation of powders or sprays
   Oral—No data

5. **Factors Affecting Release**   1, 4, 34
   Inhibitors
   > Low osmotic pressure in blood (low Na^+)
   > Ethyl alcohol
   > High extracellular fluid volume
   Stimulators
   > High blood osmotic pressure (high Na^+)
   > Acetylcholine, lobeline
   > Physostigmine
   > Cold, low fluid volume
   > Hemorrhage
   > Morphine, nicotine, ether, some barbiturates, tranquilizers, and general anesthetics
   > Ca^{2+} ion (inhibits binding to protein)
   > Stress
   > Exercise, psychic events

6. **Deficiency Symptoms**   1, 4, 37, 38, 39
   Diuresis

Polydipsia
Decreased NaCl and urea concentration in urine

7. Effects of Overdose, Toxicity   1, 4, 20, 37, 38, 39
Increased water reabsorption, blood pressure
Smooth muscle contraction—Gastrointestinal activity
Facial pallor
Uterine cramps
Coronary circulation complications

METABOLIC ROLE

1. Biosynthesis   22, 37, 39
Precursors—Eight of standard 20 amino acids; missing are Glu, Asp, Met, Lys,
   His, Leu, Prol, Try, Ile, Ala, Thr, Ser
Intermediates—Neurophysin-peptide complex

2. Production Sites   22, 37, 39
Hypothalamus, esp. supraoptic nuclei; secreted into neurohypophysis

3. Storage Areas   8, 9, 16
Hypothalamus and posterior pituitary

4. Blood Carriers   2, 8, 22, 26
Unbound, and loose association with plasma protein

5. Half-life   8, 9, 26
In plasma 15 min

6. Target Tissues   1, 22, 37, 39
Capillaries, arterioles, coronary vessels, kidney tubules, smooth muscle

7. Reactions   4, 5, 22, 25, 34, 38
Reactive intermediate: Cyclic AMP (secondary messenger) and Ca^{2+}

Organ	Enzyme System	Effect
Kidney	Hyaluronidase	Activated
Kidney (distal tubule)	Adenyl cyclase	Activated

8. Mode of Action   1, 4, 5, 8, 9, 16, 31, 37, 39

Cellular

    Anabolic—No data

    Catabolic—Depolymerizes hyaluronic acid

    Other

        Increases passive permeability of epithelium of distal segment of nephron to water; allows osmotic forces to operate more freely

        Increases intracellular water in muscle; decreases Na^+ and K^+

        Increases pore size or number in cell membrane

Organismal

    Antidiuretic—Concentrates urine

    Decreases coronary blood flow

    Increases motility of bowel

    Arterial smooth muscle sensitized to effects of norepinephrine by physiological amounts of ADH

    Renal blood flow reduced by ADH

9. Catabolism   1, 9, 22, 25, 34

Intermediates—Inactivated in kidney and liver

Excretion products—Some free in urine

MISCELLANEOUS

1. Relationship to Vitamins   8, 11, 13, 38

No data

2. Relationship to Other Hormones   8, 11, 13, 32, 38

Oxytocin, hypertensin—Structurally very similar to vasopressin but main physiological effect is very different

Aldosterone, corticosterone—Synergistic with vasopressin; related to antidiuretic activity of vasopressin

CRH—Vasopressin suggested to have CRH (corticotropin release hormone) properties

STH, T4, testosterone, prolactin—Synergistic with vasopressin

Aldosterone—ADH and aldosterone may interact in water and electrolyte conservation

Norepinephrine, prostaglandins—Norepinephrine and prostaglandins inhibit ADH activity in kidney

3. Unusual Features   29, 32, 38

Thiazides, which act as diuretics, paradoxically reduce polyuria in both pituitary diabetes insipidus and nephrogenic diabetes insipidus; may act by reducing filtration rate

Nonpregnant uterus is more sensitive to ADH than to oxytocin; rare form of diabetes insipidus is not caused by lack of ADH but by inability of kidney tubule to respond to ADH (an inborn error of metabolism)

Reverse effects in birds

Increases skin permeability in amphibians

4. **Possible Relationships of Deficiency Symptoms to Metabolic Action** 11, 13, 37

Decreased NaCl and urea concentration—Permeability of epithelium of distal segment of nephron to water is reduced, and water reabsorption is decreased by lack of ADH

5. **Relationships to Minerals** (See references in specific mineral section)

Synergism—I^- (as T4), PO_4^{3-} (as cyclic AMP)

Urinary concentration—Na^+ ($\uparrow$), K^+ $\downarrow$

Release of hormone—Ca^{2+} required, Na^+ and K^+ stimulate

Chapter 39. Thyroxine (T4)

Thyroxine, an iodine-containing hormone of the thyroid gland, is of the multi-tissue-controlling type and maintenance category. It is not vitally essential for basic existence. Its chief functions are to regulate body metabolism, temperature, growth, development, reproduction, and the nervous system. Its chief importance is in regulation of metabolism and prevention of iodine deficiency diseases. Deficiencies of T4 may cause cretinism, goiter, myxedema, and Hashimoto's and Gull's diseases.

T4 is a water-soluble amino acid containing iodine; it is exreted slowly. The hormone has been synthesized. Excess doses or conditions result in toxic symptoms including exophthalmos, thyrotoxicosis, hyperthyroidism, and Grave's disease. Its chief synergists are STH, cortisol, epinephrine, and vasopressin, while its chief antagonists are insulin and PTH.

T4 is formed in the thyroid and stored there. In the tissues it is transformed to T3 which is more potent than T4. Factors causing an increased release of T4 are TSH, low serum T4 (feedback), cold, and nerve impulses. Chief factors inhibiting release are stress, pain, high blood I^-, or T4 (feedback). T4 decreases during aging in the blood, and is similar to a vitamin in its dependence on iodine in the diet. It has been used to control blood cholesterol and lipids, but its toxic side reactions have limited its usefulness.

T4 is thought to act largely by its effect on the cell mitochondria to uncouple ATP formation from energy conversion, and to act somehow on the cell nucleus.

Please consult the minerals section listing of iodine for additional details.

GENERAL INFORMATION

1. **Synonyms**   1, 7, 18
   T4, 3,5,3′,5′-tetraiodothyronine, thyroid hormone

2. **History**   9, 10, 28, 36
   16th century—(Anon.) Cretinism described
   1825—Parry: associated enlarged thyroid with exophthalmia, tachycardia
   1874—Gull: associated atrophy of thyroid with characteristic syndrome
   1891—Murray: treated hypothyroidism with injection of thyroid extract
   1896—Baumann: showed that thyroid contains iodine
   1911—Baumann: demonstrated diiodotyrosine in thyroid
   1915—Kendall: isolated and crystallized thyroxine
   1926—Harington: determined structural formula
   1927—Harington and Barger: synthesized thyroxine
   1951—Gross et al.: isolated and identified triiodothyronine as active factor
      in thyroid

3. **Physiological Forms**   9, 26, 37, 39
   l-thyroxine, 3′,3,5-triiodothyronine (T3, TRIT), tetraiodothyroacetic acid
      (TETRAC), triiodothyroacetic acid (TRIAC)

4. **Active Analogs and Related Compounds**   17, 22, 37, 39
   d-Thyroxine (fractional activity of *l*-thyroxine)
   Triiodothyropropionic acid (very active in tadpole metamorphosis)

5. **Inactive Analogs and Related Compounds**   17, 22, 37, 39
   Deiodinated T4; T4 with esterified hydroxyl group

6. **Antagonists**   9, 17, 37, 39
   3, 3′,5′-triiodothyronine, guanethidine, 2′,6′-diiodotyrosine, insulin, PTH

7. **Synergists**   9, 17, 37, 39
   STH, cortisol, epinephrine, prolactin, MSH, oxytocin, progesterone, vaso-
      pressin, Mg^{2+}

8. **Physiological Functions**   1, 4, 14, 16, 37, 39
   Regulates growth, differentiation, oxidative metabolism, electrolytic balance
   Increases CHO metabolism, calorigenesis, protein anabolism, BMR, O_2 con-
      sumption, fat catabolism, fertility
   Sensitizes nervous system

9. **Deficiency Diseases, Disorders   1, 4, 14, 16, 37, 39**
   Deficiency—Cretinism, goiter (deficient), Hashimoto's disease, Gull's disease, myxedema
   Excess—Grave's disease, thyrotoxicosis, thyroiditis, goiter

10. **Essentiality for Life   1, 9, 38**
    Required for development and growth of all vertebrates
    Deficiency in adult shortens life span

CHEMISTRY

1. **Structure   1, 8, 9, 15, 18**

Thyroxine, $C_{15}H_{11}I_4NO_4$

2. **Reactions   1, 8, 9, 17, 18**

   Heat—Decomposes at 231°C
   Acid—Unstable (sol. in acid alc.)
   Alkali—Sol. in alk. alc.
   Water—Insol.

   Oxidation—Unstable
   Reduction—Stable
   Light—Unstable
   Enzyme action: Unstable to deiodinating enzymes

3. **Properties   1, 7, 8, 9, 17, 19**

   Appearance—White crystalline powder
   MW—776.9
   MP—231-233°C decomp.
   Crystal form—needle-like
   Salts—Sodium
   Important groups for activity
   —l-Alanine
   —O—
   —I (all 4 positions)
   —OH

   Solubility
   H_2O—Insol.
   Acet.—Insol.
   Alc.—Sol. at acid or alk. pH
   Benz., Chl., Eth.—Insol.
   Absn. max.—231 mμ
   Chemical nature
   Acidic substituted amino acid
   α_D = −4.4° (aq. alk. EtOH)
   Miscellaneous—pK_a = 2.2, (COOH), 6.45 (OH), 10.1 (NH_2); pl = 3.5

4. **Commercial Production   9, 18, 22**
   Synthetic and from pig thyroid by defatting and drying with acetone—Thyroid, U.S.P.
   Sodium salts
   Sodium levothyroxine, USP (synthroid)
   Sodium liothyronine, USP (cytomel)
   Many medicinal preparations

5. **Isolation**   22, 25
   Sources—Pig thyroid
   Method—Extraction
   > Proteolysis, pH 8.4, (pancreatin and trypsin) of thyroid, 24 hr at $37°C$
   > Extract with n-butanol saturated with N HCl
   > Paper chromatography or ion-exchange resin
   > Partition chromatography (kieselguhr in 0.5 N NaOH) separates T4 from T3

6. **Determination**   1, 14, 19a, 22, 26, 38
   Bioassay
   > Metamorphosis in tadpoles
   > Increased oxidative metabolism
   Physicochemical—Protein-bound iodine (PBI) in plasma; radioassay

MEDICAL AND BIOLOGICAL ROLE

1. **Species Occurrence, Specificity, and Antigenicity**   1, 9, 38
   Occurrence
   > All vertebrates have thyroid tissue, but follicles dispersed in lampreys and
   >   bony fish
   > Thyroxine and precursors found in various invertebrates but no follicles
   Specificity
   > Interreactive all vertebrates; no loss in potency (i.e., no specificity)
   > No response in invertebrates; different functions in lower vertebrates
   Antigenicity—No antigenicity

2. **Units**   8, 9, 14
   In mg or μg

3. **Normal Blood Levels (Man)**   2, 4, 9, 22, 39
   3.0-12.0 μg/100 ml, serum; diurnal variation—high in A.M.

4. **Administration**   8, 9, 37, 39
   Injection—No data
   Topical—No data
   Oral—Thyroid tablets, sodium levothyroxine, sodium liothyroxine

5. **Factors Affecting Release**   1, 4, 34
   Inhibitors
   > High blood I_2
   > High blood T4—Feedback via hypothalamus
   > Stress, pain
   > Antithyroid drugs—Block T4 synthesis and absorption of I_2

Stimulators
  TSH
  Low blood T4—Feedback via hypothalamus
  Cold
  Direct nervous control

6. **Deficiency Symptoms (Humans)**   1, 4, 37, 38, 39
  Tumors of pituitary
  Decreased BMR
  Accumulation of mucoprotein
  Increase in blood lipid and cholesterol
  Increase in liver gluconeogenesis
  Extracellular retention of NaCl and H_2O

7. **Effects of Overdose, Toxicity**   1, 4, 37, 38, 39
  Acceleration of growth, maturation
  Increased BMR, esp. liver, skin, kidney, smooth muscle, gastric mucosa
  Decreased tissue glycogen
  Increased blood sugar
  Exophthalmos
  Hyperthyroidism, Graves's disease
  Thyrotoxicosis

METABOLIC ROLE

1. **Biosynthesis**   22, 37, 39
  Tyrosine—Monoiodotyrosine—Diiodotyrosine—Thyroxine
  Site(s) in cell—Data not conclusive

2. **Production Sites**   22, 37, 39
  Thyroid gland

3. **Storage Areas**   8, 9, 16
  Colloid in thyroid follicles = thyroglobulin

4. **Blood Carriers**   2, 8, 22, 26
  α-Globulin
  Acid glycoprotein
  Albumin

5. **Half-life**   8, 9, 26
  6-7 days

6. **Target Tissues**   1, 22, 37, 39
Systemic—All tissues, adenohypophysis, hypothalamus

7. **Reactions**   4, 5, 22, 25, 28, 34, 38
Reactive intermediate: unknown

Organ	Enzyme System	Effect
	67 tissue enzymes affected in vivo	
Thyroid	Mitochondrial enzyme systems	Activated
Thyroid	TCA cycle—oxidative phosphorylating enzymes	Uncoupled

8. **Mode of Action**   1, 4, 5, 8, 9, 16, 31, 37, 39
Cellular
Anabolic
Increases protein synthesis on the ribosomes and mRNA synthesis in
muscle, kidney, reticulocytes, liver
Catabolic
Increases protein catabolism in brain, spleen, and testis
Increases glucose and fat catabolism generally
Other—Swells mitochondria; affects permeability; regulates redox poten-
tial; chelates metals that inhibit enzymes
Uncouples mitochondrial oxidative phosphorylation at two points
Decreases mucoprotein synthesis
Organismal
Stimulates hematopoiesis, oögenesis, spermatogenesis, lactation, intestinal
absorption
Regulates growth, differentiation, electrolyte balance, heat production, O_2
consumption, BMR
Sensitizes nervous system

9. **Catabolism**   1, 9, 22, 25, 34
Intermediates
Iodine split off in liver, kidney, salivary glands, and recycled
Residue coupled with glucuronic acid or sulfate and excreted; also oxida-
tive deamination of amino acid residues
Excretion products
Compounds containing diphenyl ether and at least two carbons of side
chain excreted as glucuronides and sulfates in bile
Very small amounts free in urine and bile

MISCELLANEOUS

1. **Relationship to Vitamins   8, 11, 13, 38**
   Vitamin A—T4; needed for vitamin A synthesis in liver
   B—Complex vitamin deficiencies develop in hyperthyroidism
   Vitamin B_{12}—T4 aids in B_{12} absorption
   Vitamin C—Synergist in cold survival
   Niacin—Synergist in mitochondrial metabolism

2. **Relationship to Other Hormones   8, 11, 13, 32, 38**
   STH, ACTH, FSH, LH, TSH, prolactin—Synergists to T4 esp. in lactation
   ACTH—Antagonist in proper relative concentration
   Insulin—T4 stimulates secretion of insulin
   TSH—Stimulates production of T4
   FSH—Inhibited by T4
   MSH, ACTH—Stimulate iodine uptake by thyroid
   PTH—Antagonist to T4
   Cortisol—Synergist to T4; increases renal clearance of iodide

3. **Unusual Features   29, 32, 38**
   Powerful chelating agent, esp. with Mg^{++}
   Free OH participates in quinonoid formation
   Regulates metamorphosis in amphibians
   Osmoregulatory in fish
   Iodinated tyrosine found in invertebrate exoskeleton—Inactive
   Diffuse thyroid gland in teleosts and other lower forms
   TRIAC—Potent stimulant for metamorphosis
   TETRAC—Potent metabolic stimulant
   Decreased activity if I is replaced with Br or Cl
   Decreased activity if OH is removed or I position changed
   T3 approx. four times as active as T4

4. **Possible Relationships of Deficiency Symptoms to Metabolic Action   11, 13, 37**
   Decreased BMR—Lack of T4 stimulus for anabolism
   Accumulation of mucoprotein—Lack of T4 control of mucoprotein synthesis
   Increase in blood lipid and cholesterol—Decreased fat catabolism
   Increase in liver gluconeogenesis—Antagonism by ACTH (cortisol)
   Extracellular retention of NaCl and H_2O—Antagonism by ACTH and aldosterone (?)

5. **Relationship to Minerals   (See references in specific mineral section)**
   Synergism—Mg^{2+}, I^- (as T4)
   Release of T4—Ca^{2+} required, Co^{2+} inhibits

I^- is part of T4
Heavy metals chelated by T4
Increases intracellular Mg^{2+}
Regulates—Bone levels PO_4^{3-} ($\downarrow$)
Synthesis of T4—Mn^{2+} involved

Chapter 40.
Parathyroid Hormone (PTH)

PTH, a hormone from the parathyroid gland, is essential to life; it is a hormone of the tissue-controlling variety. Its chief functions are to regulate (with vitamin D and TCT) Ca^{2+} and PO_4^{3-} levels in the blood, including their excretion, absorption, and bone resorption. Its chief importance lies in the extreme precision needed for blood Ca^{2+} control, since so many critical functions depend on it. PTH deficiency conditions are *tetany* and hypoparathyroidism.

PTH is a water-soluble peptide and is excreted rapidly. Excess doses result in demineralization of the skeleton, calcification of the kidney, and muscle sensitivity. Its chief synergists are vitamin D, and cortisol, while its chief antagonists are T4, TCT, STH, and estrogens (short term).

PTH is formed in the parathyroid gland, and some is stored there. Factors causing an increased release are: low serum Ca^{2+}, or Mg^{2+}, vasomotor impulses, and high TCT. Chief factors inhibiting release are: high serum Ca^{2+} or Mg^{2+}, vasomotor impulses, and high vitamin D. PTH acts by increasing Ca^{2+} uptake by target cells and by activating adenyl cyclase to form cyclic AMP, followed by cell division or by release of various agents, e.g., citrate, needed to dissolve bone or transport Ca^{2+} through kidney cells.

GENERAL INFORMATION

1. **Synonyms**   1, 7, 18
   PTH, Parathormone

2. **History**   9, 18, 28, 36
   1900—Vassale and Generali: reported convulsions and tetany from removal of parathyroids only
   1909—MacCallum and Voegtlin: reported effect of parathyroidectomy on plasma Ca^{2+}
   1924-25—Hanson, Collip: prepared active extracts from parathyroid gland
   1942—Patt and Luckhardt: demonstrated that blood Ca^{2+} level controls parathyroid secretion
   1959—Rasmussen, Aurbach: prepared pure parathyroid hormone peptides

3. **Physiological Forms**   9, 26, 37, 39
   /-Parathormone (three components—MW 9500, 7000, 4500)

4. **Active Analogs and Related Compounds**
   No data

5. **Inactive Analogs and Related Compounds**
   No data

6. **Antagonists**   9, 17, 37, 39
   T4, STH, estradiol (short term), testosterone, TCT

7. **Synergists**   9, 17, 37, 39
   Vitamin D, estrogens (birds), cortisol, Ca^{2+}, PO_4^{3-}, Mg^{2+}

8. **Physiological Functions**   1, 4, 14, 16, 37, 39
   Increases blood Ca^{2+}, kidney (Ca^{2+} and Mg^{2+}) reabsorption, PO_4^{3-} excretion, blood citrate
   Mobilizes Ca^{2+} and PO_4^{3-} from bone
   Activates Ca^{2+} and PO_4^{3-} absorption from gastrointestinal tract (requires vitamin D—1,25$(OH)_2D_3$
   Increases osteoclast formation
   Regulates synthesis of 1,25$(OH)_2D_3$

9. **Deficiency Diseases, Disorders**   1, 4, 14, 16, 37, 39
   Deficiency—Tetany, hypoparathyroidism
   Excess—von Recklinghausen's disease, hyperparathyroidism

10. **Essentiality for Life**   1, 9, 38
    One of the most essential hormones; absence rapidly leads to tetany and death of adult

CHEMISTRY

1. **Structure**   1, 8, 9, 15, 18
   Simple polypeptide (84 amino acids), sequence determined (human PTH)
   Straight chain—No S—S bridges
   Ser——Gln

2. **Reactions**   1, 8, 9, 17, 18
   Heat—No data
   Acid—Stable, dilute, acid
   Alkali—Relatively unstable
   Water—Sol., acidic

   Oxidation—H_2O_2, performic acid in-
     activate
   Reduction—Stable
   Light—No data
   Proteolysis—Loses activity

3. **Properties**   1, 7, 8, 9, 17, 19
   Appearance—No data
   MW—9500
   Important groups for activity
     Met, Try, Tyr
     Activity contained in amino
       acids—1-34

   Solubility
     H_2O—Sol.
     Acet., Alc.—Insol.
     Benz., Chl., Eth.—Insol.
   Absn. max.—Approx. 280 mμ
   Chemical nature—Acidic polypep-
     tide
   Miscellaneous—pI = 4.8

4. **Commercial Production**   9, 18, 22
   From bovine parathyroid

5. **Isolation**   22, 25
   Sources—Bovine parathyroid
   Methods
     Extraction
       Extract with 80% acetic acid
       Precipitate in 86% acetone
       Ultrafilter at pH 2.4
   Purification
     Column chromatography on Dowex 50
     Countercurrent distribution
     Gel filtration

6. **Determination**   1, 14, 19a, 22, 26, 38
   Bioassay
     Serum Ca^{2+} increase in dogs
     Increase in urine PO_4^{3-} output
   Physiochemical
     Radioimmunoassay

MEDICAL AND BIOLOGICAL ROLE

1. **Species Occurrence, Specificity, and Antigenicity**   1, 9, 38
   Occurrence—Found in all vertebrates above fish and cyclostomes
   Specificity—Interspecific potency high, e.g., bovine and human Parathormone are isoactive
   Antigenicity—Low

2. **Units**   8, 9, 14
   1 USP unit = 1/100 the amount of PTH to increase dog blood Ca^{2+} 1 mg/100 ml at 18 hr after subcutaneous injection; 1 mμg = .001 μg; 1 μg = 1 microgram

3. **Normal Blood Levels (Man)**   2, 4, 9, 22, 39
   0-25 mμg/100 ml, plasma; no diurnal rhythm

4. **Administration**   8, 9, 37, 39
   Injection—Parathyroid USP (Paroidin) usually subcutaneous; occasionally I.V.
   Topical—No data
   Oral—Destroyed by proteolytic enzymes

5. **Factors Affecting Release**   1, 4, 34
   Inhibitors—High serum Ca^{2+} or Mg^{2+}; vasomotor nerve control, high vitamin D
   Stimulators—Low serum Ca^{2+} or Mg^{2+} feedback; vasomotor nerve control, high TCT

6. **Deficiency Symptoms**   1, 4, 37, 38, 39
   Decreased blood Ca^{2+} and citrate; decreased urine PO_4^{3-} and Ca^{2+}
   Increased blood PO_4^{3-}
   Irritability of nervous system, muscle twitch, tetany, death
   Cataracts

7. **Effects of Overdose, Toxicity**   1, 4, 37, 38, 39
   Increased blood Ca^{2+}, citrate, alkaline phosphatase; increased urine PO_4^{3-}; demineralization of skeleton, osteoclast activity
   Decreased blood PO_4^{3-}, muscle sensitivity
   Metastatic deposits of Ca^{2+} in tissues, notably kidney

METABOLIC ROLE

1. **Biosynthesis**   22, 37, 39
   Precursors—18 of 20 standard amino acids; no Cys
   Intermediates—Prohormone (PRO-PTH)
   Site(s) in cell—Cytoplasmic inclusions

2. **Production Sites**   22, 37, 39
   Parathyroid gland, chief cells

3. **Storage Areas**   8, 9, 16
   Some in parathyroid gland

4. **Blood Carriers**   2, 8, 22, 26
   α-Globulin and albumin

5. **Half-life**   8, 9, 26
   20 min

6. **Target Tissues**   1, 22, 37, 39
   Bone, kidney, muscle, mammary gland, gut, thymus

7. **Reactions**   4, 5, 22, 25, 34, 38
   Reactive intermediates—Cyclic AMP (secondary messenger) and Ca^{2+}

Organ	Enzyme System	Effect
Bone and kidney	Adenyl cyclase	Activated

8. **Mode of Action**   1, 4, 5, 8, 9, 16, 31, 37, 39
   Cellular
       Anabolic—No data
       Catabolic—Bone resorption
       Other
           Mitochondrial PO_4^{3-} increased
           Regulated synthesis of $1,25(OH)_2D_3$ in kidney
           Increases Ca^{2+} uptake by target cells
           Increases cell division in thymocytes
           Mitochondrial swelling
           Increased conversion pyruvate to citrate
   Organismal
       Raises renal Ca^{2+} threshold
       Lowers renal PO_4^{3-} threshold
       Increases Ca^{2+}, Mg^{2+}, PO_4^{3-} absorption in gut via $1,25(OH)_2D_3$

9. **Catabolism   1, 9, 22, 25, 39**
   Intermediates—Partial digestion in liver
   Excretion products—1% in urine

MISCELLANEOUS

1. **Relationship to Vitamins   8, 11, 13, 38**
   Vitamin D—Synergistic with PTH in maintenance of serum calcium

2. **Relationship to Other Hormones   8, 11, 13, 32, 38**
   Estradiol—Synergizes PTH in birds
   Cortisol—Synergizes PTH in vertebrates
   T4, STH, estradiol, testosterone, calcitonin—Antagonists to PTH

3. **Unusual Features   29, 32, 38**
   Activity increased with molecular weight of analog
   Demineralization of skeleton, formation of cysts with excess PTH
   High citrate produced in bone action

4. **Possible Relationships of Deficiency Symptoms to Metabolic Action   11, 13, 37**
   Decreased blood Ca^{2+}, citrate—Lack of PTH mobilization of bone calcium
   Increased blood PO_4^{3-}—Urine threshold for PO_4^{3-} high without PTH
   Irritability of nervous system—Decrease of blood calcium
   Cataracts—?

5. **Relationship to Minerals   (See references in specific minerals section)**
   Synergism—Ca^{2+}, Mg^{2+}, PO_4^{3-}
   Excretion of Ca^{2+} ($\downarrow$), Mg^{2+} ($\downarrow$), PO_4^{3-} ($\uparrow$)
   Release of hormone—Ca^{2+}, Mg^{2+} required
   Antagonist—I^- (as T4)
   Regulates—Ca^{2+} blood levels ($\uparrow$); Ca^{2+} and Mg^{2+} in bone ($\downarrow$); Ca^{2+}, Mg^{2+}, PO_4^{3-}
   absorption ($\uparrow$) in gut

Chapter 41.
Thyrocalcitonin (TCT)

TCT, a hormone from the C cells of the thyroid gland, is a general maintenance hormone of the tissue-controlling type. It is not essential to life. Its chief functions are to regulate (with PTH and vitamin D) blood Ca^{2+} and PO_4^{3-} levels, including their excretion, absorption, and bone incorporation. Its chief importance lies in blood Ca^{2+} control by its antagonism to PTH. Extreme precision in maintenance of blood Ca^{2+} level is needed because many critical functions depend on it. Deficiencies of TCT are not reported.

TCT is a water-soluble peptide, which is destroyed and excreted rapidly. Excess doses result in blood Ca^{2+} decreases. Its chief synergists are estradiol (short term), while the chief antagonists are PTH and vitamin D.

TCT is formed in the thyroid gland (C cells), and some is stored there. Factors causing increased release are high plasma Ca^{2+}, glucagon, epinephrine, gastrin, and cholecystokinin. A factor inhibiting TCT release is low plasma Ca^{2+}.

TCT acts by stimulating osteoblastic activity and inhibiting osteoclastic activity in bone cells, via cyclic AMP.

GENERAL INFORMATION

1. **Synonyms**   1, 7, 18
   TCT, calcitonin, CT

2. **History**   9, 18, 28, 36
   1962—Copp: discovered and named hormone with effects opposite to those of Parathormone

1963—Munson: extracted thyrocalcitonin from rat thyroids
1964—Foster et al.: reported that calcitonin originated in thyroid gland in goats
1966—Pearse: identified thyroid "C" cells as source of calcitonin

3. **Physiological Forms**   9, 26, 37, 39
   /-Thyrocalcitonin

4. **Active Analogs and Related Compounds**
   No data

5. **Inactive Analogs and Related Compounds**
   No data

6. **Antagonists**   9, 17, 37, 39
   Parathyroid hormone, vitamin D

7. **Synergists**   9, 17, 37, 39
   Estradiol (short term)

8. **Physiological Functions**   1, 4, 14, 16, 37, 39
   Decreases blood Ca^{2+} [balances PTH (parathyroid hormone)]
   Inhibits bone resorption
   Increases Ca^{2+} and PO_4^{3-} incorporation into bone
   Increases PO_4^{3-} excretion
   Increases proline incorporation into bone

9. **Deficiency Diseases, Disorders**   1, 4, 14, 16, 37, 39
   Medullary carcinoma of the thyroid (excess)

10. **Essentiality for Life**   1, 9, 38
    Not demonstrated

CHEMISTRY

1. **Structure**   1, 8, 9, 15, 18
   Polypeptide, 32 amino acids, synthesized
   Straight chain, one S—S ring: Human TCT: Cys—Gly—Asn—Leu—Ser—Thr—
   Cys—Met—Leu—Gly—Thr—Tyr—Thr—Gln—Asp—Phe—Asn—Lys—Phe—
   His—Thr—Phe—Pro—Gln—Thr—Ala—Ile—Gly—Val—Gly—Ala—Pro

2. Reactions   1, 8, 9, 17, 18

Heat—Relatively stable

Acid—Sol., inactivates (conc.)

Alkali—Inactivates (conc.)

Water—Sol., acidic

Oxidation—No data

Reduction—No data

Light—No data

Proteolysis—Pepsin and trypsin inactivates

3. Properties   1, 7, 8, 9, 17, 19

Appearance—No data

MW—3600

Important groups for activity

   S—S ring 1 + 7 position

   Tyr in position 12

   Met in position 8

Solubility

  H_2O—Sol.

  Acet., Alc.—Insol.

  Benz., Chl., Eth.—Insol.

Absn. max.—Approx 280 mμ

Chemical nature—Acidic polypeptide

Miscellaneous—pI = 4.8

4. Commercial Production   9, 18, 22

Not available

5. Isolation   22, 25

Sources—Pork thyroid

Method

  Extraction

    (a) Extract with 0.2 N HCl 60-70°C for 5 min; filter after 1 hr

    (b) Dialyze, pH 4.6, against 0.1 M acetate buffer at 4°C

    (c) Precipitate from 1.5 M NaCl

  Purification

    (a) Gel filtration—Sephadex G-100, pH 4.6

    (b) Ultrafiltration—If complexed to proteins earlier

6. Determination   1, 14, 19a, 22, 26, 38

Bioassay—Effect on plasma Ca^{2+} level in rat

Physicochemical—Radioimmunoassay

MEDICAL AND BIOLOGICAL ROLE

1. Species Occurrence, Specificity, and Antigenicity   1, 9, 38

Occurrence—Found in most vertebrates

Specificity—High, great variation in interspecific potency

Antigenicity—Not antigenic

2. Units   8, 9, 14

MRC units or by weight; 1 μg = 1 microgram

5-10 MRC milliunits lowers plasma Ca^{2+} in rat by about 10%

3. **Normal Blood Levels**   2, 4, 9, 22, 39
   .002-.04 μg/100 ml plasma

4. **Administration**   8, 9, 37, 39
   Injection—Active
   Topical—Inactive
   Oral—Inactive

5. **Factors Affecting Release**   1, 4, 34
   Inhibitors—Low plasma calcium
   Stimulators—High plasma calcium level, glucagon, gastrin, dibutyryl AMP,
   epinephrine, cholecystokinin

6. **Deficiency Symptoms**   1, 4, 37, 38, 39
   Blood Ca^{2+} increase

7. **Effects of Overdose, Toxicity**   1, 4, 37, 38, 39
   Blood Ca^{2+} decrease

METABOLIC ROLE

1. **Biosynthesis**   22, 37, 39
   Precursors—18 of 20 standard amino acids
   Intermediates—Unknown
   Site(s) in cell—Unknown

2. **Production Sites**   22, 37, 39
   Thyroid, parathyroid, and thymus (man)
   Parafollicular C cells derived from ultimobranchial body

3. **Storage Areas**   8, 9, 16
   "C" cells in thyroid

4. **Blood Carriers**
   Unknown

5. **Half-life**   8, 9, 26
   10 min

6. **Target Tissues**   1, 22, 37, 39
   Bone, kidney, muscle

7. **Reactions**   4, 5, 22, 25, 34, 38
   Reactive intermediates—Cyclic AMP—secondary messenger + Ca^{2+}

Organ	Enzyme System	Effect
Thyroid (C cells)	Adenyl cyclase	Activated
	Phosphorylase b	Activated

8. **Mode of Action**   1, 4, 5, 8, 9, 16, 31, 37, 39
   Cellular
   Anabolic—Increases proline incorporation into bone; also Ca^{2+}, PO_4^{3-}
   Catabolic—No data
   Other—Stimulates osteoblasts, inhibits osteoclasts
   Organismal
   Decreases blood calcium
   Inhibits bone resorption and citrate formation
   Increases PO_4^{3-} excretion
   Decreases glucose utilization and lactate production in bone

9. **Catabolism**   1, 9, 22, 25, 34
   Intermediates—Liver proteolysis
   Excretion products—Products of protein metabolism

MISCELLANEOUS

1. **Relationship to Vitamins**   8, 11, 13, 38
   Vitamin D antagonizes TCT

2. **Relationship to Other Hormones**   8, 11, 13, 32, 38
   PTH—Antagonist to thyrocalcitonin
   Glucagon—Stimulates release of TCT
   Estradiol—Synergizes and releases TCT

3. **Unusual Features**   29, 32, 38
   Birds have a gland separate from thyroid containing TCT; salmon TCT more
   potent than human TCT for humans

4. **Possible Relationships of Deficiency to Metabolic Action**   11, 13, 37
   Blood calcium increase—Resorption of bone by PTH

5. Relationship to Minerals   (See references in specific mineral section)
Synergism—PO_4^{3-}, Ca^{2+}
Excretion of PO_4^{3-} ($\uparrow$)
Release of hormone—Ca^{2+} required
Regulates—Ca^{2+} blood level ($\downarrow$); PO_4^{3-}, bone ($\uparrow$)

Chapter 42. Insulin

Insulin, a hormone from the beta cells of the pancreas, is a general maintenance hormone of the tissue-controlling type. It is essential to life. Its chief functions are regulation of carbohydrate and fat metabolism, and stimulation of amino acid and sugar uptake by cells, as well as glycogen and mucopolysaccharide formation. Its chief importance lies in its control of diabetes mellitus, which is a deficiency disease with many causes.

Insulin is a water-soluble polypeptide that is fairly rapidly destroyed and excreted. Excess doses result in convulsions, tremor, headache, coma, and sweating. Its chief synergists are STH, testosterone, and estradiol. Antagonists are glucagon, cortisol, epinephrine, and norepinephrine.

Insulin is formed in the beta cells of the pancreas and is stored there. Factors causing increased release are: high blood amino acids and sugar, cortisol, ACTH, secretin, STH, T4, ketone bodies, sulfonyl ureas, and biguanides. Release-inhibiting factors include: low blood sugar, epinephrine, and norepinephrine. Insulin acts by altering cell membrane permeability (to K^+, amino acids, glucose) and by stimulation of RNA and protein synthesis, with probably a second messenger involved (cyclic GMP).

GENERAL INFORMATION

1. Synonyms
None

2. **History**   9, 18, 28, 36
   10 A.D.—Celsus: described diabetic syndrome
   1899—Von Mering and Minkowski: demonstrated relationship between pan-
   createctomy and diabetes mellitus
   1922—Macleod: determined that islet cells produce insulin
   1922—Banting and Best: prepared potent insulin extracts from dog pancreas
   1926—Abel et al.: isolated crystalline insulin
   1955—Sanger et al.: determined structure of insulin
   1966—Katsoyannis: synthesized insulin (human and sheep)

3. **Physiological Forms**   9, 26, 37, 39
   l-Insulin

4. **Active Analogs and Related Compounds**   17, 22, 37, 39
   Somatomedin, NSILA (non-suppressible insulin-like activity), NGF (nerve
   growth factor)

5. **Inactive Analogs and Related Compounds**   17, 22, 37, 39
   Oxidized, reduced insulin, proinsulin
   Alkali-inactivated insulin

6. **Antagonists**   9, 17, 37, 39
   Cortisol, glucagon, epinephrine, norepinephrine, STH (CHO and fat metabolism), T4

7. **Synergists**   9, 17, 37, 39
   STH (protein metabolism), testosterone, estradiol, K^+, Zn^{2+}, Cr^{3+}

8. **Physiological Function**   1, 4, 14, 16, 37, 39
   Regulates CHO and fat metabolism, esp. glucose and fat oxidations
   Stimulates amino acid and glucose transport into cells and protein synthesis
   Stimulates glycogen and mucopolysaccharide formation

9. **Deficiency Diseases, Disorders**   1, 4, 14, 16, 37, 39
   Diabetes mellitus (faulty β-cells), azoturia, hyperlipemia, ketonemia

10. **Essentiality for Life**   1, 9, 38
    Essential for survival

CHEMISTRY

1. **Structure**   1, 8, 9, 15, 18
   Structure known and synthesized—51 amino acids (human)
   Polypeptide, two parallel straight chains, three S—S bridges

Two chains insulin (human) α and β

α—21 amino acids—(acidic); Gly—Ile—Val—Glu—Glu—

Cys—Cys—Thr—Ser—Ile—Cys—Ser—Leu—Tyr—Glu—Leu—Glu—Asp—
Tyr—Cys—Asp

β—30 amino acids—(basic): Phe—Val—Asp—Glu—His—Leu—Cys—Gly—Ser—
His—Leu—Val—Glu—Ala—Leu—Tyr—Leu—Val—Cys—Gly—Glu—Arg—
Gly—Phe—Phe—Tyr—Thr—Pro—Lys—Thr

2. **Reactions**   1, 8, 9, 17, 18

Heat—Unstable

Acid—Stable

Alkali—Inactivates

Water—Soluble, acidic

Oxidation—Inactivates

Reduction—Inactivates

Light—No data

Proteolysis—Trypsin inactivates

3. **Properties**   1, 7, 8, 9, 17, 19

Appearance—White crystalline
   powder

MW—5734 monomer
   Polymer: 12,000-48,000,
      depending on pH

Crystal form—Hexagonal system

Salts—Zinc, protamine

Solubility
   H_2O—Soluble
   Acet., Alc.—Sol.
   Benz., Chl., Eth.—Insol.

Important groups for activity
   Two disulfide bridges (S—S ring)
   Active groups unknown
   Key positions—19-21 on α-chain;
      22-30 on β-chain

Tyr, Asn

Absn. max.—Approx. 280 mμ

Chemical nature—Acidic polypeptide

Miscellaneous—pl = 5.3

4. **Commercial Production**   9, 18, 22

Extraction of beef or pork pancreas

5. **Isolation**   22, 25

Sources—Pancreas—beef, pork

Method
   Extract pancreas in 80% EtOH, pH 3 (H_3PO_4)
   pH to 8 with NH_4OH precipitates impurities
   Precipitate insulin with EtOH and ether
   Dissolve in EtOH—H_3PO_4 buffer and precipitate insulin as picrate
   Dissolve in acetone HCl
   Precipitate with acetone
   Wash and dry

Purification
   Crystallization at pl in acetate buffer with 0.15-0.60% zinc
   Precipitation with alcohol

Salting out
Gel filtration and crystallization or electrophoresis

6. **Determination**   1, 14, 19a, 22, 26, 38
    Bioassay
        Isolated rat diaphragm; perfused heart; in vitro systems, for measuring
            glucose uptake
        Lowering blood sugar in rabbit
    Physicochemical
        Radioimmunoassay
        Immunoassay—Very sensitive for plasma insulin concentration

MEDICAL AND BIOLOGICAL ROLE

1. **Species Occurrence, Specificity, and Antigenicity**   1, 9, 38
    Occurrence—Found in all vertebrates
    Specificity—Moderate interspecific potency
    Antigenicity—Moderate antigenicity; pig and human sequence alike yet anti-
        genic differences exist

2. **Units**   8, 9, 14
    1 IU = 1 USP unit = 0.04167 mg international standard; 1 mU = .001 IU

3. **Normal Blood Levels**   2, 4, 9, 22, 39
    $\left\{ \begin{array}{l} .02\text{-}.10\ \mu g \\ 0.6\text{-}2.6\ mU \end{array} \right\}$ fasting $\left\{ \begin{array}{l} 0.6\ \mu g \\ 15\ mU \end{array} \right\}$ (fed)/100 ml plasma; diurnal fluctua-
    tion—higher during daytime

4. **Administration**   8, 9, 37, 39
    Injection—Subcutaneous
        Amorphous insulin, crystalline insulin—Fast-acting, short duration
        Protamine insulin, protamine Zn insulin—Slow, steady absorption
    Topical—Not used
    Oral
        Sulfonylureas—Stimulate secretion of insulin $\left. \begin{array}{l} \\ \\ \\ \end{array} \right\}$ only if functional
        Hypoglycemic agents—Stimulate secretion of insulin β cells are present
        Biguanides—Stimulate secretion of insulin

5. **Factors Affecting Release**   1, 4, 34
    Inhibitors
        Low blood sugar—Feedback
        Epinephrine
        Norepinephrine
        Somatostatin

Stimulators
  High blood sugar—Feedback
  Elevated blood amino acid level, fatty acids
  Vagal stimulation, acetylcholine
  Glucagon, ACTH, secretin, STH, gastrin, pancreozymin
  Ketone bodies, sulfonylureas, biguanides
  Hypoglycemic agents
  Cortisol, T4
  Ca^{2+}, isoproterenol, prostaglandins

6. **Deficiency Symptoms**   1, 4, 37, 38, 39
  Polyphagia
  Decrease in respiratory quotient
  Decrease in tissue protein—weight loss
  Polydipsia
  Hyperglycemia, glycosuria—Underutilization and overproduction of glucose
  Polyuria
  Hyperlipemia
  Ketonemia
  Azoturia
  Neuropathy
  Microvascular disease
  Atherosclerosis

7. **Effects of Overdose, Toxicity**   1, 4, 37, 38, 39
  Convulsions
  Increase in glycogen storage
  Mental confusion
  Coma
  Headache
  Tremor
  Sweating
  Apprehensiveness
  Hypoglycemia

METABOLIC ROLE

1. **Biosynthesis**   22, 37, 39
  Precursors—17 of 20 standard amino acids (aspartic acid, tryptophan, and
    methionine missing)
  Intermediates—Proinsulin
  Site(s) in cell—Unknown

2. **Production Sites**   22, 37, 39
  β-cells of islets of pancreas

3. **Storage Areas** 8, 9, 16
   β-granules in β-cells

4. **Blood Carriers** 2, 8, 22, 26
   Circulating proteins; α,β-macroglobulins

5. **Half-life in Plasma** 8, 9, 26
   Nonlabeled insulin, <9 min; insulin (^{131}I), 40 min

6. **Target Tissues** 1, 22, 37, 39
   Systemic, esp. liver, adipose tissue, muscle, kidney

7. **Reactions** 4, 5, 22, 25, 34, 38
   Reactive forms—Cyclic GMP (?) and Ca^{2+} (?)

Organ	Enzyme System	Effect
Liver	Lipase	Inhibited
	Adenyl cyclase	Inhibited
	Glycogen synthetase	Activated
Tissues	Hexokinase	Activated
	Phosphorylases	Activated

8. **Mode of Action** 1, 4, 5, 8, 9, 16, 31, 37, 39
   Cellular
       Anabolic—Increases mucopolysaccharide synthesis, protein synthesis, fatty acid synthesis, mRNA synthesis
       Catabolic—Inhibits gluconeogenesis; increases glucose oxidation
       Other—Increases transport of glucose and amino acids across cell membrane (does not affect glucose entrance into hepatic cells, brain, blood cells); inhibits cyclic AMP formation
   Organismal
       Inhibits moblization of fat from peripheral reservoirs
       Decreases: blood (sugar, K^+, PO_4^{3-}, ketones); liver gluconeogenesis, polyuria
       Increases liver and muscle glycogen, glucose absorption in gut, fat formation, nitrogen balance

9. **Catabolism** 1, 9, 22, 25, 34
   Intermediates—Insulinase in liver (antagonized by insulinase inhibitor) destroys insulin
   Excretion products—Metabolic products of amino acids

MISCELLANEOUS

1. **Relationship to Vitamins**   8, 11, 13, 38
   Vitamin C acts similarly to alloxan (i.e., antagonist)

2. **Relationship to Other Hormones**   8, 11, 13, 32, 38
   Cortisol, glucagon, epinephrine, norepinephrine, T4, STH (CHO and fat metabolism)—Antagonistic to insulin
   Estradiol, testosterone, STH (protein metabolism)—Synergistic with insulin

3. **Unusual Features**   29, 32, 38
   Does not depend on C-AMP for action
   Contains 0.4% zinc in crystals
   First synthetic polypeptide hormone
   Multiple insulins in rat, bonito
   Forms fibrils when heated at low pH
   Antibody sites not identical with biological activity sites
   Frog—Pancreas not active until mid-metamorphosis
   Urodeles—Only β-cells in pancreas present
   Vigorous exercise increases rate of transport of glucose into muscle cells even in absence of insulin
   NSILA (nonsuppressible insulin activity) related to somatomedin, found in blood serum

4. **Possible Relationships of Deficiency Symptoms to Metabolic Action**   11, 13, 37
   Hyperglycemia, decrease in respiratory quotient—Inability to metabolize and transport glucose into cells
   Hyperlipemia—Mobilization of fat from peripheral reserves in absence of insulin
   Ketonemia—Incomplete oxidation of mobilized fat
   Azoturia (decrease in tissue protein)—Induced gluconeogenesis producing urea and ammonia
   Polydipsia—Thirst produced by glycosuria (polyuria)
   Polyphagia—Hunger produced by loss of urinary glucose

5. **Relationship to Minerals**   (See references in specific mineral section)
   Synergism—K^+, PO_4^{3-} (cyclic GMP), Zn^{2+}, Cr^{3+}
   Release of hormone—Ca^{2+}, Mn^{2+} required, Co^{2+} inhibits
   Antagonist—I^- (as T4)
   Forms complex with Zn^{2+}

Chapter 43. Glucagon

Glucagon, a hormone from the alpha cells of the pancreas, is a general maintenance hormone of the tissue-controlling type. It is not essential to life. Its chief
function is cooperative regulation of carbohydrate metabolism (antagonist to
insulin). Its chief importance lies in its action in carbohydrate metabolism and
its relation to insulin in diabetes, i.e., action as a fuel mobilizer, and as a hyperglycemic agent. A deficiency condition is hypoglycemic coma.

Glucagon is a water-soluble polypeptide with a fairly short half-life, and is
excreted rapidly. Excess doses result in metaglucagon diabetes and high blood
sugar. Its chief synergists are epinephrine, norepinephrine, and cortisol. Its
chief antagonist is insulin.

Glucagon is formed and stored in the alpha cells of the pancreas. Factors
stimulating release of glucagon are pancreozymin, hypoglycemia, and fasting.
Factors inhibiting release of glucagon are high blood sugar and Co^{2+}.

Glucagon acts by stimulating synthesis of the second messenger cyclic AMP
in cell membranes of target tissues.

GENERAL INFORMATION

1. **Synonyms**   1, 7, 18
   HGF, HG-factor, hyperglycemic-glycogenolytic factor, glukagon

2. **History**   9, 18, 28, 36
   1922—McLeod ⎫
   ⎬ Described hyperglycemic effect of pancreatic extracts
   1923—Collip ⎭

1923—Kimball and Murlin: suggested a second pancreatic hormone; named it glucagon
1955—Staub, Sinn, and Behrens: isolated and crystallized glucagon
1956—Bromer et al.: determined structure of glucagon
1967—Wunsch: synthesized glucagon

3. Physiological Forms   9, 26, 37, 39
l-glucagon

4. Active Analogs and Related Compounds   17, 22, 37, 39
Serotonin (gastrointestinal tract, spleen, brain, skin, tongue); isoproterenol, gastrointestinal glucagon

5. Inactive Analogs and Related Compounds   17, 22, 37, 39
UV-inactivated glucagon

6. Antagonists   9, 17, 37, 39
Insulin, Cr^{3+}

7. Synergists   9, 17, 37, 39
Epinephrine (liver, muscle), norepinephrine, cortisone, Ca^{2+}

8. Physiological Functions   1, 4, 14, 16, 37, 39
Increases—Blood sugar, blood K^+, O_2 consumption, liver glycogenolysis, gluconeogenesis, nitrogen and salt excretion, glucose-1-P
Decreases—Liver glycogen, protein formation, gastric juice, fatty acid synthesis

9. Deficiency Diseases, Disorders   1, 4, 14, 16, 37, 39
Hypoglycemic coma

10. Essentiality for Life   1, 9, 38
Not essential for life of vertebrate organisms

CHEMISTRY

1. Structure   1, 8, 9, 15, 18
Polypeptide (sequence determined): human; His—Ser—Glu—Gly—Thr—Phe—Thr—Ser—Asp—Tyr—Ser—Lys—Tyr—Leu—Asp—Ser—Arg—Arg—Ala—Glu—Asp—Phe—Val—Glu—Try—Leu—Met—Asp—Thr
Straight single chain—His - - - Thr, 29 amino acids
No S—S bridges

2. Reactions   1, 8, 9, 17, 18

Heat—Stable to 100°C

Acid—Stable, pH 2

Alkali—Stable, pH 9

Water—Sol., basic

Oxidation—No data

Reduction—Stable to cysteine (removes contaminating insulin)

Light—UV inactivates

Proteolysis—Leucine, amino peptidase, pepsin, trypsin, chymotrypsin at pH = 6-8 hydrolyze

3. Properties   1, 7, 8, 9, 17, 19

Appearance—White powder

MW—3500 (29 amino acids)

Crystal form—Rhombic dodecahedra

Salts—HCl

Important groups for activity

Try, Met

Solubility

H_2O—Insol.

Acet., Alc.—Insol.

Benz., Chl., Eth.—Insol.

Absn. max.—278 mμ

Chemical nature—Basic polypeptide

Miscellaneous—pI = 7.5-8.5

4. Commercial Production   9, 18, 22

Hog pancreas

5. Isolation   22, 25

Sources—Crude pork insulin

Methods

Precipitate with acetone and salts at low pH

Crystallize from 0.033 M glycine buffer, pH 8.6, with 0.67 M urea

Purification: Starch zone electrophoresis

6. Determination   1, 14, 19a, 22, 26, 38

Bioassay

Hyperglycemic response in cats

Glycogenolysis of liver slices

Reaction of phosphorylase in liver slices

Physicochemical—Radioimmunoassay, immunoassay

MEDICAL AND BIOLOGICAL ROLE

1. Species Occurrence, Specificity, and Antigenicity   1, 9, 38

Occurrence—Found in fish through mammals

Specificity—Interspecies potency—Interactive

Antigenicity—Antigenic in rabbit or bovine x porcine glucagon, but not guinea pig glucagon

2. **Units**   9, 9, 14
By weight, also 1 I.U. = amount to increase blood sugar to 30 mg/100 ml;
   1 μg = 1 microgram

3. **Normal Blood Levels (Man)**   2, 4, 9, 22, 39
0.01-0.025 μg/100 ml plasma

4. **Administration**   8, 9, 37, 39
Injection—Glucagon HCl intravenous, intramuscular, or subcutaneous; used
   to treat insulin-induced hypoglycemia
Topical—Inactive
Oral—Inactive

5. **Factors Affecting Release**   1, 4, 34
Inhibitors—High blood sugar, $CoCl_2$ (α-cells) (large doses), insulin, somatostatin, free fatty acids, secretin
Stimulators—Hypoglycemia, fasting, pancreozymin, Co^{2+} (small doses),
   epinephrine, norepinephrine, acetylcholine, prostaglandins, gastrin

6. **Deficiency Symptoms**   1, 4, 37, 38, 39
Low blood glucose

7. **Effects of Overdose, Toxicity**   1, 4, 37, 38, 39
Metaglucagon diabetes (destroys β-cells), increased food consumption, high
   blood glucose

METABOLIC ROLE

1. **Biosynthesis**   22, 37, 39
Simple precursors—16 of standard 20 amino acids (no cysteine, isoleucine,
   proline, glutamic acid)
Intermediates—Unknown
Site(s) in cell—No data

2. **Production Sites**   22, 37, 39
α-Cells in pancreas

3. **Storage Areas**   8, 9, 16
Granules in α-cells

4. **Blood Carriers**   2, 8, 22, 26
Plasma proteins

5. **Half-life**   8, 9, 26
Less than 10 min

6. **Target Tissues**   1, 22, 37, 39
Liver, adipose tissues, kidney

7. **Reactions**   4, 5, 22, 25, 34, 38
Reactive intermediates—Cyclic AMP—secondary messenger $+ Ca^{2+}$ (probably)

Organ	Enzyme System	Effect
Liver	Glucokinase	Inhibited
	Glycogen synthetase	Inhibited
	Glycogenolysis enzymes	Activated
	Gluconeogenesis enzymes	Activated
	Adenyl cyclase	Activated
	Dephosphophosphorylase kinase	Activated
	Phosphorylase b	Activated
	Carbamoyl phosphate synthetase	Activated
	Argino-succinase	Activated
	Argino-succinic synthetase	Activated
Heart	Adenyl cyclase	Activated

8. **Mode of Action**   1, 4, 5, 8, 9, 16, 31, 37, 39
Cellular
   Anabolic—No data
   Catabolic
      Decreased protein and fatty acid synthesis
      Increased lipolysis
      Increased CHO glycogenolysis
      Increased protein catabolism
   Other
      Increased cyclic AMP formation
      Decreased adrenal ascorbic acid
Organismal
   Stimulates hepatic glycogenolysis and gluconeogenesis
   Increases adipose tissue lipolysis
   Stimulates release of catecholamines by adrenal medulla
   Increases nitrogen K, Na, Cl, PO_4 excretion
   Increases blood sugar, ketone bodies
   Decreases gastric juice flow
   Increases heart rate, ventricular contractility
   Decreases atrio-ventricular conduction time
   Retards gastrointestinal contractions

9. **Catabolism**   1, 9, 22, 25, 34
Intermediates—Proteolysis in liver, kidney, blood—glucagonase (protease), recycling
Excretion products—End products of protein metabolism (urea, CO_2)

MISCELLANEOUS

1. **Relationship to Vitamins** 8, 11, 13, 38
   Vitamin C—Depletion of adrenal ascorbic acid by glucagon

2. **Relationship to Other Hormones** 8, 11, 13, 32, 38
   Epinephrine, norepinephrine—Stimulate secretion of glucagon, also synergistic
   Cortisol, cortisone—Synergistic to glucagon
   Insulin—Antagonistic to glucagon, inhibits secretion of glucagon
   Somatostatin, secretin—Inhibit secretion of glucagon

3. **Unusual Features** 29, 32, 38
   Tissue differences in glucagon response
   More concentrated in female than male pancreas
   Gastrointestinal glucagon not identical with pancreatic glucagon
   Traces of heavy metals (Cu^{2+}, Co^{2+}) found in glucagon preparations

4. **Possible Relationships of Deficiency Symptoms to Metabolic Action** 11, 13, 37
   Low blood glucose—Lack of glucose-releasing activity by glucagon into plasma

5. **Relationships to Minerals** (See references in specific mineral section)
   Synergism—Ca^{2+}, PO_4^{3-} (as cyclic AMP)
   Hormone release—Co^{2+} (inhibited—large doses; stimulated—small doses)
   Excretion of Na^+ ($\uparrow$), K^+ ($\downarrow$)
   Antagonist—Cr^{3+}
   Trace contaminants—Cu^{2+}, Co^{2+}

Chapter 44. Aldosterone

Aldosterone, a hormone from the adrenal cortex, is a general maintenance hormone of the tissue-controlling type. It is essential to life. Its chief functions are to regulate blood electrolyte balance, kidney function, and gluconeogenesis. Its chief importance lies in the fact that it causes the kidney to retain Na^+ and excrete K^+ and H^+. Chief deficiency diseases are Addison's disease and adrenocortical insufficiency.

Aldosterone is a water-insoluble, fat-soluble steroid with a fairly short half-life in blood (20 min). Excess doses result in hypertension, congestive heart failures, and diabetes insipidus. Its chief synergists are oxytocin, STH, renin, and vasopressin, whereas its chief antagonists are cortisol, estradiol, progesterone, and vasopressin.

Aldosterone is formed in the adrenal cortex but is not stored in any tissue. Factors stimulating release are: stress, low Na^+, low blood volume, high K^+, ACTH, and high blood pressure. Factors inhibiting release include: low K^+ and high Na^+. Aldosterone acts by stimulating the Na^+ pump in the cell membrane of target tissues (kidneys).

GENERAL INFORMATION

1. **Synonyms** 1, 7, 18
   Electrocortin, mineralocorticoid, aldocortin, 18-oxocorticosterone

2. **History**   9, 18, 24, 28, 35, 36
   1953—Simpson et al. ⎱ Isolated crystalline aldosterone
   1954—Mattox et al.   ⎰ from adrenals
   1954—Wettstein and Anner: devised highly sensitive test for mineralocorticoid activity
   1954—Simpson et al.: determined structure of aldosterone
   1955—Schmidlin et al.: synthesized *dl*-aldosterone
   1956—Vischer et al.: synthesized *d*-aldosterone
   1956—Neher and Wettstein: isolated 15 more steroids similar to aldosterone and cortisol

3. **Physiological Forms**   9, 26, 35, 37, 39
   Hemiacetal form (11,18-semiacetal), aldehyde form

4. **Active Analogs and Related Forms (Mineralocorticoids)**   17, 22, 24, 35, 37, 39
   Natural—11-Deoxycorticosterone, corticosterone
   Synthetic—2α-Methylcortisol, 9α-fluorocortisol, 2α-methyl-9α-fluorocortisol

5. **Inactive Analogs and Related Forms (for Aldosterone Function)**   17, 22, 24, 35, 37, 39
   Cortexolone, dexamethasone, prednisolone

6. **Antagonists**   9, 17, 35
   Natural—Cortisol, pineal factor, estradiol, progesterone, vasopressin (kidney), prostaglandins
   Synthetic—3-Spironolactone, aldactone-A

7. **Synergists**   9, 17, 35
   11-deoxycorticosterone, vasopressin, oxytocin, angiotensin II, renin, STH

8. **Physiological Functions**   1, 4, 14, 16, 37, 39
   Maintenance of normal electrolyte blood balance
   Prolongs survival of adrenalectomized animals
   Accelerates gluconeogenesis
   Regulates kidney function

9. **Deficiency Diseases, Disorders**   1, 4, 14, 16, 37, 39
   Addison's disease, (deficiency), Cushing's syndrome (excess), adrenocortical insufficiency, primary hyperaldosteronism

10. **Essentiality for Life**   1, 9, 38
    One of the most essential of all hormones; absence can be fatal in short time period

CHEMISTRY

1. Structure   1, 8, 9, 15, 18, 35

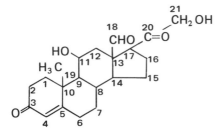

Aldosterone (aldehyde form),
$C_{21}H_{28}O_5$

2. Reactions   1, 8, 9, 17, 18

Heat—Stable
Acid—Decomposes
Alkali—Fluoresces (conc.)
    Isomerizes to 17-iso-aldosterone
Water—Slightly sol.

Oxidation—Loses aldehyde group
Reduction—Unstable
Light—Stable

3. Properties   1, 7, 8, 9, 17, 19

Appearance—Colorless crystals
MW—360.4
MP—164°C
Crystal form—Needles (acetate)
Salts, esters—Acetate
Important groups for activity
    —C(18)HO
    —C(21)H$_2$OH
    —C(11)OH

Solubility
    H$_2$O—Sparingly
    Acet., Alc.—Sol.
    Benz., Chl., Eth.—Sol.
Absn. max.—240 mμ
Chemical nature
    Hemiacetal, aldehyde
    Alc., ketone—Reducing steroid
$\alpha_D{}^{23}$ = +145 (acet.)

4. Commercial Production   9, 18, 22, 24, 35

Microbiological (stereospecific hydroxylation)

5. Isolation   22, 24, 35

Sources: Beef adrenal extract
Methods
    (1) Partition aqueous extract with pentane-methanol
    (2) Chromatograph on kieselguhr: elute with petroleum ether-benzene-
        CHCl$_3$
    (3) Rechromatograph on powdered cellulose; elute with toluene-petroleum
        ether-methanol
    (4) Recrystallize from methanol

6. Determination   1, 14, 19a, 22, 26, 38
Bioassay
  Life maintenance in adrenalectomized animals
  Increase muscular work performance
  Cold stress reactions on adrenalectomy
  In vitro incubation of perfused tissues
Physicochemical—Monitor Na/K ratios in urine

MEDICAL AND BIOLOGICAL ROLE

1. Species Occurrence, Specificity, and Antigenicity   1, 9, 38
Occurrence: All vertebrates species studied, except cyclostomes
Specificity: Same electrolyte regulator, all species
Antigenicity: None reported

2. Units   8, 9, 14
mg or μg; 1 μg = 1 microgram, 1 mμg = .001 μg

3. Normal Blood Levels (Man)   2, 4, 9, 22, 35, 39
0.1-1.0 mμg/100 ml plasma

4. Administration   8, 9, 20, 37, 39
Injection—Main route
Topical—No reports
Oral—Active

5. Factors Affecting Release   1, 4, 34
Inhibitors
  Decreased K^+ in blood
  Increased Na^+ in blood
  Hemodilution
Stimulators
  Angiotensin II—renin
  Stress, decreased Na, decreased blood volume
  Pregnancy
  ACTH (slightly)
  Increased blood pressure in carotid arteries
  Increased K^+ in blood, prostaglandins
  Ca^{2+}

6. Deficiency Symptoms (Humans)   1, 4, 37, 38, 39
Decreased—Blood: pressure, sugar, and pH; weight, liver glycogen, urinary K^+,
  temperature, reproductive functions

Increased—Urinary: Na^+, Cl^-, HCO_3^-
Kidney failure, muscular weakness, gastrointestinal disturbances, hemoconcentration, stress intolerance, acidosis

7. Effects of Overdose, Toxicity   1, 4, 20, 37, 38, 39
Hypertension
Congestive heart failure
Increased Na and H_2O in blood, muscles
Hemodilution
Hypokalemia
Edema
Alkalosis
Diabetes insipidus (type of)

METABOLIC ROLE

1. Biosynthesis   20, 21, 22, 23, 37, 39
Acetate $\rightarrow$ Mevalonate $\rightarrow$ Squalene $\rightarrow$ Cholesterol $\rightarrow$ Pregnenolone $\rightarrow$ Progesterone $\rightarrow$ deoxycorticosterone $\rightarrow$ 18-hydroxycorticosterone $\rightarrow$ Aldosterone
Site(s) in cell—Membranes

2. Production Sites   20, 21, 22, 23, 37, 39
Adrenal cortex (zona glomerulosa), embryonic rest cells

3. Storage Areas   8, 9, 16
None

4. Blood Carriers   2, 8, 22, 26
Lipoproteins, albumin
Conjugates, free steroid—Combined with above proteins

5. Half-life   8, 9, 26
25 min

6. Target Tissues   1, 20, 22
Distal renal tubules, sweat and salivary glands, intestinal mucosa, gills (fish), skin (amphibians), nasal gland (birds), rectal gland (sharks)

7. Reactions   4, 5, 22, 25, 33, 34, 38
Reactive form—Equilibrium (hemiacetal-aldehyde) redox couple

Organ	Enzyme System	Effect
Kidney	1. Unknown enzymes involved in sodium transport	Activated
	2. Also enzymes similar to cortisol (glucocorticoid function)	Activated
	3. RNA polymerase	Activated
Liver, muscle, plasma, general	Similar to cortisol; see cortisol	Activated

8. **Mode of Action**   1, 4, 5, 8, 9, 16, 31, 37, 39
   Cellular
   Anabolic—Liver (proteins, CHO, nucleic acids)
   Catabolic—Extrahepatic (proteins, fats, CHO, nucleic acids)
   Other—Increases Na^+ active transport in renal tubules, activates redox pump; H_2O transported with Na^+
   Organismal
   Increases blood (Na^+, volume, pressure); urinary (K^+, H^+); cold tolerance, muscle work performance, liver glycogen
   Decreases blood (K^+, H^+); urine (Na^+, H_2O, volume); eosinophils, lymphocytes

9. **Catabolism**   1, 9, 22, 25, 33, 34
   Intermediates—Tetrahydro derivative (inactive)
   Excretion products—30-40% glucuronides, 4-8% free, 52-66% other conjugates

MISCELLANEOUS

1. **Relationship to Vitamins**   8, 11, 13, 38
   Vitamin C—Adrenal cortex depleted of vitamin C on production of aldosterone
   Niacin—NADPH involved in synthesis of aldosterone
   Biotin—Prolongs life in adrenalectomized rats

2. **Relationship to Other Hormones**   8, 11, 13, 32, 38
   Cortisol—Synergistic to aldosterone in glucocorticoid activity; antagonistic to aldosterone in water metabolism
   ACTH—Trigger for small release of aldosterone
   Vasopressin, oxytocin—Synergists for aldosterone action in water metabolism
   Angiotensin II, renin—Stimulate production of aldosterone
   Other hormones antagonistic or synergistic with cortisol (glucocorticoid action)—See cortisol

3. **Unusual Features**   29, 32, 38

   Not a glucocorticoid even though it has —OH on C-11 and 1/3 of glucocorticoid power of cortisol

   Redox couple—Hemiacetal-aldehyde equilibrium

   No nervous controls

   Active on oral administration

   Most water-soluble of all steroids

   Largely independent of ACTH control

4. **Possible Relationships of Deficiency Symptoms to Metabolic Action**   11, 13, 20, 37

   Decreased—Blood: pressure and pH; urinary K^+ ⎫ Loss of mineralocorticoid
   Increased—Urinary: Na^+, Cl^-, HCO_3^- ⎪ function; failure of Na^+
   Acidosis, kidney failure   ⎬ pump and Na^+-H_2O reab-
   Hemoconcentration   ⎪ sorption mechanisms in
   Weight loss   ⎭ kidney tubules

   Muscular weakness   ⎫
   Gastrointestinal disturbances   ⎪
   Stress intolerance   ⎬ Loss of glucocorticoid functions
   Decreased blood sugar   ⎪ and decreased gluconeogenesis
   Decreased liver glycogen   ⎪
   Decreased temperature   ⎭

5. **Relationship to Minerals**   **(See references in specific mineral section)**

   Excretion of K^+, Na^+ by kidney

   Release of hormone—Ca^{2+} required; Na^+ inhibits; K^+ stimulates

Chapter 45. Cortisol

Cortisol, a hormone (glucocorticoid) from the adrenal cortex, is a general maintenance hormone of the tissue-controlling type. It is readily convertible to cortisone. It is systemic in action and essential to life. Its chief functions are to maintain stress reactions, capillary permeability, release of other hormones, liver anabolism, and extrahepatic catabolism. Its chief importance is in maintenance of stress reactions. Chief deficiency conditions are Addison's disease, adrenal insufficiency, rheumatic arthritis, and inflammation.

Cortisol is a water-insoluble, fat-soluble steroid with a fairly long half-life in blood. Excess doses result in diabetes, atherosclerosis, osteoporosis, buffalo obesity, and adrenal regression. Its chief synergists are epinephrine, Cu^{2+}, Mn^{2+}, norepinephrine, PTH, and T4, whereas its chief antagonists are STH, estrogens, and testosterone.

Cortisol is formed in the adrenal cortex, and a small amount is stored there. Factors stimulating release are: glucagon, vasopressin, insulin, estrogens, stress, and ACTH. Factors inhibiting release are: high glucocorticoids, low ACTH, and low pituitary hormones.

Cortisol acts by interaction with the DNA in the nucleus after traversing the cell membrane, resulting in various enzyme syntheses and actions (e.g., gluconeogenesis in extrahepatic tissues).

GENERAL INFORMATION

1. **Synonyms**   1, 7, 18

   Hydrocortisone, Compound F, 17-hydroxycorticosterone, Substance M, glucocorticoid

2. **History**   9, 18, 24, 28, 35, 36
   1937—Reichstein: isolated cortisol from adrenal glands
   1942—Von Euw, Reichstein: determined configuration of cortisol
   1948—Mason, Sprague: isolated cortisol from urine
   1950—Reich et al.: isolated cortisol from blood
   1950—Wendler et al.: synthesized cortisol
   1951—Zaffaroni et al.: demonstrated biosynthesis of cortisol in adrenals

3. **Physiological Forms**   9, 26, 35, 37, 39
   Cortisol, cortisone (glucocorticoids)

4. **Active Analogs and Related Compounds (Glucocorticoids)**   17, 22, 24, 35, 37, 39
   Natural—Deoxycorticosterone, cortexolone, cortisone ("E"), corticosterone ("B"), dehydrocorticosterone ("A")
   Synthetic—Dexamethasone, 9α-F-cortisol, prednisone, prednisolone

5. **Inactive Analogs and Related Compounds**   17, 22, 24, 35, 37, 39
   Estrone, progesterone, 17-α-hydroxyprogesterone, cortexolone, adrenosterone

6. **Antagonists**   9, 17, 35
   Protein and CHO metabolism—Insulin, STH, estrogens, testosterone

7. **Synergists**   9, 17, 35
   Fat metabolism—STH, epinephrine, norepinephrine, PTH, T4

8. **Physiological Functions**   1, 4, 14, 16, 37, 39
   Increases—Protein catabolism (exc. liver) (gluconeogenesis), carbohydrate anabolism (liver), blood sugar, glucose absorption, brain excitation, spread of infections, urinary glucose and nitrogen, stress tolerance, lactation, water diuresis
   Decreases—Fat anabolism, growth rate, inflammation, eosinophils, lymphocytes, antigen sensitivity, respiratory quotient, ketosis, wound healing, skin pigmentation, RBC hemolysis
   Regulates—General adaptation syndrome, water balance, blood pressure, hormone release

9. **Disorders and Deficiency Diseases**   1, 4, 14, 16, 37, 39
   Addison's disease (deficiency), Cushing's syndrome (excess), adrenal insufficiency, adrenogenital syndrome, rheumatic arthritis, inflammation

10. **Essentiality for Life**   1, 9, 38
    Absence causes shortening of life span due to inability to respond to stress situations

CHEMISTRY

1. Structure   1, 8, 9, 15, 18, 35

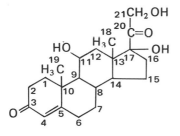

Cortisol, $C_{21}H_{30}O_5$

2. Reactions   1, 8, 9, 17, 18

Heat—Oxidizes
Acid—Esterifies
    Fluorescent in H_2SO_4 (conc.)
Alkali—Stable (dilute)
    Fluorescent (conc.)
Water—Very sl. sol.

Oxidation—Forms cortisone
    C-11 Hydroxyl → Keto
Reduction—Stable
Light—Stable

3. Properties   1, 7, 8, 9, 17, 19

Appearance—White powder
MW—362.5
MP—217-220°C
Crystal form—Rectilinear plates
Salts, esters—Acetate
Important groups for activity
    —C(17)OH
    —C(11)OH
    —C(21)H_2OH

Solubility
    H_2O—0.28 mg/ml
    Acet., Alc.—15, 6.2 mg/ml
    Chl., Eth.—9.3, 0.35 mg/ml
Absn. max.—242 mμ
Chemical nature
    Reducing agent
    Alcohol, ketone
α_D^{20} = 167 (EtOH)

4. Commercial Production   9, 18, 22, 24, 35

Extraction and isolation from beef and hog adrenals

5. Isolation   22, 24, 35

Sources—Adrenal cortex
Methods
    Free
        Extract with dilute alkali; partition between two solvents
        Chromatography—Glass, paper, thin layer, gas, liquid
        Columns—Florasil
        Countercurrent distribution
    Conjugates—Extract tissue, paper chromatography, alumina columns

6. **Determination**   1, 14, 19a, 22, 26, 38
   Bioassay:
      Increased—Liver glycogen, life span in cold, tolerance to trauma, isotope
         uptake
      Decreased—Eosinophils, lymphocytes
   Physicochemical
      Reduction to red formazan
      Oxidation to 17-oxosteroids
      Phenylhydrazone formation
      Fluorescence at 550 or 570 mμ
      Polarography

MEDICAL AND BIOLOGICAL ROLE

1. **Species Occurrence, Specificity, and Antigenicity**   1, 9, 38
   Occurrence—Cortisol major form of glucocorticoids in primates, dog, fish,
      decreasing in activity in lower forms. Corticosterone major glucocorticoid
      in rodents, birds, amphibians, reptiles
   Specificity—Can cross species lines without loss of activity
   Antigenicity—Not antigenic

2. **Units**   8, 9, 14
   By weight, μg (microgram)

3. **Normal Blood Levels**   2, 4, 9, 22, 35, 39
   5-25 μg/100 ml, plasma; diurnal variation (higher in A.M.)

4. **Administration**   8, 9, 20, 37, 39
   Injection—Intramuscular
   Oral—Active; prednisone form used
   Topical—Acetonides in creams, lotions

5. **Factors Affecting Release**   1, 4, 34
   Inhibitors
      Pituitary hypofunction
      Diurnal rhythm—Low in afternoon
      Decreased ACTH
      Increased plasma glucocorticoids
   Stimulators
      Pregnancy, infancy, stress
      ACTH ingestion and ACTH increase
      Adrenal hyperfunction
      Angiotensin II, insulin, estrogens

Glucagon, vasopressin
Decreased plasma glucocorticoids
Thyroxin (T4)
Ca^{2+}

6. **Deficiency Symptoms (Humans)**   1, 4, 37, 38, 39
   Decreased
       Growth, secondary sex characteristics
       Blood pressure, body temperature
       Kidney function, leading to death
       Liver glycogen, gluconeogenesis
       Intestinal absorption, blood sugar
       Stress response—Ultimately death
   Increased
       Glucose oxidation, ACTH levels, respiratory quotient
       Fat anabolism, hemoconcentration
       Muscular weakness
       Skin pigmentation
       Insulin sensitivity

7. **Effects of Overdose, Toxicity**   1, 4, 20, 37, 38, 39
   Buffalo obesity, bruisability, moon-face
   Osteoporosis (demineralization of bone)
   Adrenal regression
   Anesthesia
   Atherosclerosis, hypercholesterolemia, lipemia
   Diabetes
   Alkalosis
   Decreased growth
   Inhibition of inflammatory responses and wound healing

METABOLIC ROLE

1. **Biosynthesis**   20, 21, 22, 23, 37, 39
   Acetate → Mevalonate → Squalene → Cholesterol → Pregnenolone → Proges-
       terone → 17α-Hydroxyprogesterone → deoxycortisol → Cortisol
   Sites in cell—Mitochondria, microsomes

2. **Production Sites**   20, 21, 22, 23, 37, 39
   Adrenal cortex, placenta, embryonic rest cells

3. **Storage**   8, 9, 16
   Adrenal cortex (small amount)

4. **Blood Carriers   2, 8, 22, 26**
   Lipoproteins, conjugates, α-globulins (transcortin), albumin; also free

5. **Half-life   8, 9, 26**
   110 min

6. **Target Tissues   1, 20, 22**
   Liver, central nervous system, hypothalamus, thymus, lymph nodes, intestine,
   connective tissues, skin, mammary gland, vascular system, general systemic

7. **Reactions   4, 5, 22, 25, 33, 34, 38**
   Reactive Form: Cortisol ⇌ cortisone (redox couple)

Organ	Enzyme Systems	Effect
Liver	Phosphoenolpyruvate carboxykinase	Activated
	Pyruvate carboxylase	Activated
	Tryptophan pyrrolase	Activated
	Glycolytic cycle enzymes	Activated
	Krebs cycle enzymes	Activated
	Urea cycle enzymes	Activated
	Deaminases and transaminases	Activated
Liver, kidney	Glucose-6-phosphatase	Activated
	Glycogen synthetase	Activated
	Arginase	Activated
Liver, plasma	Alkaline phosphatase	Activated
Muscle	Aminopeptidase	Activated
General	Histidine decarboxylase	Inhibited
	Hexokinase	Inhibited

8. **Mode of Action   1, 4, 5, 8, 9, 16, 31, 37, 39**
   Cellular
       Anabolic—Increases liver (protein, nucleic acid, CHO, fat) synthesis
       Catabolic—Increases extrahepatic (protein, lipid, and nucleic acid) break-
           down; decreases extrahepatic CHO breakdown
       Other—Redox mechanisms maintained; water and sodium membrane
           transport regulated in kidney glomerulus (with aldosterone), effects on
           DNA template in nucleus, new RNA synthesis
   Organismal
       Maintains circulation and blood pressure (with aldosterone)
       Maintains fluid balance (with aldosterone)
       Maintains renal function (with aldosterone)
       Releases other hormones
       Maintains stress reactions

Regulates ACTH output of pituitary
Maintains collagen, capillary permeability

9. **Catabolism**   1, 9, 22, 25, 33, 34
Intermediates—Bile salts, 17-hydroxy steroids
Excretion products
Urine
100 (approx.) different steroids in urine
87% Glucuronides or sulfates—Cortols, cortolones, 17-hydroxy steroids
4% Free metabolites—Cortols, cortolones, 17-hydroxy steroids
1% Free cortisol—Cortols, cortolones, 17-hydroxy steroids
Feces—Bile salt derivatives

MISCELLANEOUS

1. **Relationship to Vitamins**   8, 11, 13, 38
Vitamin C—May be needed for steroid hormone biosynthesis; depleted from
adrenal cortex on cortical secretion
Niacin—NADPH required for steroid hormone biosynthesis
Vitamin D—Action antagonized by cortisol, i.e., reduces Ca absorption in
intestine
Pantothenic acid, folic acid maintain secretions of steroids by adrenal cortex
Biotin—Adrenocortical insufficiency noted in biotin deficiency
Vitamin A—Deficiency of vitamin A causes cortical necrosis

2. **Relationship to Other Hormones**   8, 11, 13, 32, 38
Estradiol-17β—Antagonist to cortisol protein metabolic effects
Insulin—Antagonist to cortisol (CHO, protein, lipid) metabolic effects
STH—Antagonist to cortisol protein metabolic effects
Testosterone—Antagonist to cortisol protein metabolic effects
Cortisone—Converted to cortisol in body (redox couple)
T4, norepinephrine, epinephrine—Potentiated by cortisol, synergistic
ACTH—Production stopped via feedback mechanism of cortisol
PTH—Synergist to cortisol in bone resorption
Vasopressin, oxytocin—Antagonists to cortisol water balance effects; stimu-
lants for production of glucocorticoids
Glucagon—Stimulant for production of cortical hormones

3. **Unusual Features**   29, 32, 38
Production of euphoria, anesthetic action
Decreased activity if side chain is lengthened
Substituents on C-20, C-18, determine antihemolytic activity

Suppression of mast cell activity, migration of lymphocytes and phagocytes
Inhibition of wound healing and collagen formation by fibroblasts
Inhibition of antibody production, regression of thymus tissue
Suppression of mitosis in lymphoid tissue
Species difference in sensitivity

4. **Possible Relationships of Deficiency Symptoms to Metabolic Action   11,
    13, 20, 37**
    Osteoporosis—Antagonism to vitamin D; synergism with PTH
    Diabetes—Inhibition of glucose oxidation
    Alkalosis—Retention of sodium
    Bruisability—Depletion of vitamin C (?)
    Buffalo obesity, moon face—Antagonism to insulin (?)
    Adrenal regression—Shut-off of ACTH production
    Anesthesia—Effects on membranes (?)
    Atherosclerosis—Diabetogenic effect (?)

5. **Relationships to Minerals   (See references in specific mineral section)**
    Excretion of Na^+ (↓), K^+ (↑), Zn^{2+} (↑)
    Release of hormone—Ca^{2+} required, I^- (as T4)
    Synergism—I^- (as T4), Mn^{2+}
    Regulates
        Serum levels—Na^+ (↑), K^+ (↓), Zn^{2+} (↓), Fe^{2+} (↓), Cu^{2+} (↓)
        Bone levels—PO_4^{3-} (↓)

Chapter 46. Estradiol

Estradiol, which is the major female sex hormone (an estrogen), falls into the reproductive hormone category, and is also a systemic hormone. It is in equilibrium with estrone and estriol in the blood. It is not essential to life but is essential for reproduction and female characteristics. Its chief functions are to maintain and regulate female sex organs in menstrual cycles and pregnancy and to regulate female sex characteristics and behavior. Its chief importance is as the major female sex hormone with its command of female sex development and maintenance of female body characteristics and behavior. Estradiol is also a major active ingredient in the birth control pill.

Deficiency conditions include menopause and delayed maturation.

Estradiol is a water-insoluble, fat-soluble steroid with a fairly short half-life (2-4 min) in blood. Excess doses can produce tumors and permanent sterility, as well as vomiting, thrombophlebitis, dizziness, and water retention. Its chief synergists are oxytocin, relaxin, progesterone, and prolactin, whereas its chief antagonists are testosterone, cortisol, and aldosterone.

Estradiol is formed in the ovary (corpus luteum), and smaller amounts are formed in the adrenal cortex (male and female); small amounts are also made in the male by the testes. Small quantities may be stored in the corpus luteum. Factors stimulating release of estradiol are: FSH, LH, and low blood estrogen. Factors inhibiting release are: high blood estrogen and melatonin.

Estradiol acts (after transportation by cytoplasmic receptor) by interaction with the DNA of the nucleus of target cell tissue. It causes formation of enzymes and other chemicals needed to carry on the function of estradiol.

GENERAL INFORMATION

1. **Synonyms**   1, 7, 18

   Estradiol-17β, female hormone, β-estradiol, dihydrotheelin, dihydrofollicular hormone, dihydrofolliculin, estrogen

2. **History**   9, 18, 24, 28, 35, 36

   1929—Doisy, Butenandt, et al.: isolated and crystallized estrone from pregnancy urine
   1930—Marrian: isolated estriol from pregnancy urine
   1932—Marrian, Butenandt: determined structure of estrone and estriol
   1936—McCorquodale: isolated crystalline estradiol from pregnancy urine and sow ovaries
   1940—Inhoffen: synthesized estradiol from cholesterol
   1948—Anner and Miescher: totally synthesized estrone

3. **Physiological Forms**   9, 26, 35, 37, 39

   Estrone, estriol, estradiol (estrogens)

4. **Active Analogs and Related Compounds (Estrogens)**   17, 22, 24, 35, 37, 39

   Synthetic—Diethylstilbesterol, hexestrol, dienestrol, benzestrol, ethinylestradiol, chlorotrianisene
   Natural—Estriol, estrone, equilin

5. **Inactive Analogs and Related Compounds**   17, 22, 24, 35, 37, 39

   Pregnanediol, lumiestrone, progesterone, 17α-estradiol, 17α-hydroxyprogesterone, 17α-hydroxypregnenolone

6. **Antagonists**   9, 17, 35

   [Progesterone, cortisol, testosterone (all concentration-dependent)] ; uterine factor, melatonin, ethanoxytriphetol, aldosterone, clomiphene, nafoxidine

7. **Synergists**   9, 17, 35

   Prolactin, progesterone, androgens, corticoids, STH, oxytocin, T4, relaxin, insulin

8. **Physiological Functions**   1, 4, 14, 16, 37, 39

   Regulates menstrual cycle, female sex behavior
   Maintains secondary sex characteristics
   Affects antibody properties
   Induces estrus, uterine hypertrophy, vaginal cornification; potentiates and stimulates calcitonin secretion

9. **Deficiency Diseases, Disorders**   1, 4, 14, 16, 37, 39
   Menopause (natural deficiency) gonadal dysgenesis, delayed maturation

10. **Essentiality for Life**   1, 9, 38
    Not for life of organism, but for reproduction of organism

CHEMISTRY

1. **Structure**   1, 8, 9, 15, 18, 35

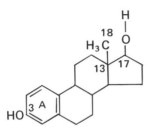

Estradiol-17β, $C_{18}H_{24}O_2$

2. **Reactions**   1, 8, 9, 17, 18

Heat—Stable	Oxidation—Unstable; forms estriol
Acid—Stable (dilute)	or estrone
Fluoresces (conc.)	Reduction—Unstable
Alkali—Sol., stable	Light—No data
Water—Insol.	

3. **Properties**   1, 7, 8, 9, 17, 19

Appearance—Colorless powder
MW—272.4
Salts, esters—Acetate, benzoate,
   propionate, heptanoate, valerate
Important groups for activity
   Aromatic Ring A
   —C(3)OH, —C(17)OH

MP—173-179°C
Crystal form—Prisms
Solubility
   H_2O—Insol.
   (Estriol—3 mg/100 cc H_2O)
   Acet., Alc.—Sol.
   Benz., Chl., Eth.—Sol.
Absn. max.—225, 280 mμ
Chemical nature—Alcohol, aro-
   matic, phenolic
α_D^{22} = 76-83

4. **Commercial Production**   9, 18, 22, 24, 35
   Extract pregnant mare's urine
   Total synthesis

5. **Isolation**   22, 24, 35
   Sources—Pregnancy urine of mares, follicular liquor of sow ovaries
   Method
   Protein-bound or conjugated steroids 15% HCl, 60 min 100°C, or sepha-
   dex G-25 with H_2O elution, or amberlite column LA-2, elution with
   ethyl acetate at pH = 2; saponification
   Free steroids-ether extraction
   Purification
   Countercurrent distribution
   Column chromatography
   High-voltage electrophoresis

6. **Determination**   1, 14, 19a, 22, 26, 38
   Bioassay
   Vaginal cornification
   Increase in uterine weight in ovariectomized animals
   Topical application in vagina; vaginal smear of exfoliated cells
   Physicochemical
   Fluorescence assay
   Colorimetry—Kober reaction
   Chromatography
   Radioimmunoassay

MEDICAL AND BIOLOGICAL ROLE

1. **Species Occurrence, Specificity, Antigenicity**   1, 9, 38
   Occurrence—All vertebrates, but different distribution of activities for three
   physiological forms; some plants (derivatives of estradiol)
   Specificity—Species difference in sensitivity
   17β-Estradiol, estrone (human, dog, pig, rat)
   Estrone, equilin, equilinin (horse)
   17α-Estradiol (sheep, goat, beef)
   17-Epiestriol (mouse)
   Antigenicity—No antigenicity reported

2. **Units**   8, 9, 14
   1 mg = 10,000 I.U.; 1 μg = 1 microgram

3. **Normal Blood Levels (Man)**   2, 4, 9, 22, 35, 39
   Male—.008-.02 μg/100 ml (estradiol and estrone), plasma
   Females—.005-.07 μg/100 ml or less (estrone and estriol)—cyclic in females
   during 28-day period
   Pregnant females (av.)—2.1 μg/100 ml estradiol, 6.5 μg/100 ml estrone, 10.9
   μg/100 ml estriol (varies with stage of pregnancy)

4. **Administration**   8, 9, 20, 37, 39
Injection—Subcutaneous, intramuscular
Topical—In creams and cosmetics
Oral—Inactive free form; active as esters or synthetic analogs; various synthetic estrogens used in small quantity with synthetic progestogens in contraceptive pills

5. **Factors Affecting Release**   1, 4, 34
Inhibitors—Feedback via blood to hypothalamus, melatonin, high plasma estrogen
Stimulators—FSH and LH (cyclic via hypothalamus), low plasma estrogen, Ca^{2+}

6. **Deficiency Symptoms (Humans)**   1, 4, 37, 38, 39
Delayed maturation
Female accessory and reproductive organs regress
Decreased female behavioral pattern
Senescence
Menopause

7. **Effects of Overdose, Toxicity**   1, 4, 20, 37, 38, 39
Inhibition of gonads (decrease FSH, LH) → permanent sterility; vomiting; dizziness; thrombophlebitis; water retention; tumors (long term)

METABOLIC ROLE

1. **Biosynthesis**   20, 21, 22, 23, 37, 39
Acetate ⇀ Mevalonate ⇀ Squalene ⇀ Cholesterol ⇀ Pregnenolone ⇀ Progesterone ⇀ 17α-Hydroxyprogesterone ⇀ Androstenedione ⇀ Testosterone ⇀ 19-Hydroxytestosterone → Estradiol
Site(s) in cell—Mitochondria, microsomes

2. **Production Sites**   20, 21, 22, 23, 37, 39
All vertebrates
Ovarian follicles (membrane granulosa, theca interna)
Testes (interstitial cells)
Corpus luteum, adrenal cortex (fasciculata reticularis)
Placenta, embryonic rest cells

3. **Storage Areas**   8, 9, 16
Small amounts—corpus luteum (?)

4. **Blood Carriers**   2, 8, 22, 26
   Plasma proteins—Estriol glucuronides, free estrone and estradiol
   Plasma lipoprotein, estroprotein, serum albumin, red cell proteins

5. **Half-life**   8, 9, 26
   2-4 min

6. **Target Tissues**   1, 20, 22
   Systemic; uterus, mammary gland, vagina, ovary (corpus luteum), secondary
   female sex organs, skin, CNS, thyroid, thymus, long bones, anterior pituitary, hypothalamus

7. **Reactions**   4, 5, 22, 25, 33, 34, 38
   Reactive forms (Redox couple)
   Estradiol $\rightleftharpoons$ estrone $\rightarrow$ estriol (oxidation product)

Organ	Enzyme System	Effect
Uterus	Lactic acid dehydrogenase	Activated
	Phosphorylase b $\rightarrow$ a	Activated
	RNA polymerase	Activated
Placenta	Isocitric dehydrogenase	Activated
Endometrium	Glucose-6-phosphate dehydrogenase	Activated
Kidney	Kynurenine aminotransferase	Inhibited
Liver	Kynureninase	Inhibited
	N^1-Methylnicotinamide oxidase	Inhibited

8. **Mode of Action**   1, 4, 5, 8, 9, 16, 31, 37, 39
   Cellular
       Anabolic
           RNA and protein synthesis (uterus) increased
           CHO synthesis (uterus) increased
           Increased growth (uterus)
       Catabolic—CHO glycolysis (uterus) increased
       Other
           Direct action on nucleus
           Increases mitosis (uterus)
           Transcription of RNA affected
           Hyperpolarization of cell membranes
   Organismal
       Uterus
           Increases glycolysis, respiration, H_2O permeability, hyperemia
           Releases histamine

Potentiates and stimulates TCT in calcium bone deposition
Development of female characteristics
Growth of female $1°$ and $2°$ sex organs
    Estradiol, estrone—Act on corpus luteum
    Estriol—Acts on sex organs
Regulates menstrual cycle and sex behavior
Maintains secondary sex characteristics
Affects antibody properties

9. **Catabolism**   1, 9, 22, 25, 33, 34
Intermediates—Estriol
Excretion products

$$\text{Urine—Mainly conjugated,} \quad \frac{\text{estrone glucuronide or SO}_4}{\text{estriol glucuronide or SO}_4} = 1/3$$

    Free—As estriol or 16-epiestriol
    Pregnancy—Estrone + estradiol increases 100X; estriol increases 1000X
Feces—Enterohepatic circulation

MISCELLANEOUS

1. **Relationship to Vitamins**   8, 11, 13, 38
Folic acid—Involved in mitotic effect of estradiol
Niacin (TPN)(DPN)—Involved in increased respiration and in cholesterol precursor synthesis
Vitamin E—Essential for gonadotropin production or release
Vitamin B_6—Competes as cofactor with estrogen sulfate in kynurenine aminotransferase activity
Vitamin D—Synergistic in calcium metabolism with estradiol

2. **Relationship to Other Hormones**   8, 11, 13, 32, 38
Progesterone, cortisol, testosterone—Antagonistic or synergistic to estradiol, depending on relative concentrations of estradiol and other hormone
Prolactin, STH, oxytocin, T4, relaxin—Synergistic to estradiol
TCT—Potentiated and stimulated by estradiol
FSH, LH—Stimulate release or production of estradiol

3. **Unusual Features**   29, 32, 38
Estradiol-$17\beta \rightleftharpoons$ estrone $\rightarrow$ estriol (activity 1000:100:1)
Aromatic ring—Carcinogenicity implicated
Redox couple: estradiol $\rightleftharpoons$ estrone
Derived from testosterone in biosynthesis
Occurrence of estrogens in plants—Genistein, Coumestrol (active)

Tumor formation enhanced by estradiol
Enterohepatic circulation of estradiol
Variable species forms
Synthetic estrogens not steroids

4. **Possible Relationships of Deficiency to Metabolic Action**   11, 13, 20, 37
Ovarian regression—Decrease of mitosis in sex tissues
Regression of female sex organs and secondary sex characteristics—Decrease
   of mitosis in sex tissues
Decreased female sex behavior patterns—Decrease of estradiol in central ner-
   vous system
Senescence, menopause—Decrease in mitosis in sex organs (?)

5. **Relationships to Minerals   (See references in specific mineral section)**
Release of hormone—Ca^{2+} required
Synergism—I^- (as T4), Ca^{2+} (via TCT)
Serum levels regulated—Cu^{2+} ($\uparrow$), Mn^{2+} ($\uparrow$), I^- ($\uparrow$)

Chapter 47. Progesterone

Progesterone, a female sex hormone (a progestin), is in the reproductive hormone category. It is indirectly systemic in action and is indirectly essential for life, since it is a precursor to aldosterone and cortisol, which are essential. Its chief functions are to synergize the actions of estradiol in the female organs, especially in pregnancy. Its importance stems from the fact that it is a precursor to all the steroid hormones and that estradiol requires its presence for many of its actions. It is also a major ingredient of the birth control "pill." Deficiency conditions include acne, pseudopregnancy (animals), and dysfunctional uterine bleeding.

Progesterone is a water-insoluble, fat-soluble steroid with a short half-life (5 min). Excess doses produce inhibition of uterine growth and increased Na^+, K^+ excretion, and prolongation of pregnancy. Its chief synergists are: estradiol, prolactin, relaxin, oxytocin, cortisol, and T4. Its chief antagonists are: testosterone, aldosterone, and, under certain conditions, estradiol and oxytocin.

Progesterone is formed in the corpus luteum (ovary), testicles, adrenal cortex, and placenta. It is a precursor to all steroid hormones and is stored in the adrenal cortex, corpus luteum, and body fat. Factors stimulating release of progesterone are: LH, prolactin, nerve impulses (psychic), and estrogen. Some factors inhibiting release include: high levels of plasma progestins, uterine factors, and environmental factors. Progesterone action is by way of action on the DNA of the cell nucleus after transport by cytoplasmic receptors. New RNA and proteins are then synthesized, to carry on effects of progesterone.

GENERAL INFORMATION

1. **Synonyms**   1, 7, 18
   Progestin, luteosterone, corpus luteum hormone

2. **History**   9, 18, 24, 28, 35, 36
   1903—Fraenkel: demonstrated that removal of corpora lutea in pregnant rabbits terminates pregnancy, prevents attachment of ovum to uterus
   1928—Corner and Allen: restored progestational changes in above rabbits with extracts of corpora lutea
   1930—Fels and Slotta ⎫
   1932—Allen   ⎬ Obtained crude crystalline concentrates containing progestational activity
   1932—Fevold and Hisaw ⎭
   1934—Butenandt et al. ⎫
       Slotta et al.   ⎪ Isolated pure crystalline
       Allen et al.   ⎬ corpus luteum hormone
       Hartmann et al. ⎭
   1934—Slotta et al.: proposed formula for corpus luteum hormone
   1934—Butenandt, Fernholz: synthesized progesterone from stigmasterol

3. **Physiological Forms**   9, 26, 35, 37, 39
   Progesterone, 17α-hydroxyprogesterone (progestins)

4. **Active Analogs and Related Compounds (Progestins, progestogens)**   17, 22, 24, 35, 37, 39
   Natural
       20α-Hydroxypregnenone
       20β-Hydroxypregnenone
       11-Dehydroprogesterone
       Cortexone
       17α-Hydroxyprogesterone
   Synthetic
       A-Norprogesterone
       19-Norprogesterone
       21-Norprogesterone
       Ethisterone
       17α-Methyltestosterone
       6α-Methyl-17α-acetoxyprogesterone
       Δ^1-Dehydro-6α-methyl-17α-acetoxyprogesterone

5. **Inactive Analogs and Related Compounds**   17, 20, 21, 22, 24, 35, 37, 39
   5α-Pregnane-3β-ol-20-one, 21-ethylprogesterone, 11β-hydroxyprogesterone, pregnanediol, pregnanetriol

6. **Antagonists**   9, 17, 35
(Estradiol, testosterone, oxytocin, aldosterone) all concentration-dependent

7. **Synergists**   9, 17, 35
Estradiol, prolactin, testosterone, cortisol, STH, T4, relaxin, oxytocin

8. **Physiological Functions**   1, 4, 14, 16, 37, 39
Low concentrations
Prepare uterus for blastocyst implantation; promote ovulation and mammary gland development
Regulate female sex accessory organs, weak corticosteroid properties, precursor to sex hormones
Higher concentrations
Maintain pregnancy; repress ovulation and sex activity; inhibit vaginal cornification and parturition; decrease myometrial excitation

9. **Deficiency Diseases, Disorders**   1, 4, 14, 16, 37, 39
Pseudopregnancy (laboratory animals), acne, dysfunctional uterine bleeding

10. **Essentiality for Life**   1, 9, 38
Indirectly essential for life via corticosteroid requirement
Essential for aldosterone and glucocorticoid formation
Essential for reproduction in female vertebrates

CHEMISTRY

1. **Structure**   1, 8, 9, 15, 18, 35

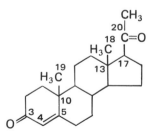

Progesterone, $C_{21}H_{30}O_2$

2. **Reactions**   1, 8, 9, 17, 18

Heat—Stable	Oxidation—Unstable
Acid—Unstable; fluoresces in H_2SO_4	Reduction—Unstable; reduces to
Alkali—Unstable	pregnanediol
Water—Insol.	Light—Unstable

3. Properties   1, 7, 8, 9, 17, 19

Appearance—white powder
MW—314.5
MP—α = 128°C; β = 121°C
Crystal form
   α—Orthorhombic prisms
   β—Orthorhombic needles
Salts, esters-Acetate, caproate
Important groups for activity
   —C(3)=O,
   —C(4)=C(5)—
   —C(20)—CH$_3$
    ‖
    O

Solubility
   H_2O—Insol.
   Acet., Alc.—Sol.
   Benz., Chl., Eth'—Sol.
Absn. max.—240 mμ
Chemical nature
   Ketone, steroid
α_D = 172-182 (dioxane)

4. Commercial Production   9, 18, 22, 24, 35

Synthesis from cholesterol, stigmasterol, or diosgenin
Isolation from sow ovary corpora lutea

5. Isolation   22, 24, 35

Sources—Sow ovary corpora lutea
Methods
   Extract with alkali
   Extract with ether or ether-ethanol (1:3) or methyl acetate-benzene
   Partition between hexane (or petroleum ether) and 70% methyl alcohol
   Purify by chromatography: celite column, thin layer, paper or counter-
    current distribution

6. Determination   1, 14, 19a, 22, 26, 38

Bioassay
   Decidual responses
   Change of progesterone in endometrium
Physicochemical
   Absorption at 240 mμ or at 290 mμ in H_2SO_4
   Yellow fluorescence with $SbCl_3$
   Blue absorption with phosphomolybdic acid
   Protein-binding assay

MEDICAL AND BIOLOGICAL ROLE

1. Species Occurrence, Specificity, Antigenicity   1, 9, 38

Occurrence—Found in plants, all vertebrates
Specificity—Activity crosses species lines
Antigenicity—No antigenicity reported

2. **Units**   8, 9, 14
μg or mg; rabbit unit = 0.6 mg progesterone

3. **Normal Blood Levels**   2, 4, 9, 22, 35, 39
Normal males—0.01-0.03 μg/100 ml plasma
Normal females—0.1-1.1 μg/100 ml plasma; cyclic variation in females, 28-day period
Pregnant females—10-28 μg/100 ml plasma

4. **Administration**   8, 9, 20, 37, 39
Injection—Intramuscular
Topical—Not reported
Oral—As caproate or acetate of 17α-hydroxyprogesterone; various synthetic progestogens used in contraceptive pills in combination with small amounts of estrogens

5. **Factors Affecting Release**   1, 4, 34
Inhibitors
   Psychic phenomena
   Uterine factor
   Feedback mechanisms via hypothalamus
   Environmental factors
Stimulators
   Hypothalamic agent—LRH (human)—via pituitary and LH
      Males—Continuous secretion (low levels)
      Females—Continuous secretion in nonspontaneous ovulators (rabbit, ferret, cat); rhythmic in spontaneous ovulators (dog, human)
   Psychic and environmental controls
   Prolactin or LH, depending on species
   Ca^{2+}

6. **Deficiency Symptoms (Humans)**   1, 4, 37, 38, 39
Termination of pregnancy
Decreased production of steroids
Decreased ovulation
Loss of normal cyclic changes
Decreased development for implantation and gestation

7. **Effects of Overdose, Toxicity**   1, 4, 20, 37, 38, 39
Progestational changes
Pregnancy prolongation
Inhibition of uterine growth
Increased Na and K excretion

METABOLIC ROLE

1. **Biosynthesis**   20, 21, 22, 23, 37, 39
   Acetate → Mevalonate → Squalene → Cholesterol → Pregnenolene → Proges-
   terone
   Cell Site: Microsomes

2. **Production Sites**   20, 21, 22, 23, 37, 39
   Ovary (follicles, corpus luteum)
   Testicles (interstitial cells)
   Adrenal cortex (reticularis fasciculata)
   Placenta (syncytical trophoblast)

3. **Storage Sites**   8, 9, 16
   Corpora lutea
   Adrenal cortex
   Body fat

4. **Blood Carriers**   2, 8, 22, 26
   Plasma lipoproteins—Albumin, transcortin

5. **Half-life**   8, 9, 26
   About 5 min

6. **Target Tissues**
   Uterus, vagina, cervix, pubic symphysis, ovary, hypothalamus, mammary
   gland, female sex accessory organs, kidney, adrenal cortex, adenohypophysis

7. **Reactions**   4, 5, 22, 25, 33, 34, 38
   Reactive form—Unknown

Organ	Enzyme System	Effect
Uterus	Acid phosphatase	Activated
	Carbonic anhydrase	Activated

8. **Mode of Action**   1, 4, 5, 8, 9, 16, 31, 37, 39
   Cellular
   Anabolic: Increases glycoprotein (uterus); increases glycogen (uterus)
   Catabolic: Increases protein catabolism; increases galactose oxidation
   Other: Increases membrane potential; immediate precursor for other sex
   hormones; thermogenic action; effects on DNA template, new RNA
   synthesis

Organismal
> Increases kidney filtration rate (glomerulus)
> Promotes development and growth of uterus and mammary gland
> Promotes ovulation and development of sex accessories (female)
> Promotes excitation of uterus
> Inhibits release of LH

9. Catabolism   1, 9, 22, 25, 33, 34
Intermediates—Pregnanediol, 17α-hydroxyprogesterone
Excretion products
> Urine—Mainly as glucuronates of pregnanediol, pregnanetriol
> Feces—Androgens (cow, rat)

MISCELLANEOUS

1. Relationship to Vitamins   8, 11, 13, 38
Niacin—DPN involved in progesterone synthesis
Vitamin C—Depleted from adrenal cortex or ovary on progesterone formation

2. Relationship to Other Hormones   8, 11, 13, 32, 38
Estradiol—Antagonist or synergist to progesterone, depending on concentration; made from progesterone
Prolactin, LH—Stimulant for production of progesterone, depending on species
Testosterone—Antagonist or synergist to progesterone, depending on concentration; made from progesterone
Cortisol, aldosterone—Made from progesterone
STH, T4—Synergist in growth aspects of progesterone
ACTH—Releaser of steroids from adrenal cortex; stimulator of progesterone production
FSH—Synergist with LH in production of progesterone
Relaxin, oxytocin—Synergists with progesterone in parturition
LRH—Hypothalamic agent stimulating release of LH

3. Unusual Features   29, 32, 38
Concentration dependence of effects
Primitive type of hormone
Causes maternal behavior in rabbit
Causes pseudopregnancy in nonspontaneous ovulators
Inhibits estrogenic tumors
Anesthetic effects
Androgenic or antiandrogenic, depending on species
Cyclic release in certain species but not in others

4. **Possible Relationships of Deficiency Symptoms to Metabolic Action   11, 13, 20, 37**

Loss of pregnancy—Lack of growth and developmental stimulus to uterus by progesterone

Decreased steroid production—Serves as precursor to all other steroid hormones

Decreased ovulation—No progesterone stimulus for development of follicle in ovary

Loss of normal cyclic changes—Feedback mechanisms of progesterone on hypothalamus not controlling (?)

Decreased development for implantation and gestation—Loss of growth and development stimulating action on uterus due to lack of progesterone

5. **Relationships with Minerals   (See references in specific mineral section)**

Synergism—I^- (as T4)

Release of hormone—Ca^{2+} required

Serum levels regulated—Zn^{2+} ($\downarrow$), Ca^{2+} ($\uparrow$)

Chapter 48. Testosterone

Testosterone is the major male sex hormone (an androgen) and falls into the category of reproductive hormones. It is systemic in action but not essential for life. It is essential for reproduction and maintenance of male characteristics. Its chief functions are: development and maintenance of the male organs, male sex characteristics, and behavior, as well as stimulation of growth (anabolic), and metabolism of muscles, liver, and kidney. The chief importance of testosterone lies in its major command of male sex development, body characteristics, and behavior. Deficiencies include eunuchoidism, and male hypogonadism.

Testosterone is a water-insoluble fat-soluble steroid with a short half-life (10-20 min). Excess doses produce virilization, acne, hypertrophy of sex organs, increased libido, and hirsutism. Its chief synergists are STH, insulin, Zn^{2+}, and low concentrations of estrogens. Its chief antagonists are estrogens (except low concentrations), progesterone, and methylcholanthrene.

Testosterone is formed mainly in the testes (interstitial cells) but also in small amounts in the adrenal cortex and ovary. Small amounts may be stored in the testes. Factors stimulating release are: low androgen or estrogen levels in blood, FSH, LH, LRH, ACTH, Melatonin, and increased blood flow to the testis. Some factors inhibiting release are: cortisol, high blood androgen levels, and nerve impulses (psychic effects). Testosterone acts by its effects on nuclear DNA, producing new RNA followed by new enzymes and proteins, then by increased secretions and cellular changes.

GENERAL INFORMATION

1. **Synonyms**   1, 7, 18

   17β-Hydroxy-4-androsten-3-one, Δ^4-androsten-17β-ol-3-one, androgen

2. **History**   9, 18, 24, 28, 35, 36

   1849—Berthold: demonstrated effects of castration prevented by testis transplants

   1889—Brown-Sequard: claimed rejuvenative powers of testicular extracts

   1911—Pezard: showed comb growth in capons by injection of testicular extracts

   1927—McGee: found extracts of bull testis highly potent for male sex hormone activity

   1931—Butenandt: isolated androsterone from human urine

   1935—Laqueur: crystallized testosterone from testicular extracts

   1935—Butenandt, Ruzicka: determined structure and synthesized testosterone

3. **Physiological Forms (Androgens)**   9, 26, 35, 37, 39

   Androstenedione, testosterone, 11β-hydroxyandrostenedione, adrenosterone, dihydrotestosterone

4. **Active Analogs and Related Compounds (Androgens)**   17, 22, 24, 35, 37, 39

   Natural

   11-Hydroxyandrosterone, adrenosterone, 7-hydroxyprogesterone

   11-Keto-androsterone

   11β-Hydroxyandrostenedione

   Synthetic

   Ethynyl testosterone, methyltestosterone

   6α-chlorotestosterone, 19-nortestosterone, 17α-ethyl-19-nortestosterone

5. **Inactive Analogs and Related Compounds (for Androgenic Activity)**   17, 20, 21, 22, 24, 35, 37, 39

   Cortisone, cortisol, 17-hydroxyprogesterone, lumiandrosterone, 17α-hydroxy-11-desoxycorticosterone, 17β-methyl/epitestosterone, etiocholanolone

6. **Antagonists**   9, 17, 35

   Estrogens, (except in low concentrations), progesterone, norethandrolone, 11α-hydroxyprogesterone,   methylcholanthrene,   A-norprogesterone, cyproterone acetate, diethylstilbesterol

7. **Synergists**   9, 17, 35

   STH, insulin, other androgens, estrogens (in low concentrations), Zn^{2+}, Co^{2+}

8. **Physiological Functions**   1, 4, 14, 16, 37, 39
Controls secondary male sex characteristics
Maintains functional competence of male reproductive ducts and glands
Increases protein anabolism; maintains spermatogenesis; inhibits gonado-
  trophin
Increases male sex behavior; increases closure of epiphyseal plates

9. **Deficiency Diseases, Disorders**   1, 4, 14, 16, 37, 39
Male hypogonadism, eunuchoidism
Feminizing testes, hyperplasias of adrenals and testes

10. **Essentiality for Life**   1, 9, 38
Not essential for life of the organism, but essential for reproduction in all
  (male) vertebrates

CHEMISTRY

1. **Structure**   1, 8, 9, 15, 18, 35

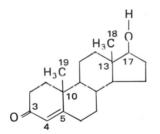

Testosterone, $C_{19}H_{28}O_2$

2. **Reactions**   1, 8, 9, 17, 18

Heat—Stable
Acid—Esterifies
Alkali—Fluoresces (conc.)
Water—Insol.

Oxidation—Oxidizes to androstene-
  dione
Reduction—Unstable
Light—Stable

3. **Properties**   1, 7, 8, 9, 17, 19

Appearance—White powder
MW—288.4
MP—155°C
Crystal form—Needles
Salts, esters—Propionate, acetate,
  butyrate, palmitate, stearate,
  benzoate
Important groups for activity
  —C(3)=O, C(17)—OH
  —C(4)=C(5)

Solubility
  H_2O—Insol.
  Acet., Alc.—Sol.
  Benz., Chl., Eth.—Sol.
Absn. max.—238 mμ
Chemical nature
  Alcoholic ketone, steroid
$\alpha_D^{24} = 109°$

4. **Commercial Production**   9, 18, 22, 24, 35
Microbiological conversion of dehydroandrosterone
Synthesis from cholesterol

5. **Isolation**   22, 24, 35
Sources—Urine, blood
Method: Urine
    Hydrolyze with H_2SO_4, extract with organic solvents
    Precipitate with digitonin or Girard's reagent T
    Chromatography: $MgSiO_4$ column or paper or gas
Method: Blood
    Complex with methyl green; transesterify with acetic acid
    Chromatography on Florisil alumina columns

6. **Determination**   1, 14, 19a, 22, 26, 38
Bioassay
    Growth of capon comb
    Increase in various muscles
    Increase in weight of prostate
    Increase in fructose, citric acid in semen
    Maintenance of spermatogenesis in hypophysectomized rat
Physicochemical—Zimmerman reaction-(17-oxosteroids); Pettenkofer reaction

MEDICAL AND BIOLOGICAL ROLE

1. **Species Occurrence, Specificity, and Antigenicity**   1, 9, 38
Occurrence—Vertebrates (cyclostomes and higher forms), variable types of androgens
Specificity—Variable
    Mammals and birds—Testosterone and androsterone active; pregnenolone inactive
    Rat—Pregnenolone active (not in mammals or birds)
Antigenicity—None reported

2. **Units**   8, 9, 14
0.015 mg = I.U.

3. **Normal Blood Levels (Man)**   2, 4, 9, 22, 35, 39
Males—.45-.75 μg/100 ml plasma, androsterone and dehydroepiandrosterone, diurnal rhythm in males
Females—.025-.040 μg/100 ml plasma

4. **Administration**   8, 9, 20, 37, 39
Injection—Intramuscular preferred
Topical—Some cutaneous absorption
Oral—Active, but less than injected or implanted hormones; more active as esters or synthetic androgens

5. **Factors Affecting Release**   1, 4, 34
Inhibitors
Cortisol
Psychic effects
Androgens
Feedback to hypothalamus
Stimulators
Photoperiodicity
Temperature increase, within limits
Melatonin
FSH, ACTH, LH, LRH
Increased blood flow to testis
Decreased blood levels of androgens or estrogens
Ca^{2+}

6. **Deficiency Symptoms (Humans)**   1, 4, 37, 38, 39
Involution of accessory organs (prostate, seminal vesicles)
Decreased male behavior patterns and libido
Decreased secondary sex traits
Poor muscle development and function
Delayed closure of epiphyses
Decreased excretion of 17-keto-steroids in urine

7. **Effects of Overdose, Toxicity**   1, 4, 20, 37, 38, 39
LD_{100} = 325 mg/kg in female rats
Increases libido
Virilization, acne
Increases fat catabolism
Increases androgen and estrogen excretion (17-keto-steroids)
Precocious sex development
Hypertrophy of accessory sex organs
Increases skeletal growth until epiphyses close
Increases muscle mass, hirsutism
Decreases scalp hair growth (?)
Decreases weight—chick, rat

METABOLIC ROLE

1. **Biosynthesis**   20, 21, 22, 23, 37, 39
   Acetate $\rightarrow$ Mevalonate $\rightarrow$ Squalene $\rightarrow$ Cholesterol $\rightarrow$ Pregnenolone $\rightarrow$ Progesterone $\rightarrow$ 17α-hydroxyprogesterone $\rightarrow$ Androstenedione $\rightarrow$ Testosterone

2. **Production Sites**   20, 21, 22, 23, 37, 39
   Interstitial cells of ovary and testis (Leydig and Sertoli cells): Agranular cytoplasm
   Adrenal cortex (reticularis fasciculata), embryonic placenta
   Skin, salivary glands

3. **Storage Areas**   8, 9, 16
   Testes—Small amounts

4. **Blood Carriers**   2, 8, 22, 26
   Albumin, and a specific β-globulin

5. **Half-life**   8, 9, 26
   10-20 min

6. **Target Tissues**   1, 20, 22
   Systemic, fat deposits, muscles, hypothalamus, kidney
   Male sex organs, adenohypophysis, hair follicles
   Epiphyses of long bones, vocal cords

7. **Reactions**   4, 5, 22, 25, 33, 34, 38
   Reactive form—Dihydrotestosterone
   　　Redox couples—Testosterone $\rightleftharpoons$ androstenedione $\rightleftharpoons$ androsterone

Organ	Enzyme System	Effect
Kidney	β-Glucuronidase	Activated
	d-Aminooxidase	Activated
	Arginase	Activated
	Alkaline phosphatase	Inhibited
Prostate	Succinic dehydrogenase	Activated
Seminal vesicle	Amino acid activating enzymes	Activated

8. **Mode of Action**   1, 4, 5, 8, 9, 16, 31, 37, 39
   Cellular
   　　Anabolic—Increases incorporation of amino acids and protein synthesis in muscles, liver, kidney
   　　Catabolic—Increases fat catabolism; decreases amino acid catabolism

Other
    Redox couple regulation of oxidation
    Increases mitosis in certain tissues
    Increases creatine storage
    Membrane effects; effects on DNA template in nucleus, new RNA
      synthesis
Organismal
    Increases development of male secondary sex organs and characteristics
    Increases growth of muscles, liver, kidney
    Androgenic, increases libido
    Has effects on CNS, male behavior
    Increases folliculoid and luteoid activity in immature females
    Increases basal metabolism
    Maintains positive balances of N, K^+, Ca^{2+}, PO_4^{3-}
    Decreases creatinuria
    Promotes closure of bone epiphyses
    Stimulates red cell production

9. **Catabolism**   1, 9, 22, 25, 33, 34
Intermediates—Androstanolone, androstanedione
Excretion products—Androsterone, etiocholanolone, 17-keto-steroids, dehydroepiandrosterone; in urine, bile, feces—free or conjugated with sulfate
or glucuronide; enterohepatic circulation

MISCELLANEOUS

1. **Relationship to Vitamins**   8, 11, 13, 38
Vitamins A, E, C, folic acid—Synergists with testosterone for maturation of
germ cells and increased anabolic activity
Vitamin B complex—Male accessory gland maintenance in rat (involution on
vitamin B deficiency, similar to castration); synergistic in increased metabolic rate
Vitamin D—Synergist with testosterone in bone metabolism

2. **Relationship to Other Hormones**   8, 11, 13, 32, 38
Estradiol—Formed from testosterone
LH, LRH, FSH—Stimulators of testosterone formation or release
Estradiol, STH, insulin—Synergists for action of testosterone (in proper con-
centrations)
ACTH—Stimulates formation of adrenal androgens
Progesterone, estrogens—Antagonists to testosterone (in proper concentra-
tions)
Cortisol, estrogens, androgens—Act as release inhibitors in high concentra-
tions

3. **Unusual Features**   29, 32, 38
   Multiple sources of production
   Fetal sex determination to male via hypothalamus by testosterone
   Sensitivity of capon comb to testosterone
   Insensitivity of certain muscles to testosterone
   Female birds produce testosterone in ovary
   Immediate precursor in estrogen synthesis
   Two major synthetic routes, three minor ones in adrenals and testes
   Social functions in seals affected by androgens
   Species differences in effects of testosterone on sperm maturation rate
   Dietary effect—Vitamin B deficiency or protein deficiency similar to castration
   Active form in tissues is dihydrotestosterone, more potent than testosterone

4. **Possible Relationships of Deficiency Symptoms to Metabolic Action**   11, 13, 20, 37
   Involution of male accessory organs, decreased secondary sex traits—Withdrawal of anabolic effect of testosterone
   Decreased male behavior and libido—Decreased effect on CNS
   Poor muscle development and function—Withdrawal of anabolic effect of testosterone
   Delayed closure of epiphyses—Withdrawal of anabolic effect of testosterone
   Decreased excretion of 17-keto-steroids in urine—Decreased production of androgens

5. **Relationship to Minerals**   (See references in specific mineral section)
   Synergism—Zn^{2+}, Co^{2+}
   Release of hormone—Ca^{2+} required
   Increased tissue uptake of K^+, Ca^{2+}, $PO_4{}^{3-}$
   Regulates serum levels—Cu^{2+} ($\uparrow$), I^- ($\downarrow$)
   Excretion—Se ($\uparrow$)
   Impotency of aging—MoO_4 (?)

Chapter 49. Relaxin

Relaxin is a minor female sex hormone, which falls into the category of reproductive hormones. It is localized in action, and is not essential for life. It is essential for reproduction of certain mammals, but its need is not demonstrated for humans, although its presence has been shown. Its chief functions are: maintenance of pregnancy, synergism with other female hormones, separation of pubic symphysis, mammary gland stimulation, and inhibition of uterine contraction. The chief importance of relaxin lies in its role as an accessory female hormone that acts cooperatively with all the other hormones to achieve a successful pregnancy. No deficiencies are reported.

Relaxin is a slightly water-soluble polypeptide with a relatively long half-life (1 hr). No data are available on toxicity. Its chief synergists are estradiol, progesterone, and oxytocin. The chief antagonists are androgens and corticosterone.

Relaxin is formed mainly in the ovary (corpora lutea). It is also found in the placenta. Factors stimulating release are pregnenolone and low plasma levels of estradiol, or progesterone. Factors inhibiting release include androgens and corticosterone. Relaxin acts by activating enzymes (collagen depolymerases) in the pubic symphysis.

GENERAL INFORMATION

1. **Synonyms**   1, 7, 18
   Releasin, Cervilaxin

2. **History**   9, 18, 28, 36
   1926—Hisaw: cited evidence for a pregnancy hormone that causes relaxation of pelvic ligaments in preparation for parturition
   1930—Fevold et al.: extracted relaxin from corpora lutea
   1942—Abramowitz: isolated relaxin from pregnant-rabbit serum
   1955—Lehrman et al.: isolated and purified relaxin from ovaries of pregnant sows
   1966—Struck and Bhargava: isolated first homogeneous preparations of relaxin

3. **Physiological Forms**   9, 26, 37, 39
   l-relaxin

4. **Active Analogs and Related Compounds**   17, 22, 37, 39
   Peptides in relaxin family

5. **Inactive Analogs and Related Compounds**   17, 20, 21, 22, 37, 39
   Oxidized or reduced forms of relaxin

6. **Antagonists**   9, 17, 37, 39
   Androgens, corticosterone, high levels of estradiol and progesterone

7. **Synergists**   9, 17, 37, 39
   Low levels of estradiol and progesterone, oxytocin, T4

8. **Physiological Functions**   1, 4, 14, 16, 37, 39
   Enlargement of birth canal in preparation for parturition
   Separation of symphysis pubis, loss of rigidity in pelvic bones
   Decreases uterine motility
   Maintenance of pregnancy (progesterone + estrogen sparing)
   Increases sensitivity to oxytocin
   Releases oxytocin
   Stimulates mammary gland
   Stimulates imbibition of water in uterus
   Inhibits uterine contraction

9. **Deficiency Diseases, Disorders**
   None known

10. **Essentiality for Life**   1, 9, 38
   Not essential for human female reproduction, but is essential for other mammalian reproduction; otherwise not essential for life

CHEMISTRY

1. **Structure**   1, 8, 9, 15, 18
   Polypeptide (two subunits); 49-53 amino acid residues contains Ala, Asp,
   Cys, Glu, Gly, Lys, Ser, Val, guanidine

2. **Reactions**   1, 8, 9, 17, 18

   Heat—Stable in neutral solution
   Acid—Stable—Sol.
   Alkali—Inactivates—Sol.
   Water—Sol.

   Oxidation—Inactivates
   Reduction—Inactivates
   Light—No data
   Proteolysis—Trypsin
   inactivates

3. **Properties**   1, 7, 8, 9, 17, 19

   Appearance—Amorphous powder
   MW—6300-9000
   MP—No data
   Crystal Form—Amorphous
   Salts—No data
   Important groups for activity
   Guanidine, S—S, Cys

   Solubility
   H_2O—Sl. sol.
   Acet., Alc.—Insol.
   Benz., Chl., Eth.—Insol.
   Absn. max.—277.5 mμ
   Chemical activity—Polypeptide
   Miscellaneous—pI = 7.0 (approx.)

4. **Commercial Production**   9, 18, 22
   Isolation from pregnant-sow ovaries

5. **Isolation**   22, 25
   Source—Pregnant-sow ovaries
   Method—Extraction with trichloroacetic acid, glacial acetic acid, acid-acetone;
   chromatography on columns of DEAE cellulose, IRC-50; gel filtration on
   sephadex G-50

6. **Determination of Potency and Concentration**   1, 14, 22, 26, 38
   Bioassay
   Measure length of interpubic ligament in mice
   X-Ray photograph of innominate bones in estrogen-primed guinea pig
   Inhibition of motility of mouse uterine segments in vitro
   Physicochemical—None

MEDICAL AND BIOLOGICAL ROLE

1. **Species Occurrence, Specificity, and Antigenicity**   1, 9, 38
   Occurrence—Found in mammals, birds, sharks; relaxin-like substances have
   been isolated from elasmobranch ovaries and bird testes
   Specificity—High; species differences pronounced
   Antigenicity—Moderate; can be antigenic

2. Units   8, 9, 14
Guinea pig units (GPU), minimal amount necessary to cause appreciable separation of symphysis in guinea pig (est. 50-300 GPU/mg)

3. Normal Blood Levels   2, 4, 9, 22, 39
200 GPU/100 ml (pregnant sow), plasma (est. 0.6-4.0 mg/100 ml); no human values available

4. Administration   8, 9, 37, 39
Injection—Usually used
Topical—Not active
Oral—Not active

5. Factors Affecting Release   1, 4, 34
Inhibitors
    Androgens
    Corticosterone
    High progesterone level
    High estradiol level
Stimulators
    Low estradiol level
    Low progesterone level
    Pregnenolone

6. Deficiency Symptoms
Humans—Unknown

7. Effects of Overdose, Toxicity
Unknown

METABOLIC ROLE

1. Biosynthesis   22, 37, 39
Precursors
    11 of 20 standard amino acids. Missing: Try, Asn, Gln, Met, Leu, Ile, Phe, Thr, Pro—progesterone (cofactor)
    Reducing sugars
Intermediates—Unknown
Site(s) in Cell—Unknown

2. Production Sites   22, 37, 39
Corpus luteum in pregnancy; possibly placenta, uterus in some species

3. **Storage Areas**
   None

4. **Blood Carriers**
   Unknown

5. **Half-life**   8, 9, 26
   Approx. 1 hr

6. **Target Tissues**   1, 22, 37, 39
   Connective tissue of pubic symphysis
   Uterus (diminution of contractions and softening of cervix)
   Mammary gland
   Vagina

7. **Reactions**   4, 5, 22, 25, 34, 38
   Reactive forms: Unknown

Organ	Enzyme System	Effect
Public symphysis	Collagen depolymerases	Activated
Liver	Cholesterol biosynthesis	Inhibited
Uterus	Alkaline phosphatase	Increased

8. **Mode of Action**   1, 4, 5, 8, 9, 16, 31, 37, 39
   Cellular
       Anabolic—Increases uterine glycogen synthesis
       Catabolic—No data
       Other—Decreases membrane potential of myometrium; enzyme activator
   Organismal
       Increases vascularity of pubic symphysis
       Imbibition of water, disaggregation and depolymerization of mucoproteins in ground structure of symphysis
       Increases glycogen and water content of uterus, also dry weight and N content
       Decreases uterine motility
       Softens cervix of uterus
       Increases uterine sensitivity to oxytocin
       Stimulates release of oxytocin
       Relaxes interpubic ligament

9. **Catabolism**   1, 9, 22, 25, 34
   Intermediates—Peptides, amino acids
   Excretion products—Ammonia, CO_2, H_2O, amino acids, 1-4% relaxin in urine

MISCELLANEOUS

1. **Relationship to Vitamins**   8, 11, 13, 38
   Vitamin C—Maintains mucoprotein ground substance in connective tissue, affected by relaxin

2. **Relationship to Other Hormones**   8, 11, 13, 32, 38
   Estradiol—Relaxin works in conjunction with estrogens—Synergistic or antagonistic, depending on concentration (requires estrogen "priming")
   Oxytocin—Relaxin may initiate oxytocin release
   STH—Relaxin may require growth hormone for relaxation of interpubic ligament
   Progesterone—Synergistic or antagonistic, depending on concentration
   TSH—Increased biosynthesis of TSH stimulated by relaxin
   Testosterone, corticosterone—Act as release inhibitors

3. **Unusual Features**   29, 32, 38
   Hormone of pregnancy only
   Strictly female hormone, although general effects noted in body
   Found in rooster testes—No known function
   Inhibits cholesterol biosynthesis, hypocholesteremic
   Increases hydrolysis of collagen

4. **Possible Relationships of Deficiency Symptoms to Metabolic Action**   11, 13, 37
   Unknown

5. **Relationship to Minerals**   (See references in specific mineral section)
   Synergism—I⁻ (as T4)

Chapter 50. Epinephrine

Epinephrine, a hormone (catecholamine) from the adrenal medulla, is a general maintenance hormone of the tissue-controlling type. It is systemic in its effects. It is not directly essential for life, but is indirectly essential, since it is involved in stress responses via cortisol, which is essential. Its chief functions are: to increase cardiac output, blood flow, and metabolic rate; to decrease kidney function, and motility of lung, intestine, and genital systems; to excite the nervous system; and to stimulate release of ACTH and cortisol. Its chief importance lies in its very rapid and potent vasopressor response to stressful stimuli, which enables the organism to respond to emergency and stress situations. No major deficiencies are reported.

Epinephrine is a water-soluble amine with a very short half-life in blood (2 min). Excess doses can be toxic and can cause ventricular fibrillation, hypertension, tachycardia, fatigue, pallor, and increased heart rate and respiration. Synergistic agents include glucagon, cortisol, ACTH, and T4. Some antagonists are insulin, oxytocin, ergotamine, and nitrites.

Epinephrine is formed mainly in the gut and adrenal medulla, and is stored in the liver and gut chromaffin cells. Factors stimulating release of epinephrine are: hormones (cortisol, ACTH, insulin), drugs (nicotine, morphine, reserpine, histamine, acetylcholine, ether), and nervous factors (trauma, exercise, psychic). Release-inhibitors include: nerve controls and high catecholamines. Epinephrine acts by stimulating adenyl cyclase in the cell membrane, with resulting effects due to cyclic AMP.

GENERAL INFORMATION

1. **Synonyms** 1, 7, 18

    Adrenaline, Adrenin, Suprarenin, Vasotonin, Vasoconstrictine, Adrenamine, Levorenine, catecholamine

2. **History** 9, 18, 28, 36

    1895—Oliver and Shafer: demonstrated pressor effect of suprarenal extracts
    1899—Abel: named pressor agent epinephrine
    1901—Takamine, Aldrich: isolated epinephrine from animal adrenal glands
    1904—Stolz }
    1905—Dakin } synthesized *dl*-epinephrine
    1908—Flacher: responsible for resolution of *dl*-form of epinephrine
    1910—Barger and Dale: defined sympathomimetic amines and their properties
    1958—Pratesi: determined configuration of epinephrine

3. **Physiological Forms (Catecholamines)** 9, 26, 37, 39

    l-Epinephrine

4. **Active Analogs and Related Compounds (Catecholamines and others)** 17, 22, 37, 39

    d-Epinephrine (1/15 as active as *l*-isomers), norepinephrine, dopamine, ephedrin, benzedrine, paredrine, tyramine, isoproterenol

5. **Inactive Analogs and Related Compounds** 17, 22, 37, 39

    DOPA

6. **Antagonists** 9, 17, 37, 39

    Insulin, ergotamine, dibenamine, oxytocin, dibenzyline, tetraethylammonium chloride

7. **Synergists** 9, 17, 37, 39

    Glucagon, T4, cortisol, ACTH

8. **Physiological Functions** 1, 4, 14, 16, 37, 39

    Blood circulation—Increases: blood pressure (pressor agent), heart output and rate, flow in brain, liver, and skeletal muscle; peripheral vasodilator
    Kidney—Reduces glomerular filtration rate
    Lung, intestine, genital system—Inhibits motility
    Metabolic effects—Increases: O_2 consumption, temperature, BMR, gluconeogenesis
    CNS effects—Increases restlessness, anxiety, LRH release from hypothalamus
    Pituitary effects—Stimulates production and release of ACTH and corticoids
    Emergency hormone—Initiates stress reactions

9. **Deficiency Diseases, Disorders**   1, 4, 14, 16, 37, 39
   Pheochromocytoma (chromaffin cells)

10. **Essentiality for Life**   1, 9, 38
    Not absolutely essential for life of organism; possible shortening of life span
    due to decreased response to emergencies

CHEMISTRY

1. **Structure**   1, 8, 9, 15, 18

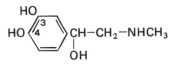

   l-Epinephrine, $C_9H_{13}NO_3$

2. **Reactions**   1, 8, 9, 17, 18
   Heat—Decomposes at 215°C
   Acid—Inactivates—Soluble
   Alkali—Unstable—Very sol. in dil.
     NaOH; insol. in NH_4OH
   Water—Sol., basic

   Oxidation—Oxidizes easily
   Reduction—Stable
   Light—Fluorescent in UV; darkens
     on exposure, forms adreno-
     chrome

3. **Properties**   1, 7, 8, 9, 17, 19
   Appearance—White crystalline
     powder
   MW—183.2
   MP—211-212°C
   Crystal form—No data
   Salts—HCl
   Important groups for activity
     Phenol, amine, alcohol
     —C(4)OH, —NH—, —CHOH

   Solubility
     H_2O—Sparingly
     Acet., Alc.—Insol.
     Benz., Chl., Eth.—Insol.
   Absn. max.—279 mμ
   Chemical nature
     Catecholamine
     Secondary amine
   $\alpha_D{}^{25} = -53.5°$ (0.5 N HCl)

4. **Commercial Production**   9, 18, 22
   Adrenal gland extractions
   Synthetic production

5. **Isolation**   22, 25
   Sources—Adrenal medulla, urine, blood
   Methods
     Hydrolysis of conjugates, if any, boiling at pH 2, 20 min
     Extraction with acidic ethanol or *n*-butanol
     Purification via paper chromatography

6. **Determination**   1, 14, 22, 26, 38
   Bioassay
      Inhibition of movement of isolated rat uterus
      Constrictor action on artery of denervated rabbit ear
   Physicochemical
      Iodochrome oxidation to distinguish norepinephrine from epinephrine
      Fluorescence in alkali
      Color reaction with ferric chloride

MEDICAL AND BIOLOGICAL ROLE

1. **Species Occurrence, Specificity, and Antigenicity**   1, 9, 38
   Occurrence—Found in all vertebrates and some invertebrates
   Specificity—None, full interspecific potency
   Antigenicity—None

2. **Units**   8, 9, 14
   By weight; 1 μg = 1 microgram

3. **Normal Blood Levels (Man)**   2, 4, 9, 22, 39
   .002-.008 μg/100 ml, plasma (venous)

4. **Administration**   8, 9, 37, 39
   Injection—Subcutaneous, intramuscular
   Topical—Active (electrophoretic application)
   Oral—Possible, but slow

5. **Factors Affecting Release**   1, 4, 34
   Inhibitors—Nerve controls, excess catecholamines
   Stimulators—Nicotine, histamine, reserpine, acetylcholine, morphine, ether,
      ACTH, glucocorticoids, low blood sugar, stress, insulin, psychic (hypo-
      thalamus) nerve controls, trauma, exercise, Ca^{2+}

6. **Deficiency Symptoms**   1, 4, 37, 38, 39
   Not fatal, but organism cannot respond to emergency, hard work, tempera-
      ture extreme, emotional disturbance

7. **Effects of Overdose, Toxicity**   1, 4, 37, 38, 39
   Decreases oxygen consumption, BMR, clotting time
   Tachycardia, restlessness, anxiety, fatigue, inhibited gastrointestinal tract
   Increases heart rate, respiration, pallor, blood sugar, sweat, blood flow
      (muscle)
   Ventricular fibrillation, paroxystic or sustained hypertension

METABOLIC ROLE

1. **Biosynthesis**   22, 37, 39
   Phenylalanine $\rightarrow$ Tyrosine $\rightarrow$ 3,4-Dihydroxyphenylalanine (DOPA) $\rightarrow$ 3,4-Di-hydroxyphenylethylamine (Dopamine) $\rightarrow$ Norepinephrine $\rightarrow$ Epinephrine
   Site(s) in cell: In golgi (osmiophilic granules)

2. **Production Sites**   22, 37, 39
   Chromaffin cells in gut and adrenal medulla

3. **Storage Areas**   8, 9, 16
   Chromaffin cells in liver and gut

4. **Blood Carriers**   2, 8, 22, 26
   Free in blood or conjugated with sulfate or glucuronides, or combined with albumin

5. **Half-life**   8, 9, 26
   About 2 min

6. **Target Tissues**   1, 22, 37, 39
   Systemic, vascular system, liver, muscles

7. **Reactions**   4, 5, 22, 25, 33, 38
   Reactive intermediate—Cyclic AMP—(secondary messenger) and Ca^{2+} (?)

Organ	Enzyme System	Effect
Muscle and liver	Phosphorylase b	Activated
	Adenyl cyclase	Activated
	Phosphorylase b kinase	Activated
	Synthetase I kinase	Activated
	Synthetase I	Inhibited
Adipose tissue	Lipase	Activated
	Adenyl cyclase	Activated

8. **Mode of Action**   1, 4, 5, 8, 9, 16, 31, 37, 39
   Cellular
      Anabolic—No data
      Catabolic—Increases glycogenolysis in liver, increases fat catabolism
   Other
      Decreases glucose entry into cells of skeletal muscle
      Increases glucose entry into heart, brain and adipose tissue cells
      Increases cyclic AMP

Suppresses mitosis
Calorigenic action
Organismal
   Increases—Systolic pressure; blood flow to skeletal muscles, liver; blood
      sugar; lipolysis; blood K^+; O_2 consumption (BMR), glucose absorption
      from gut, mental alertness, sweating
   Decreases—Glucose tolerance, eosinophils, blood flow to capillaries of
      skin and kidney, plasma volume
   Lightens chromatophores

9. **Catabolism**   1, 9, 22, 25, 34
   Intermediates—3,4-Dihydroxymandelic acid
   Excretion products—Free (0.5 to 2%) or as metanephrine (3-methoxy, 4-
      OH-mandelic acid)

MISCELLANEOUS

1. **Relationship to Vitamins**   8, 11, 13, 38
   Vitamin C—maintains reduced state of epinephrine
   Vitamins C, B_6, B_{12}, folic acid—cofactors in synthesis of epinephrine from
      phenylalanine

2. **Relationship to Other Hormones**   8, 11, 13, 32, 38
   LH, ACTH—Released by epinephrine
   Norepinephrine—Immediate precursor to epinephrine
   Insulin—Antagonist to epinephrine
   Glucagon, T4, ACH—Synergists to epinephrine
   TSH—Released by epinephrine
   Prolactin—Blocking of milk ejection by epinephrine
   Cortisol, cortisone—Synergistic in stress response with epinephrine
   Oxytocin—Epinephrine antagonistic in milk ejection

3. **Unusual Features**   29, 32, 38
   Active at 1.4 parts per billion
   Absent in developing fetus; proportion of NOR/EP = 1:4 in adult human
      adrenal (reverse in chick); blocks milk ejection; rabbit most sensitive;
      behavioral effects
   Proportion of NOR/EP varies in invertebrates
   Increases mental alertness
   Calorigenic action

4. **Possible Relationships of Deficiency Symptoms to Metabolic Action**   11,
   13, 37
   Decreased emergency response—Decreased lipolysis in adipose tissue results
      in decreased glucose energy (ATP) available for stress reaction

Decreased response to emotional disturbances, temperature extremes, hard work—As in the previous symptom

5. **Relationships to Minerals**   (See references in specific mineral section)
Synergists—I^- (as T4), PO_4^{3-} (as cyclic AMP)
Release of hormone—Ca^{2+} required
Blood K^+ increased
Cu^{2+} and Fe^{2+} enzymes required for synthesis, also Mn^{2+}

Chapter 51. Norepinephrine

Norepinephrine is a hormone (catecholamine) and a neurotransmitter from the adrenal medulla and adrenergic nerve endings. It is a general maintenance hormone of the tissue-controlling type, which is systemic in its effects. It is not directly essential for life unless other similar neurotransmitters are absent, in which case it becomes essential. Its chief functions are: increase in blood pressure by vasoconstriction; decrease in kidney function, and motility of lung, gut, and genital system; small increase in metabolic rate; and use as precursor to epinephrine. No major deficiencies are reported.

Norepinephrine is a water-soluble amine with a very short half-life in blood (2 min). Excess secretion or doses can be toxic and cause bradycardia and pheochromocytoma. Synergistic agents are epinephrine, cortisol, glucagon, and serotonin. Antagonists are insulin and vasopressin.

Norepinephrine is formed mainly in the adrenal medulla at chromaffin cells and adrenergic nerve endings. It is stored in chromaffin cells in the liver and gut, as well as in the adrenal medulla. Factors stimulating release of norepinephrine are: drugs (nicotine, histamine, reserpine, morphine), nervous factors (stress, trauma, nerve controls), and physiological agents (acetylcholine, tyrosine, phenylalanine, low blood glucose, and T4).

Norepinephrine acts by stimulating cell membrane receptors to produce cyclic AMP, which then causes release or synthesis of various new cell products.

GENERAL INFORMATION

1. **Synonyms** 1, 7, 18

   Noradrenaline, arterenol, levarterenol, sympathin, catecholamine

2. **History**   9, 18, 28, 36

    1898—Lewandowsky ⎫ Noted similarity of effects of adrenal gland extracts

    1901—Langley   ⎭ and stimulation of sympathetic nerves, on tissues

    1904—Eliot: proposed sympathetic nerve endings release epinephrine-like substance

    1910—Barger and Dale: synthesized norepinephrine

    1927—Cannon and Uridil: noted that liver releases epinephrine-like substance called sympathin on stimulation of sympathetic nerves

    1948—Tullar: resolved *dl*-form of norepinephrine

    1951—Euler: demonstrated sympathin to be norepinephrine

    1959—Pratesi: established configuration of norepinephrine

3. **Physiological Forms (Catecholamines)**   9, 26, 37, 39

    l-Norepinephrine

4. **Active Analogs and Related Compounds (Catecholamines and others)**   17, 22, 37, 39

    Dopamine, ephedrine, *d*-norepinephrine, *d*-epinephrine (1/15 as active as *l*-isomers)

5. **Inactive Analogs and Related Compounds**   17, 22, 37, 39

    DOPA

6. **Antagonists**   9, 17, 37, 39

    Insulin, vasopressin

7. **Synergists**   9, 17, 37, 39

    Epinephrine, serotonin, cortisol, cortisone, glucagon

8. **Physiological Functions**   1, 4, 14, 16, 37, 39

    Blood circulation—Increases blood pressure, peripheral vasoconstrictor, without change or slight decrease in output and heart rate; no flow increase in brain, liver, or muscle

    Kidney—Decreases glomerular filtration rate

    Lung, intestine, genital system—Inhibited

    Metabolic effects—Weak epinephrine effect

    CNS effects—Adrenergic transmitter agent at synapses, no brain excitation

    Pituitary effects—None

    Maintenance hormone—Diurnal regulation

    Immediate precursor of epinephrine

9. **Deficiency Diseases, Disorders   1, 4, 14, 16, 37, 39**
   Neuroblastoma (excess)
   Pheochromocytoma (excess)

10. **Essentiality for Life   1, 9, 38**
    Not absolutely essential for life of organism, except if other neurotransmitters not available

CHEMISTRY

1. **Structure   1, 8, 9, 15, 18**

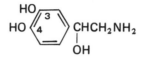

   l-Norepinephrine, $C_8H_{11}NO_3$

2. **Reactions   1, 8, 9, 17, 18**

Heat—Unstable	Oxidation—Easily oxidizes to nor-
Acid—Inactivates	adrenochrome
Alkali—Very sol. dil. NaOH;	Reduction—Stable
Insol. NH_4OH	Light—No fluorescence in UV
Water—Soluble, alkaline	

3. **Properties   1, 7, 8, 9, 17, 19**
   Appearance—Colorless crystals
   MW—169.2
   MP—145-146°C
   Crystal form—No data
   Solubility
     H_2O—Sparingly
     Acet., Alc.—Sl. sol.
     Benz., Chl., Eth.—Sl. sol.
   Absn. max.—279 mμ

   Salts—HCl
   Important groups for activity
     —CHOH (alcohol), —C(4)OH
     (phenol), —NH_2 (amine)
   Chemical nature—Catecholamine;
     primary amine
   $\alpha_D^{25} = -37.3$ (HCl)
   Misc.—pK = 8.8, 9.98

4. **Commercial Production   9, 18, 22**
   Synthetic production

5. **Isolation   22, 25**
   Sources—Adrenal medulla, blood, urine
   Methods
     Hydrolysis of conjugates, if any—Boil at pH 2, 20 min
     Extraction with acidic ethanol or *n*-butanol

6. **Determination**   1, 4, 22, 26, 38
Bioassay—Pressor effect in cat, rat
Physicochemical
    Colorimetric—Ferric chloride complex
    Fluorometric—Condense with ethylenediamine

MEDICAL AND BIOLOGICAL ROLE

1. **Species, Occurrence, Specificity, and Antigenicity**   1, 9, 38
Occurrence—Found in all vertebrates and some invertebrates
Specificity—None; full, interspecific potency
Antigenicity—None

2. **Units**   8, 9, 14
By weight; 1 μg = 1 microgram

3. **Normal Blood Levels (Man)**   2, 4, 9, 22, 39
.012-.028 μg/100 ml plasma (venous)

4. **Administration**   8, 9, 37, 39
Injection—Usual
Topical—By electrophoresis through skin
Oral—Inactive

5. **Factors Affecting Release**   1, 4, 34
Inhibitors—Nerve controls, excess catecholamines
Stimulators—ACH, nicotine, histamine, Tyr, Phe, low blood sugar, low T4,
    nerve controls, stress, trauma, reserpine, morphine

6. **Deficiency Symptoms**   1, 4, 37, 38, 39
Poor nerve condition
Orthostatic hypotension—Fainting on standing up, dizziness, lightheadedness

7. **Effects of Overdose, Toxicity**   1, 4, 37, 38, 39
Bradycardia, pheochromocytoma

METABOLIC ROLE

1. **Biosynthesis**   22, 37, 39
Phenylalanine $\rightarrow$ Tyrosine $\rightarrow$ 3,4-Dihydroxyphenylalanine (dopa) $\rightarrow$ 3,4-Di-
    hydroxyphenylethylamine (dopamine) $\rightarrow$ Norepinephrine
Site(s) in cell—Osmiophilic granules in Golgi apparatus

2. Production Sites   22, 37, 39
Adrenal medulla
Adrenergic nerve endings
Chromaffin cells—Sympathetic nerves and ganglia, gut

3. Storage Areas   8, 9, 16
Chromaffin cells in liver and gut, intraaxonal spaces, adrenal medulla

4. Blood Carriers   2, 8, 22, 26
Free or sulfate, glucuronide esters

5. Half-life   8, 9, 26
2 min or less

6. Target Tissues   1, 22, 37, 39
Systemic, esp. vascular system, lung, eye

7. Reactions   4, 5, 22, 25, 34, 38
Reactive intermediate: Cyclic AMP (secondary messenger) and Ca^{2+} (?)

Organ	Enzyme System	Effect
Muscle and liver	Adenyl cyclase	Activated
	Phosphorylase b	Activated
	Phosphorylase b kinase	Activated
	Synthetase I kinase	Activated
	Synthetase I	Inhibited
Adipose tissue	Adenyl cyclase	Activated
	Lipase	Activated

8. Mode of Action   1, 4, 5, 8, 9, 16, 31, 37, 39
Cellular
    Anabolic—No data
    Catabolic
        Increased CHO catabolism
        Increased glycogen to glucose conversion
        Increased fat catabolism
    Other—No data
Organismal
    Decreases—Pulse, blood flow, gastrointestinal and genital activity, respiration, kidney function
    Increases—Diastolic and systolic pressure, vasodilation of coronary arteries, lipid mobilization, glucose absorption from gut
    Bradycardia
    Vasoconstrictor

9. **Catabolism**   1, 9, 22, 25, 34
   Intermediates—3,4-Dihydroxymandelic acid
   Excretion products—Free in urine (3-6%), normetanephrine, 3-methoxy, 4-hydroxymandelic acid

MISCELLANEOUS

1. **Relationship to Vitamins**   8, 11, 13, 38
   Vitamin C protects against oxidation of norepinephrine
   Vitamins B_6, C, folic acid—cofactors in synthesis of norepinephrine from phenylalanine

2. **Relationship to Other Hormones**   8, 11, 13, 32, 38
   Epinephrine—Derivative of norepinephrine; synergist also
   Insulin—Antagonist to norepinephrine, secretion inhibited by norepinephrine
   Serotonin, cortisol, cortisone—Synergists to norepinephrine
   T4, ACH—Stimulators for release of norepinephrine

3. **Unusual Features**   29, 37, 38
   Neurohumor—Much carried intraaxonally
   EPA/NOR = 4/1 in medulla (man)
   Diurnal (higher in day)
   No behavioral effects
   Increases pigment concentration in skin
   Main amine in fetus
   Anticipatory type, i.e., normal plasma maintenance

4. **Possible Relationships of Deficiency Symptoms to Metabolic Action**   11, 13, 37
   Poor nerve conduction—Lack of transmitter-agent
   Dizziness, light-headedness, fainting—Low blood pressure

5. **Relationships to Minerals**   (See references in specific mineral section)
   Synergism—PO_4^{3-} (as cyclic AMP)
   Release of hormone—Low I^- (as T4)
   Cu + Fe enzymes required for synthesis; also Mn^{2+}

PRINCIPAL REFERENCES, Part III

GENERAL—HORMONES, VITAMINS, etc.

1. Altman, P. L., and Dittmer, D. S. (Eds.), *Biology Data Book*, Vols. II and III, 2nd ed., Fed. Am. Soc. Exp. Biol., Washington, D.C. (1974).
2. Altman, P. L., and Dittmer, D. S. (Eds.), *Human Health and Disease*, Fed. Am. Soc. Exp. Biol., Washington, D.C. (1977).
3. Altman, P. L. and Dittmer, D. S. (Eds.), *Metabolism*, Fed. Am. Soc. Exp. Biol., Washington, D.C. (1968).
4. Berkow, R. (Ed.), *The Merck Manual*, 13th ed., Merck & Co., Rahway, N.J. (1977).
5. Boyer, P. D., and Snell, E. E. (Eds.), *Annual Reviews of Biochemistry*, Vols. 36-47, Annual Reviews, Inc., Palo Alto, Calif. (1967-78).
6. Conn, E. E., and Stumpf, P. K., *Outlines of Biochemistry*, 3rd ed., Wiley, New York (1976).
7. Dawson, R. M. C., Elliott, D. C., Elliot, W. H., and Jones, K. M. (Eds.), *Data for Biochemical Research*, 2nd ed., Oxford University Press, New York and Oxford (1969).
8. Diem, K. (Ed.), *Documenta Geigy Scientific Tables*, 6th ed., Geigy Pharmaceuticals, Ardsley, N.Y. (1962).
9. Goodman, L. S. and Gilman, A. (Ed.), *The Pharmaceutical Basis of Therapeutics*, 5th ed., Macmillan, New York (1975).
10. Greenberg, D. M. (Ed.), *Metabolic Pathways*, 3rd ed., Vol. VII, Academic Press, New York and London (1975).
11. Harris, R. S., and Thimann, K. (Eds.), *Vitamins and Hormones*, Vols. 25-34, Academic Press, New York and London (1967-76).
12. Long, C. (Ed.), *Biochemists' Handbook*, Van Nostrand Reinhold, New York (1961).
13. Needham, A. E., *The Growth Process in Animals*, Van Nostrand Reinhold, New York (1964).
14. Oser, B. L. (Ed.), *Hawk's Physiological Chemistry*, 14th ed., McGraw-Hill (Blakiston Div.), New York (1965).
15. Weast, R. C. (Ed.), *Handbook of Chemistry and Physics*, 57th ed., The Chemical Rubber Co., Cleveland, Ohio (1976).
16. West, E. S., Todd, W. R., Mason, H. S., and Van Bruggen, J. T., *Textbook of Biochemistry*, 4th ed., Macmillan, New York (1966).
17. Wilson, C. O., Gisvold, O., Doerge, R. E. (Eds.), *Textbook of Organic Medicinal and Pharmaceutical Chemistry*, 6th ed., Lippincott, Philadelphia (1971).
18. Windholz, M. (Ed.), *The Merck Index* 9th ed., Merck & Co., Inc., Rahway, N.J. (1976).

SPECIFIC—HORMONES

19. Back, N., Martini, L., and Paoletti, R. (Eds.), Pharmacology of hormonal polypeptides and proteins, in *Advances in Exp. Med. Biol.*, Vol. 2, Plenum Press, New York (1968).

19a. Breuer, H., Hamel, D., Krüskemper, H. L., *Methods of Hormone Analysis*, Wiley, New York (1976).

20. Briggs, M. H. (Ed.), *Advances in Steroid Biochemistry and Pharmacology*, Vols. 1-5, Academic Press, New York and London (1970-76).

21. Briggs, M. H., and Brotherton, J., *Steroid Biochemistry and Pharmacology*, Academic Press, London and New York (1970).

22. Butt, W. R., *Hormone Chemistry*, Vol. I, 2nd ed., Wiley, New York (1976).

23. Eisenstein, A. B. (Ed.), *The Adrenal Cortex*, Little, Brown and Co., Boston (1967).

24. Fieser, L. F., and Fieser, M., *Steroids*, Van Nostrand Reinhold, New York (1959).

25. Frieden, E., *Chemical Endocrinology*, Academic Press, New York (1976).

26. Gray, C. H., and Bacharach, A. L. (Eds.), *Hormones in Blood*, Vols. 1 and 2, 2nd ed., Academic Press, London and New York (1967).

27. Hafez, E., and Reel, J. R. (Eds.), *Hypothalamic Hormones*, Vol. I, Ann Arbor Sci. Pub., Ann Arbor, Mich. (1975).

28. Harland, W. A., and Orr, J. S. (Eds.), *Thyroid Hormone Metabolism*, Academic Press, New York (1975).

29. Krüskemper, H. L., *Anabolic Steroids*, Academic Press, New York and London (1968).

30. Labrie, F., Meites, J., and Pelletier, G. (Eds.), *Hypothalamus and Endocrine Functions*, Plenum Press, New York (1976).

31. Litwack, G. (Ed.), *Biochemical Actions of Hormones*, Vols. I, II, and III, Academic Press, New York and London (1970-75).

32. Martini, L., and Ganong, W. F. (Eds.), *Neuroendocrinology*, Vols. I and II, Academic Press, New York and London (1967).

33. McKerns, K. W., *Steroid Hormones and Metabolism*, Appleton-Century-Crofts (Meredith Corp.), New York (1969).

34. Sawin, C. T., *The Hormones*, Little, Brown and Co., Boston (1969).

35. Schulster, D., Burstein, S., and Cooke, B., *Molecular Endocrinology of the Steroid Hormones*, Wiley, New York (1976).

36. Tepperman, J., *Metabolic and Endocrine Physiology*, 3rd ed., Year Book Medical Publishers, Chicago (1973).

37. Thomas, J., and Mawhinney, M., *Synopsis of Endocrine Pharmacology*, University Park Press, Baltimore, Md. (1973).

38. Turner, C. D. and Bagnara, J. T., *General Endocrinology*, 6th ed., Saunders, Philadelphia (1976).

39. Williams, R. H. (Ed.), *Textbook of Endocrinology*, 5th ed., Saunders, Philadelphia (1974).

Summarizing Tables

Table 1. Characteristics of Vitamins

(+ = present in structure or function ± = slightly)
(− = catabolic or inhibiting effect)

Structural Component or Function	A	B_1	B_2	B_6	B_{12}	C	D	E	K	Biotin	F.A.[a]	Niacin	P.A.[b]
Amino acid										+	+		+
Purine, pyrimidine (derivative)		+	+		+								
Benzene ring			+					+	+		+		
Pyridine ring				+								+	
Isoprene group (derivative)	+						+	+	+				
Sugar (derivative)			+		+	+							
Alcohol groups	+	+	+	+	+	+	+	+			+		+
Double bonds (−C=C−)	+	+	+	+	+	+	+	+	+		+	+	+
Elements other than CHON		S			Co					S			
Redox agent			+		+	+		+	+		+	+	
PO$_4$ complex in vivo		+	+	+	+	+	+				+	+	+
Antioxidant			+			+		+					

Property												
Biosynthesis via cholesterol pathway	+									+	+		
Anabolic functions	+	+	+	+	+	+	+	+	+	+	+		
Catabolic functions	+	+	±	+	+	+	+	+	+	+	+		
Stored in organism (man)	+	±	±	±	+	±	±	+	±	+	±		
Available from intestinal bacteria (man)	±	±	+	+					+				
Toxic in excess (man)	+	+	+	±	+	+	+			+			
Mitosis effect			+	−	+						+		
Mitochondrial sites	+	+	+	+	+	+	+			+			
Chloroplast sites	+g	+	+							+			
Microsomal sites					+					+			
Membrane sites	+	+	+	+	+	+	+			+			
Protein synthesis				+	±		+						
Amino acid synthesis		−	−					±	±	±	−		
CHO synthesis	+	−	+	+	+	−	+			+			

a Folic acid.　　b Pantothenic acid.　　g Carotenoids.

Table 1. Characteristics of Vitamins (continued)

(+ = stimulating effect or present in organelles)

Structural Component or Function	A	B_1	B_2	B_6	B_{12}	C	D	E	K	Biotin	F.A.[a]	Niacin	P.A.[b]
TCA cycle effect		+	+									+	+
Lipid synthesis					+							±	±
Fatty acid synthesis				+						+			±
Nucleic acid synthesis					+								
Purine pyrimidine synthesis					+					+	+		
Mineral metabolism	ZnCa,P	Mg,P	Fe,P	Zn,P	Co,Ca,P	Fe,Ca	Ca,P,Se		Mn	Mn	Fe,Cu	ZnCr	Zn
H₂O metabolism													+
Hormone synthesis	Prog.[e] Cortic.[c] Andro.[d]	ACH[f]		ACH[f] Nor. Serot.		Serot. Gluc.						+	ACH[f]
Sterol synthesis	+			+		+						+	+

[a]Folic acid. [b]Pantothenic acid. [c]Corticosterone. [d]Androstenedione. [e]Progesterone. [f]Acetylcholine.

Table 2.　Synergisms (+) and Antagonisms (−) Among the Vitamins

Vitamins	A	B_1	B_2	B_6	B_{12}	C	D	E	K	Biotin	F.A.[a]	Niacin	P.A.[b]
A			+	+	+			±					
B_1			+	+	+							+	+
B_2	+	+		+	+					+	+	+	+
B_6		+	+			+		+		+	+	+	
B_{12}	+	+	+			+		+		+	+	+	+
C	+			+	+			+	+		+		+
D												+	
E	±			+	+	+			+		+		
K						+		+					
Biotin		+	+	+							+		+
F.A.[a]		+	+	+	+			+		+		+	+
Niacin		+	+	+	+		+				+		+
P.A.[b]		+	+		+	+				+	+	+	

[a]Folic acid.　[b]Pantothenic acid.

Table 3. Characteristics of Hormones

Hormones[a]	Amino Acid Units (Proteins, Peptides)	S—S Bonds	CHO Component	Steroid Unit	Catecholamine	Elements Other Than CHON	Redox Couple in Vivo	Mediated Via Cyclic AMP	CHO Anabolism + / Catabolism −	Lipid Anabolism + / or Fat Catabolism −	Protein (Amino Acid) Anabolism + / Catabolism −	Nucleic Acid (or Purine, pyrim.) Anabolism + / Catabolism −	Steroid Anabolism + / Catabolism −	Mineral and H₂O Balance	Mitotic Effect (Increase +, Decrease −)	Membrane Effect	Kidney Function	Blood Pressure	Nerve Function
ACTH	+					S		+	−	−			+[b]						
Aldos.				+			+		±	−	±	±		+	−	+	+		
Cort.				+			+		±	±	±	±		+	−	+	+		
Epi.					+		+	+	−	−	+	+	+[b]	+	+	+	+	+	+
Est.				+			+		±	+	+	+			+	+			+
FSH	+	+	+			S		+	+		+		+			+			
Gluc.	+					S		+	+	−	−			+		+	+		
GH (STH)	+	+				S		+	+	−	+	+		+	+	+	+		
(HRH)	+	+				S		+								+			

465

[a]				[b]												
In.	+	+		S		±	+	+	+	+	+	+	+	+	+	+
LH	+	+	+	S		−	+	+	+	+	+	+	+	+	+	+
MSH	+		+	S		−	+				+			+		
Norepi.	+	+	+	S		−	−	+			+	+	+	+	+	+
Oxy.	+	+		S		+					+	+	+	+	+	+
PTH	+			S		−					+	+	+	+	+	
Prog.	+			S	+	±	±			+	+	+	+	+	+	
Prol.	+	+		S		+	−	+	+	+	+	+	+	+	+	+
Relax.	+	+		S		±			+		+	+	+	+	+	
Test.				S	+	−	−	+	+	+	+	+	+	+	+	+
TCT	+	+		S		+	+	+	+	+	+	+	+	+	+	
T4	+			−		−	−	+	+	+	+	+	+	+	+	
TSH	+	+	+	S		−	−	±	+	+	+			+		
Vaso.	+	+		S		−	−	+	+	+	+	+	+	+	+	+

[a]See list of abbreviations for full name.

[b]Release.

466

Table 4.   Synergisms (+) and Antagonisms (−) Among the Hormones

Hormones[a]	ACTH	Aldos.	Cort.	Epi.	Est.	FSH.	Gluc.	GH (STH)	HRH	In.	LH
ACTH			±	+				±		−	
Aldos.			−		−			+			
Cort.	±	−		+	±		+	±		−	
Epi.	+		+				+			−	
Est.		−	±					+	+		
FSH								+			+
Gluc.			+	+						−	
GH (STH)	±	+	±		+	+				±	
HRH											
In.	−		−	−	+	−	−	±			±
LH						+				±	
MSH			±	−				+			
Norepi.			+	+			+			−	
Oxy.		+	±	−	+			+			
PTH			±		±[b]			−			
Prog.		−	+		±			+			
Prol.			+		±			+			±
Relax.		−			±						
Test.		−			±			+		+	
TCT					+						
T4	±		+	+	+	+		+		−	+
TSH	+							+			
Vaso.		±	−	+				+			

[a]See list of abbreviations for full name.   [b]Birds.

Table 4. (continued)   Synergisms and Antagonisms Among the Hormones

Hormones[a]	MSH	Norepi.	Oxy.	PTH	Prog.	Prol.	Relax.	Test.	TCT	T4	TSH	Vaso.
ACTH									±	+		
Aldos.			+		−							.±
Cort.	±	+	±	±	+	+	−	−		+		−
Epi.	−	+	−							+		−
Est.			+	±[b]	±	±	±	±	+	+		
FSH										+		
Gluc.		+										
GH (STH)	+		+	−	+	+		+		+	+	+
HRH												
In.		−						+		−		
LH					±					+		
MSH										+	+	
Norepi.												−
Oxy.					±	+	+			+		
PTH					+				−	−	−	
Prog.			±			+	±	±		+		
Prol.			+	+	+			−		+		+
Relax.			+		±			−		+		+
Test.			−		±	−	−					+
TCT			−									
T4	+		+	−	+	+	+				+	+
TSH	+								+			
Vaso.		−			+		+		+			

[a]See list of abbreviations for full name.   [b]Birds.

Table 5.   Synergisms (+) and Antagonisms (−) Between Vitamins and Hormones

Hormones[a]	A	B₁	B₂	B₆	B₁₂	C	D	E	K	Biotin	F.A.[b]	Niacin	P.A.[c]
ACTH	+						+					+	+
Aldos.													
Cort.					±	−							
Epi.				+	+								
Est.	−		−			+	+			+			
FSH													
Gluc.				+									
GH (STH)	+	+	+	+	+	+	+	+	+	+	+	+	+
					All related to growth								
HRH													
In.		+	+		−								
LH							+						
MSH	+												
Norepi.				+	+								
Oxy.													
PTH						±							
Prog.													
Prol.[e]	+	+	+	+	+	+	+	+	+	+	+	+	+
Relax.													
Test.	+	+	+			+	+	+		+	+		
TCT						−							
T4	±[d]	+	+	−		+		−				+	
TSH	−[d]		+										
Vaso.													

[a]See list of abbreviations for full name.   [b]Folic acid.   [c]Pantothenic acid.   [d]Large Doses.
[e]All synergistic when acting as a growth hormone.

Table 6.   Principal Functional Relationships of Vitamins and Hormones

( ) = indirect effect   ___ = Major Effect

Function	Vitamin(s)[a]	Hormone(s)[a]
Bone and Ca metabolism	A, C, D	Cort., (ACTH), Est., GH PTH, Test., TCT, T4, (TSH)
Circulation, blood cells	B$_6$, B$_{12}$, C, E, K, Bio., F.A., P.A.	Cort., (ACTH), Epi., Norepi., Vaso.
Digestion and absorption	B$_1$, B$_{12}$, D, E, F.A., Nia.	Cort., (ACTH), Gluc., In., PTH, T4 (TSH)
Epithelium, skin (membrane effect)	A, B$_2$, B$_{12}$, D, Bio., P.A.	Aldos., Cort., (ACTH), Epi., Est., GH, In., Norepi., Oxy., Prog., Relax., Test., T4 (TSH), Vaso.
Fat and CHO metabolism	B$_1$, B$_2$, B$_6$, B$_{12}$, Bio., Nia., P.A.	(ACTH), Aldos., Cort., Epi., Est., Gluc., GH, In., Norepi., T4 (TSH), Test.
Growth	All, by definition	All, by definition; Esp.: Est., GH, In., T4 (TSH), Test.
Metabolic rate, temperature (TCA Cycle)	B$_1$, B$_2$, C, E, K, Nia., P.A.	Epi., Norepi., Prog., T4, (TSH), Test.
Nerve function, psyche	A, B$_1$, B$_2$, B$_{12}$, C, Bio., Nia., F.A., P.A.	Cort., (ACTH), Epi., Norepi., Prol., Test., T4, (TSH), Est.
Pigmentation	B$_6$, C, F.A., Nia.	(ACTH), Cort., MSH
Pregnancy, lactation	All required at higher levels	Cort., (ACTH), Est. (FSH), GH, In., (LH), Oxy., Prol., Prog., Relax., T4, (TSH)
Salt (Na) and H$_2$O metabolism	B$_6$, P.A. (A, C, E, Nia.)	Aldos., Cort., (ACTH), Epi., Gluc., GH., (In.), Norepi., Oxy., Prog., T4, (TSH), Vaso.
Stress, immunity	C, P.A., A (B$_1$, B$_2$, B$_6$, K, Bio., F.A.)	Aldo., Cort., (ACTH), Est.
Visual mechanisms	A, B$_2$	

[a]See list of abbreviations for full name.

1980 REVISED RECOMMENDED DIETARY ALLOWANCES

The following tables have been approved by the National Academy of Sciences for distribution. They included tables on (a) recommended energy intakes, together with mean heights and weights; (b) the Recommended Dietary Allowances for protein, fat-soluble vitamins, water-soluble vitamins, and minerals; and (c) estimates of adequate and safe intakes of selected vitamins, trace elements, and electrolytes.

For further information, write or call: Myrtle L. Brown, PH.D., Executive Secretary, Food and Nutrition Board, 2101 Constitution Avenue, Washington, D.C. 20418; 202–389-6366.

Table 7.   Mean Heights and Weights and Recommended Energy Intake*

Age and Sex Group	Weight kg	Weight lb	Height cm	Height in	Energy Needs MJ	Energy Needs kcal	Energy Range in kcal
Infants							
0.0-0.5 yr	6	13	60	24	kg × 0.48	kg × 115	95-145
0.5-1.0 yr	9	20	71	28	kg × 0.44	kg × 105	80-135
Children							
1-3 yr	13	29	90	35	5.5	1,300	900-1,800
4-6 yr	20	44	112	44	7.1	1,700	1,300-2,300
7-10 yr	28	62	132	52	10.1	2,400	1,650-3,300
Males							
11-14 yr	45	99	157	62	11.3	2,700	2,000-3,700
15-18 yr	66	145	176	69	11.8	2,800	2,100-3,900
19-22 yr	70	154	177	70	12.2	2,900	2,500-3,300
23-50 yr	70	154	178	70	11.3	2,700	2,300-3,100
51-75 yr	70	154	178	70	10.1	2,400	2,000-2,800
76+ yr	70	154	178	70	8.6	2,050	1,650-2,450
Females							
11-14 yr	46	101	157	62	9.2	2,200	1,500-3,000
15-18 yr	55	120	163	64	8.8	2,100	1,200-3,000
19-22 yr	55	120	163	64	8.8	2,100	1,700-2,500
23-50 yr	55	120	163	64	8.4	2,000	1,600-2,400
51-75 yr	55	120	163	64	7.6	1,800	1,400-2,200
76+ yr	55	120	163	64	6.7	1,600	1,200-2,000
Pregnancy						+300	
Lactation						+500	

*From Recommended Dietary Allowances, Revised 1980, Food and Nutrition Board, National Academy of Sciences—National Research Council, Washington, D.C. The data in this table have been assembled from the observed median heights and weights of children, together with desirable weights for adults for mean heights of men (70 in.) and women (64 in.) between the ages of eighteen and thirty-four years as surveyed in the U.S. population (DHEW/NCHS data).

Energy allowances for the young adults are for men and women doing light work. The allowances for the two older age groups represent mean energy needs over these age spans, allowing for a 2 percent decrease in basal (resting) metabolic rate per decade and a reduction in activity of 200 kcal per day for men and women between fifty-one and seventy-five years; 500 kcal for men over seventy-five years; and 400 kcal for women over seventy-five. The customary range of daily energy output is shown for adults in the range column and is based on a variation in energy needs of ±400 kcal at any one age, emphasizing the wide range of energy intakes appropriate for any group of people.

Energy allowances for children through age eighteen are based on median energy intakes of children of these ages followed in longitudinal growth studies. Ranges are the 10th and 90th percentiles of energy intake, to indicate range of energy consumption among children of these ages.

Table 8.   Recommended Dietary Allowances, Revised 1980*
Designed for the maintenance of good nutrition
of practically all healthy people in the U.S.A.
FOOD AND NUTRITION BOARD,
NATIONAL ACADEMY OF SCIENCES-NATIONAL RESEARCH COUNCIL

Age and Sex Group	Weight kg	Weight lb	Height cm	Height in	Protein	Fat-soluble Vitamins Vitamin A	Fat-soluble Vitamins Vita-min D	Fat-soluble Vitamins Vitamin E	Water-soluble Vitamins Vita-min C	Water-soluble Vitamins Thia-min	Water-soluble Vitamins Ribo-flavin
						μg R.E.†	μg‡	mg αT.E.#	◄————	mg	————►
Infants											
0.0-0.5 yr	6	13	60	24	kg × 2.2	420	10	3	35	0.3	0.4
0.5-1.0 yr	9	20	71	28	kg × 2.0	400	10	4	35	0.5	0.6
Children											
1-3 yr	13	29	90	35	23	400	10	5	45	0.7	0.8
4-6 yr	20	44	112	44	30	500	10	6	45	0.9	1.0
7-10 yr	28	62	132	52	34	700	10	7	45	1.2	1.4
Males											
11-14 yr	45	99	157	62	45	1,000	10	8	50	1.4	1.6
15-18 yr	66	145	176	69	56	1,000	10	10	60	1.4	1.7
19-22 yr	70	154	177	70	56	1,000	7.5	10	60	1.5	1.7
23-50 yr	70	154	178	70	56	1,000	5	10	60	1.4	1.6
51+ yr	70	154	178	70	56	1,000	5	10	60	1.2	1.4
Females											
11-14 yr	46	101	157	62	46	800	10	8	50	1.1	1.3
15-18 yr	55	120	163	64	46	800	10	8	60	1.1	1.3
19-22 yr	55	120	163	64	44	800	7.5	8	60	1.1	1.3
23-50 yr	55	120	163	64	44	800	5	8	60	1.0	1.2
51+ yr	55	120	163	64	44	800	5	8	60	1.0	1.2
Pregnancy					+30	+200	+5	+2	+20	+0.4	+0.3
Lactation					+20	+400	+5	+3	+40	+0.5	+0.5

*The allowances are intended to provide for individual variations among most normal persons as they live in the United States under usual environmental stresses. Diets should be based on a variety of common foods in order to provide other nutrients for which human requirements have been less well defined. See text for detailed discussion of allowances and of nutrients not tabulated. See preceding table for weights and heights by individual year of age and for suggested average energy intakes.

†Retinol equivalents; 1 retinol equivalent = 1μg retinol or 6μg β-carotene. See text for calculation of vitamin activity of diets as retinol equivalents.

‡As cholecalciferol: 10 μg cholecalciferol = 400 I.U. vitamin D.

#αtocopherol equivalents: 1 mg d-α-tocopherol = 1αT.E. See text for variation in allowances and calculation of vitamin E activity of the diet as α tocopherol equivalents.

¶1 N.E. (niacin equivalent) = 1 mg niacin or 60 mg dietary tryptophan.

‖The folacin allowances refer to dietary sources as determined by *Lactobacillus casei* assay

Water-soluble Vitamins				Minerals					
Niacin	Vita-min B$_6$	Fola-cin[||]	Vita-min B$_{12}$	Cal-cium	Phos-phorus	Magne-sium	Iron	Zinc	Iodine
mg N.E.[¶]	mg	⟵ µg ⟶		⟵ mg ⟶					µg
6	0.3	30	0.5**	360	240	50	10	3	40
8	0.6	45	1.5	540	360	70	15	5	50
9	0.9	100	2.0	800	800	150	15	10	70
11	1.3	200	2.5	800	800	200	10	10	90
16	1.6	300	3.0	800	800	250	10	10	120
18	1.8	400	3.0	1,200	1,200	350	18	15	150
18	2.0	400	3.0	1,200	1,200	400	18	15	150
19	2.2	400	3.0	800	800	350	10	15	150
18	2.2	400	3.0	800	800	350	10	15	150
16	2.2	400	3.0	800	800	350	10	15	150
15	1.8	400	3.0	1,200	1,200	300	18	15	150
14	2.0	400	3.0	1,200	1,200	300	18	15	150
14	2.0	400	3.0	800	800	300	18	15	150
13	2.0	400	3.0	800	800	300	18	15	150
13	2.0	400	3.0	800	800	300	10	15	150
+2	+0.6	+400	+1.0	+400	+400	+150	[††]	+5	+25
+5	+0.5	+100	+1.0	+400	+400	+150	[††]	+10	+50

after treatment with enzymes ("conjugases") to make polyglutamyl forms of the vitamin available to the test organism.

**The RDA for vitamin B$_{12}$ in infants is based on average concentration of the vitamin in human milk. The allowances after weaning are based on energy intake (as recommended by the American Academy of Pediatrics) and consideration of other factors, such as intestinal absorption.

††The increased requirement during pregnancy cannot be met by the iron content of habitual American diets or by the existing iron stores of many women; therefore, the use of 30 to 60 mg supplemental iron is recommended. Iron needs during lactation are not substantially different from those of non-pregnant women, but continued supplementation of the mother for two to three months after parturition is advisable in order to replenish stores depleted by pregnancy.

Table 9. Estimated Safe and Adequate Daily Dietary Intakes of Additional Selected Vitamins and Minerals*

Age Group	Vitamins			Trace Elements†						Electrolytes		
	Vitamin K (μg)	Biotin (μg)	Panto-thenic Acid	Copper (mg)	Man-ganese	Fluoride	Chromium	Selenium	Molyb-denum	Sodium	Potassium	Chloride
Infants												
0.0-0.5 yr	12	35	2	0.5-0.7	0.5-0.7	0.1-0.5	0.01-0.04	0.01-0.04	0.03-0.06	115-350	350-925	275-700
0.5-1.0 yr	10-20	50	3	0.7-1.0	0.7-1.0	0.2-1.0	0.02-0.06	0.02-0.06	0.04-0.08	250-750	425-1,275	400-1,200
Children and adolescents												
1-3 yr	15-30	65	3	1.0-1.5	1.0-1.5	0.5-1.5	0.02-0.08	0.02-0.08	0.05-0.1	325-975	550-1,650	500-1,500
4-6 yr	20-40	85	3-4	1.5-2.0	1.5-2.0	1.0-2.5	0.03-0.12	0.03-0.12	0.06-0.15	450-1,350	775-2,325	700-2,100
7-10 yr	30-60	120	4-5	2.0-2.5	2.0-3.0	1.5-2.5	0.05-0.2	0.05-0.2	0.1-0.3	600-1,800	1,000-3,000	925-2,775
11+ yr	50-100	100-200	4-7	2.0-3.0	2.5-5.0	1.5-2.5	0.05-0.2	0.05-0.2	0.15-0.5	900-2,700	1,525-4,575	1,400-4,200
Adults	70-140	100-200	4-7	2.0-3.0	2.5-5.0	1.5-4.0	0.05-0.2	0.05-0.2	0.15-0.5	1,100-3,300	1,875-5,625	1,700-5,100

*From Recommended Dietary Allowances, Revised 1980. Food and Nutrition Board, National Academy of Sciences—National Research Council. Because there is less information on which to base allowances, these figures are not given in the main table of the RDAs and are provided here in the form of ranges of recommended intakes.

†Since the toxic levels for many trace elements may be only several times usual intakes, the upper levels for the trace elements given in this table should not be habitually exceeded.

Index

(Entries followed by T denote Tables)

relationship of deficiency to metabolic action, 112; relative organ concentrations, 103; relationships to hormones, 112; relationships to other minerals, 112; relationships to vitamins, 112; specific functions, 110; storage, 110; synergists, 102; target tissues, 110; units, 106; unusual features, 112.

CoR. *See* Biotin.

Corpus luteum hormone. *See* Progesterone.

Corpus luteum-ripening hormone. *See* Luteinizing hormone.

Cortical-releasing factor. *See* Corticotrop(h)in-releasing hormone.

Corticotrop(h)ic hormone. *See* Adrenocorticotrophic hormone.

Corticotrop(h)in-releasing hormone (CRH), 300.

Cortisol: active analogs and related forms, 408; administration, 410; antagonists, 408; biosynthesis, 411; blood carriers, 412; catabolism, 412; commercial production, 409; deficiency diseases, disorders, 408; deficiency symptoms, 411; determination, 410; effects of overdose, 411; enzyme systems, 412; essentiality for life, 408; factors affecting release, 410; half-life, 412; history, 408; inactive analogs and related forms, 408; isolation, 409; mode of action, 412; normal blood levels, 410; physiological forms, 408; physiological functions, 408; possible relationships of deficiency symptoms to metabolic action, 414; production (sites), 411; properties, 409; reactions, 409, 412; relation to other hormones, 413; relation to vitamins, 413; species occurrence, 410; storage, 411; structure, 409; synergists, 408; synonyms, 407; target tissues, 412; units, 410; unusual features, 413.

CRF. *See* Corticotrop(h)in-releasing hormone.

Cyanocobalamin. *See* Vitamin B$_{12}$.

Daily dietary allowances, 473-4T.

Dihydrofollicular hormone. *See* Estradiol.

Dihydrotheelin. *See* Estradiol.

6,7-Dimethyl-9-(d-1′-ribityl)isoalloxazine. *See* Riboflavin.

Egg white injury factor. *See* Biotin.

Electrocortin. *See* Aldosterone.

Ephynol. *See* Vitamin E.

Epinephrine: active analogs and related forms, 446; administration, 448; antagonists, 446; biosynthesis, 449; blood carriers, 449; catabolism, 450; commercial production, 447; deficiency diseases, disorders, 447; deficiency symptoms, 448; determination, 448; effects of overdose, 448; enzyme systems, 449; essentiality for life, 447; factors affecting release, 448; half-life, 449; history, 446; inactive analogs and related forms, 446; isolation, 447; mode of action, 449; normal blood levels, 448; physiological forms, 446; physiological functions, 446; possible relationships of deficiency symptoms to metabolic action, 450; production (sites), 449; properties, 447; reactions, 447, 449; relation to other hormones, 450; relation to vitamins, 450; species occurrence, 448; storage, 449; structure, 447; synergists, 446; synonyms, 446; target tissues, 449; units, 448; unusual features, 450.

Epsilan. *See* Vitamin E.

Estradiol: active analogs and related forns, 416; administration, 419; antagonists, 416; biosynthesis, 419; blood carriers, 420; catabolism, 421; commercial production, 417; deficiency diseases, disorders, 417; deficiency symptoms, 419; determination, 418; effects of overdose, 419; enzyme systems, 420; essentiality for life, 417; factors affecting release, 419; half-life, 420; history, 416; inactive analogs and related forms, 416; isolation, 418; mode of action, 420; normal blood levels, 418; physiological forms, 416; physiological functions, 416; possible relationships of deficiency symptoms to metabolic action, 422; production (sites), 419; properties, 417; reactions, 417, 420; relation to other hormones, 421; relation to vitamins, 421; species occurrence, 418; storage, 419; structure, 417; synergists, 416; synonyms, 416; target tissues, 420; units, 418; unusual features, 421.

β-Estradiol. *See* Estradiol.

Factor X. *See* Vitamin E.

Female hormone. *See* Estradiol.

Fluorine: analytical methods, 150; antago-